The Prevention® Guide to SURGERY and Its ALTERNATIVES

The Prevention® Guide to SURGERY and Its ALTERNATIVES

By
Rebecca Christian
Sharon Faelten
James Nechas
Emrika Padus
of the Staff of Prevention Magazine

Carol Baldwin, Research Chief
Carol Matthews, Carol Munson,
Eileen Mazer, Research Associates

Rodale Press Emmaus, Pa.

Book design by Kim E. Morrow

Printed in the United States of America on recycled paper, containing a high percentage of de-inked fiber.

Library of Congress Cataloging in Publication Data
Main entry under title:
The Prevention guide to surgery and its alternatives.

Includes index.
1. Surgery—Popular works. I. Christian, Rebecca.
II. Baldwin, Carol, 1947- III. Prevention.
[DNLM: 1. Surgery—Popular works. W075 P944]
RD31.3.P73 617 80-13686
ISBN 0-87857-304-6 hardcover

4 6 8 10 9 7 5 3 hardcover

• Notice •

This book is meant to supplement the advice and guidance of your physician. No two medical conditions are the same. Surgical practice varies from region to region and is changing constantly. Therefore, we urge you to seek out the best medical resources available to help you make informed decisions.

Contents

Preface

Why should *Prevention,* a magazine devoted to explaining how we can *avoid* illness, assign a group of editors to produce a major book on—of all things—surgery?

One answer is simply that 25 million operations are performed in this country each year. The chances are that some day, you will have surgery performed on you. And unfortunately, chances are that you will understand very little about it—including how you might have prevented your problem from reaching the stage where surgery was necessary.

But there is another reason for a book like this. During my years as editor of *Prevention* magazine, I've become aware of a strange paradox of behavior. When it comes to protecting our health through nutrition, exercise and other means, many of us are quite knowledgeable and active. We put a lot of time and energy into shopping for and preparing what we consider to be the very best possible diet for our families. We read about new scientific discoveries concerning vitamins and minerals. We attend classes to learn yoga or aerobic dancing, how to relax or lose weight. We take vitamin supplements and put a couple of quarters in the machine at the shopping mall to see how the blood pressure is doing. The result is that we're doing a tremendous amount of good for ourselves when it comes to preventing all sorts of health problems. But what happens when out best efforts aren't good enough and we suddenly find ourselves confronted with the possibility of surgery?

The answer, too often, is that the same person who had so much knowledge and motivation suddenly forgets all about his ability to control his destiny just when he needs it most—at the moment of crisis.

Many of us, I suppose, feel that when surgery seems to be in the offing, the only thing to do is to put ourselves into the hands of our local surgeons and pray for the best. Today, that notion is definitely out of step with the times—and reality. As you will learn in this book, there is a great deal you can do to bring about the most favorable possible outcome from your health crisis. In fact, you might very well come out of it much better off than you were before—in more ways than one.

Most important, perhaps, you will learn about *natural* alternatives to certain common operations and whether such alternatives are appropriate for your particular condition (every case is different, of course). You will learn about treatments involving physical therapy or drugs rather than surgery, and what research has shown about the effectiveness of these less radical approaches. If surgery seems to be the only route, you will learn about the various *kinds* of surgery that may be available to you; which, you may be surprised to learn, vary considerably in their side effects. You will also learn about changes in health habits that can prevent your problem from returning after you have surgery, how to bring about healing as rapidly as possible, and many other good things you can do for yourself.

The Prevention Guide to Surgery and Its Alternatives is not a scary book—it is overwhelmingly positive and reassuring. This book, we feel, can bring an end to your needless fears about surgery. When you understand something, there is no longer any reason to be afraid of it. While reading this book certainly won't give you the knowledge of your doctor, it will, at the very least, enable you to discuss your situation with him with far greater mutual understanding and benefit. Hopefully, this will make it easier for you to get the very best medical care available, along with the best information to guide your decisions.

Robert Rodale
Editor, *Prevention*

Acknowledgments

The authors are indebted to many people for helping to make this book more accurate, objective and complete. While each chapter has been reviewed for accuracy by an expert in the field, the authors assume all responsibility for any errors which may exist. And the authors, of course, are responsible for the judgments, evaluations and opinions expressed herein.

We wish especially to thank the following people who are among those who provided major information or critical reviews:

M. Alexander, M.B., B.S., staff surgeon, Shouldice Hospital Limited, Thornhill, Ontario, Canada; Samuel J. Arnold, M.D., attending urologist, Memorial Hospital, Morristown, N.J.; Stanley J. Birnbaum, M.D., professor of obstetrics and gynecology, The New York Hospital-Cornell Medical Center, New York City; Peter C. Block, M.D., director, Cardiac Catheterization Laboratory, Department of Medicine, Massachusetts General Hospital, Boston, Mass.; Denis P. Burkitt, M.B., B.Ch., M.D., St. Thomas's Hospital Medical School, London, England; Irving M. Bush, M.D., senior consultant, Center for Study of Genitourinary Diseases, Burlington, Ill. and professor of urology, The Chicago Medical School, Chicago, Ill.; Robert A. Buyers, M.D., general surgeon, Norristown Surgical Associates, Inc., Norristown, Pa.; Stanley Z. Cowen, M.D., Department of Surgery, Encino Hospital, Encino, Calif.; Joel Freeman, M.D., chief, Division of General Surgery, Department of Surgery, Ottawa General Hospital and associate professor of surgery, University of Ottawa, Ottawa, Ontario, Canada; Franz Goldstein, M.D., professor of medicine, Jefferson Medical College and chief, Division of Gastroenterology, Lankenau Hospital, Philadelphia, Pa.; Robert M. Goldwyn, M.D., associate clinical professor of surgery, Harvard Medical School, Boston, Mass.; Morton I. Grossman, M.D., Ph.D., Center for Ulcer Research and Education, VA Wadsworth Hospital, Los Angeles, Calif.; Ruth Haase, assistant vice-president, Blue Cross and Blue Shield of Greater New York, New York City; Charles P. Hall, Jr., Ph.D., professor, Department of Health Administration and Insurance and Risk, Temple University, School of Business Administration, Philadelphia, Pa.; Marian Kennedy, R.N., director of nursing, Center for Ambulatory Surgery, Inc., Washington, D.C.; Mark Littman, M.D., National Institutes of Health, Bethesda, Md.; John Mikuta, M.D., chief of the Department of Gynecological Oncology, Hospital of the University of Pennsylvania, Philadelphia, Pa.; Donald E. Reiner, M.D., general surgeon, Santa Maria, Calif.; David Seitzman, M.D., executive director, Center for Ambulatory Surgery, Inc., Washington, D.C.; John F. Seybolt, M.D., clinical professor of pathology, director of The Papanicolaou Cytology Laboratories, The New York Hospital-Cornell Medical Center, New York City; Doris Walsh, director of merchandising, Ruthton Corporation, Los Angeles, Calif.; Robert Wertz, M.D., ophthalmologist, Chicago, Ill.

In addition, we would like to thank the following people for their assistance and guidance:

Edgardo S. Alday, M.D., associate professor of surgery, Department of Surgery, Jefferson Medical College, Philadelphia, Pa.; Robert Henry Barter, M.D., professor of gynecology, George Washington University School of Medicine, Washington, D.C. and member of the Society of Vaginal Surgeons; Evalyn Gendel, M.D., Director of Human Sexuality Program, Department of Psychiatry, University of California, San Francisco, Calif.; Richard Costlow, Ph.D., Chief of Preventive Medicine Branch, Division of Cancer Control and Rehabilitation, National Cancer Institute, Bethesda, Md.; Sonya Cohen, screening administrator, Guttman Institute, New York City; Morton Comess, M.D., general surgeon, Phoenix, Ariz.; John W. Cones, J.D., executive vice-president, PIMA (Professional Independent Mass-Marketing Administrators), Chicago, Ill.; Frank Glenn, M.D., professor of surgery, emeritus, Cornell University Medical College, and attending surgeon, The New York Hospital, New York City; James Hefflin, former vice-president, Delaware Valley Hospital Council, Philadelphia, Pa.; Samuel Hellman, M.D., professor and chairman, Department of Radiation Therapy, Harvard Medical School, Boston, Mass.; Alan Kaplan, M.D., chief, Division of Gynecological Oncology, Baylor College of Medicine, Houston, Texas; Lucienne Lanson, M.D., San Francisco, Calif.; Robert S. London, M.D., director, Obstetric and Gynecologic Endocrine Research Laboratory, Sinai Hospital of Baltimore, Inc., and assistant professor, obstetrics and gynecology, The Johns Hopkins University School of Medicine, Baltimore, Md.; Myron R. Melamed, M.D., chairman of the Department of Pathology, Memorial Sloan-Kettering Cancer Center, New York City; C.B. McVay, M.D., Ph.D., emeritus chairman and professor of surgery, University of South Dakota School of Medicine, Yankton, S.D.; Harry M. Nelson Jr., M.D., vascular surgeon, Norristown Surgical Associates, Inc., Norristown, Pa.; Lloyd M. Nyhus, M.D., chief, Department of Surgery, The Abraham Lincoln School of Medicine, Chicago, Ill.; Pat O'Conner, PRESSO (Program for Elective Surgical Second Opinion), Blue Cross-Blue Shield of Greater New York City; Allen Paris, M.D., epidemic intelligence officer, Center for Disease Control, Atlanta, Ga.; Carlos Perez-Mesa, M.D., professor of pathology, University of Missouri Medical Center, Columbia, Mo.; Dennis Smith, M.D., gynecologist and psychiatrist, Case Western Reserve University Medical School, Cleveland, Ohio; James O. Stallings, M.D., plastic surgeon, Plastic Surgery Institute, West Des Moines, Iowa; Carl W. Tyler, Jr., M.D., director of the Family Planning Evaluation Division, Bureau of Epidemiology, Center for Disease Control, Atlanta, Ga.; Eugene Vayda, M.D., professor and chairman, Department of Health Administration, University of Toronto, Ontario, Canada; Mildred Hope Witkin, Ph.D., assistant clinical professor, Department of Psychiatry, Cornell University Medical College and associate director of the Human Sexuality Program, The New York Hospital-Cornell Medical Center, New York City; Robert Williams, executive director, FASA (Freestanding Ambulatory Surgical Association); Susan Wolfe, marketing coordinator for Eastern Pennsylvania Health Maintenance Organization (HMO), Allentown, Pa.

In addition, we would like to express our gratitude to the following agencies for their cooperation:

American Hospital Association
Center for Disease Control
Commission on Professional and Hospital Activities
Joint Commission on Hospital Accreditation
National Center for Health Statistics
National Cancer Institute
National Institutes of Health

Part I

Getting the Best in Surgical Care

1
How This Book Can Help You

With nearly 25 million operations performed on Americans each year, the chances are quite good that surgery will be recommended to you sometime in your life. And about 80 percent of those procedures are elective, that is, optional, not immediately necessary to preserve life.

Many people believe that indications for surgery—even elective surgery—are black and white. Either you need it or you don't. And if you need it, you rely on your doctor to arrange everything. All you need to do is show up at the hospital. In reality, surgery is not that simple.

Answers to your questions concerning discomfort, possible complications and the procedure itself traditionally have come from the surgeon. Some doctors, however, feel it's impossible to explain fully any type of surgery—or the need for it—without sending the patient to medical school. Or they tend to softsell the possibility of postoperative complications because they don't want to frighten patients so much that they refuse treatment for conditions far more dangerous than the complications themselves. That's because "surgery," like "divorce" or "cancer," is a scare word. It makes many people panic.

One woman confessed:

> I know my doctor tried to describe the operation to me when he recommended it, but after I heard him say "surgery" I couldn't concentrate. My mind went blank. I couldn't repeat what he said for anything.

The information exchange between your surgeon and you, the patient, is further limited by the fact that you aren't likely to have the ongoing relationship with your surgeon that you have with your regular family doctor. The visits are likely to be brief, the patient tense and the surgeon busy.

Or you may not be satisfied with the standard spiel the surgeon gives you before presenting a legalistic consent slip for you to sign. He may say something like: "This operation is a common one. Like any, it has risks, but for a person of your age and in your condition, I don't anticipate any problems."

This book is meant to fill the communications gap between you and your surgeon; that is, to supplement, not challenge your surgeon's advice, by addressing the uncertainties common to patients facing elective surgery. The information in this book can be digested calmly and thoughtfully, outside the doctor's office setting, in light of what you're told about your individual case. You'll probably want to know:

How does anesthesia work? What are its risks?
How long will the operation take?
What complications might arise?
How much pain will I have? How can that be managed?
What difference will surgery make in my condition?
What will happen if I don't have the operation?
What will be the effects on my job or family and living arrangements?
Are there any nonsurgical alternatives to consider?

Compounding those questions are the fears of mutilation, threat to life, and fear of what the surgeon may find during the operation.

Many patients told us how much emotional trauma they would have been spared if they had only had more elementary information before entering the hospital. Some sample comments:

> My doctor never mentioned how swollen and stiff my arm would be after the mastectomy (operation for breast cancer). I thought something was terribly wrong . . .

> I was really scared when I looked down after gallbladder surgery and saw a tube full of greenish-yellow stuff coming out of my belly. It wasn't until later that I learned a tube is routinely put in after that operation to drain bile . . .
>
> I was in bed for 3 days after surgery with intense pain. No one ever offered me any pain pills. I finally asked and learned that on my chart the doctor has ordered pain medication for me upon request. If I hadn't been too timid to say something, I would have been spared that pain . . .

Some psychologists feel that providing the patient with as much factual information as possible about what to expect can minimize the stress of surgery and facilitate recovery. Malcolm A. Marshall, Ph.D., a Canadian psychologist, feels that well-informed patients "require less specialized emergency nursing care, less medication and less help in controlling feelings of panic . . . will be easier to work with and are less likely to be labelled as unreasonable and troublesome by both physicians and nursing staff, because they will be less demanding of staff time and energy. In addition, less time in expensive intensive care units and shorter stay in the hospital result in considerable savings . . ." (*Canadian Medical Association Journal,* July 8, 1978).

Affirming the belief that an informed patient is a healthier patient is Joseph B. Furst, M.D., assistant professor of clinical psychiatry at the School of Medicine, State University of New York at Stony Brook. "For most patients, avoidance of discussion is not bliss," Dr. Furst points out. He contends that dealing with patient uncertainties before surgery can actually lessen the physical consequences of the operation and probably cut convalescence time. One study cited by Dr. Furst, which dealt with hysterectomies, revealed that "The amount of vomiting, the level of pain medication required, the speed of recovery from the anesthetic, and the general cooperativeness of the patient are influenced by their preoperative level of anxiety and by their attitudes toward the present illness and surgical treatment" (*New York State Journal of Medicine,* June, 1978).

If surgery is recommended to you, you're entitled to an explanation of specific details. Surgery has become commonplace—if you have never had it, chances are that someone close to you has. But familiarity, or even repeated surgery, does not lessen fears and uncertainties in a patient. If your family doctor thinks you may need elective surgery, our advice is to learn all you can about your condition, find the best surgeon you can and listen carefully to his suggestions. It's unfair for the doctor to exclude you from decisions about your treatment. You should be partners in maintaining and restoring your health.

It's important for the patient to have the knowledge and the right to make the decision on his or her own behalf regarding treatment, according to Allan J. Ryan, M.D., former editor of a leading medical journal. "As a practicing surgeon I never answered in the affirmative the common question, 'Do I have to have this operation?' I explained as fully as possible to the patient, family, or both the possible consequences of the surgery or of the failure to accept it. The decision was theirs and they could change their mind, as I pointed out. Many times they found help and guidance from a second or third opinion" (*Postgraduate Medicine,* September, 1978).

You may not know how to select a surgeon, what specific questions to ask about your individual gallbladder operation or hysterectomy, for instance, or how to evaluate the hospitals where the surgeon has operating privileges. It is even less likely that it will occur to your surgeon to tell you what you need to bring to the hospital, how to interpret your itemized bill, or how to build yourself up nutritionally ahead of time. That's where this book comes in.

You may have heard that your insurance policy entitles you to a second opinion, but you may not know how to go about getting one without insulting your surgeon.

Many thoughtful people will want to explore more conservative treatments before going into the operating room. That's another reason this book was written—to help you to find less drastic alternatives that could spare you the expense and trauma of surgery.

Researchers who believe that at least some of the surgery performed in the U.S. is unnecessary, point out that where there are more surgeons, there is more surgery. Certain operations are performed so much more often in particular regions of the country than in others that the higher rate can hardly be considered coincidental.

The U.S., like most countries, has its pet operations. While tonsillectomy and hysterectomy ride high on the surgical hit parade here, a West German is more likely to be surgically relieved of his appendix.

The problem of so-called "unnecessary" surgery is generally conceded to be unjustifiably high. But even researchers and statisticians who agree that there may be too much surgery, argue over how much is too much and why. One study shows that physicians and their spouses undergo surgery more often than nonmedical families, casting doubt on the idea that unscrupulous surgeons talk the medically ignorant into undergoing operations they don't need. Some doctors blame patients who go from surgeon to surgeon until one agrees to operate; others say the high rates are the fault of unhealthful lifestyles that lead to problems which must be surgically solved.

"Unnecessary surgery," some surgeons argue, is an unfair term because it is nearly impossible to define. Some examples of cases where the need for surgery is debatable include:

- An operation for peptic ulcer on a patient who has failed to respond to medical treatment. He has no perforation or bleeding, which are among the life-threatening conditions that would make the surgery no longer elective but mandatory. While there is the disturbing possibility that the surgery will have side effects and his ulcer will recur after surgery, there is also a good chance that the pain that has been making him miserable will be relieved. *Is his surgery necessary?*

- An operation for varicose veins on a woman who still may have more children. Although her leg veins pose no threat to her overall circulation, they are unattractive and often uncomfortable. Her legs give her considerable pain after a vigorous day at her job as a waitress. The more conservative medical treatments of wearing support hose and elevating her legs periodically give her some, but only temporary, relief. Her symptoms would be relieved by surgery, but a later pregnancy could influence the development of more varicosities in veins not removed during the operation. So if she has surgery and then decides to have another child, she may develop the same problem all over again. *Is her operation necessary?*

- An operation for a 70-year-old man with a hernia of the groin. He is wearing a truss but the truss bothers him, especially in hot weather. There is always the chance that the hernia will strangulate, necessitating an emergency operation at a time when he is in poorer condition than he is now. But since he is diabetic, the operation is riskier for him than for a disease-free patient of comparable age. *Is his operation necessary?*

Even if there is too much surgery in the U.S., it's not our purpose in this book to harangue the medical establishment because of it. What we would like to do is help readers evaluate the pros and cons of surgery in *individual* cases. When a doctor tells you that a diseased organ needs to come out, it matters little to you if there are more tonsillectomies per capita in Rhode Island than in Vermont. What does matter to you is whether the operation you have been advised to undergo is necessary. That's a question that doesn't always have an absolute answer. Basing your decision on the best information you can get from your surgeon and family doctor, it's up to you to weigh costs, risks and benefits.

When all other methods of treatment fail, surgery can be a godsend. Techniques in operating and administering anesthesia have improved so much in recent decades that with good care in a good hospital, surgery can be reasonably safe. In some cases it may relieve the pain and discomfort of a patient who has suffered for years.

In order to seek out good care and a good hospital, you'll

have to put in some time and effort. You should familiarize yourself with your rights as a patient. You'll need to learn about anesthesia in order to help the anesthesiologist decide what kind you'll have. You'll need to pay attention to your diet to be sure you are nutritionally prepared. You'll want to study your insurance policy to learn what expenses will have to come out of your own pocket. You'll have to be willing to ask the surgeon questions like, "What will happen if I don't have the operation?" This book will show you why—and how.

2
Choosing and Communicating with Your Surgeon

You've seen the television medical dramas where a simple but noble laborer in Indiana declaims he wants "the best" for his daughter's brain surgery, even if it takes him the rest of his hard-working life to pay off the surgeon's fees.

The concerned family physician furrows his kindly brow and phones "the best brain man" in the U.S., who just happened to be his roommate in medical school. "The best" drops everything in New York and immediately jets to Indiana where he successfully operates on the brave and sassy patient, free of charge.

The assumptions are that "the best" is as easily identifiable as the only bald man in a police lineup. He charges the most, except in cases of need (for which he waives fees entirely, collecting his thank yous with an embarrassed nod). He works in a teaching hospital on the metropolitan East Coast. And he may operate at any hospital to which he is summoned.

The patient who has had the contents of his prostate gland scooped out or fibroids removed from her uterus can tell you that the scene described above is far removed from their experiences with elective surgery.

Most people don't exercise half the care in choosing a surgeon that they do in choosing a washing machine. A number of doctors and public health experts interviewed for this chapter lamented the fact that patients are so passive and uninformed that they don't choose at all—they just go to the surgeons their family doctors or internists recommend.

What ought to happen is something like this:

Noticing disturbing symptoms, you call your doctor. The

nurse or receptionist answers the phone and inquires about your problem. An appointment is made for you within the week.

On the scheduled day, you go to the doctor and you're ushered right in. The doctor asks questions, listens thoughtfully to your answers and conducts the necessary examination and tests. The examination includes questions about your chief complaint and current illness, examination of your body by organ systems, and reference to your medical history previously gathered and on file.

The doctor suggests you may need surgery and advises consulting a surgeon—perhaps suggesting a specialist or two who have good records regarding frequency with which they perform the prospective operation, and the mortality, complication and success rates for that type of surgery.

After you're satisfied that the surgeon's credentials are adequate, you make an appointment to consult him. The surgeon conducts a thorough exam of his own (without adding to the expense by repeating tests the primary care physician made) and concurs the procedure is needed.

Then you seek an opinion from a second qualified surgeon; you inform this second surgeon that he will not be asked to perform the operation. The second surgeon agrees the surgery is needed. Your insurance company pays for all three consultations and hospitalization in full.

But what could happen is something like this:

After spending several hours in the waiting room, you finally get your turn. The nurse whispers, "Doctor will see you now," curiously referring to her boss by profession rather than name.

The hurried doctor at first confuses you with a patient of similar build and age. He waves away your account of minor symptoms and past illnesses which you think may be related. After a thump here and a blood test there, the doctor says surgery might be needed.

The surgeon he calls in for consultation is a friend from across the hall. On the basis of the first doctor's "exam," the surgeon agrees the surgery is needed. Frightened, you quickly agree to have him operate and the procedure is scheduled and performed without further ado. Later, you discover that anesthesiologists in your area charge more than is reimbursed by your insurance plan. You must pay additional anesthesiology fees out of your own pocket.

Ironically, the man or woman in the first example could die of shock on the operating table while the person in the second example could sail through with a routine recovery and smooth scar. *Choosing a surgeon with care does not guarantee that the result will be successful. But it can reduce your chances for failure.*

Because of the lack of hard, published data, it is difficult to evaluate members of the medical profession. Surgical patients, unless they have a particularly cooperative family doctor and/or surgeon, will have to sleuth out information on their own. The only way to find out basic information about a surgeon—such as how often he performs specific procedures and with what success, mortality and complication rates—is to ask him or his colleagues.

Such information should be available, according to Richard Egdahl, M.D., a surgeon specializing in endocrine problems, who gets calls from patients asking for a good surgeon in the Boston area. But Dr. Egdahl, who is director of Boston University Medical Center and a professor of surgery, admits, "At the current time, I don't see how a patient can check on a doctor's success rate. I think the American College of Surgeons should provide some guidance to patients about surgeons' experience. Right now, patients go to the surgeon their internist recommends. It's like going to a car mechanic to ask which dealer you should go to—you ask because he knows about them.

"I think the time is coming when surgeons' track records will be available," continues Dr. Egdahl. "Right now there is no sophisticated system to which patients can refer. There are a few places where the whistle has been blown on unequipped hospitals in which incompetent doctors were doing major surgery. But systematically gathered data is hard to find."

In wholehearted agreement with Dr. Egdahl about the need for published information about surgeons is George J. Annas, attorney, Boston University professor of health law, a pioneer in patients' rights and author of *The Rights of Hospital Patients* (the Basic American Civil Liberties Guide to Hospital Patients' Rights, Avon, 1975). Annas disputes the argument used by some doctors who are against providing such information—that patients are unable to digest the surgeon's record meaningfully. He added that patients won't have an opportunity to view surgeons' records until they demand it. Annas suggests:

> You can ask the doctor himself how often he does the procedure. Then you can ask another surgeon how often a surgeon ought to do that procedure to keep his skills up. Some of the things a patient should know are how often the doctor does the procedure, where he does it, what his complication rate is and what his death rate is. If he gets angry about this, then get another doctor.
>
> This kind of information isn't public, although someday it might be. If the patient is embarrassed to ask this kind of question, he can find another doctor who will talk about the surgeon's record in confidence. Most people have an acquaintance who is a doctor or have a friend who can put them in touch with one.
>
> I think eventually we'll have a rating system where a patient can call a consumer agency and ask for a surgeon's rating. The rating system could be set up in points assigned by the agency. Maybe each surgeon could have two ratings—one done by a group of surgeons and one by the agency.
>
> Of course, this idea is being fought vigorously by doctors who say that some doctors will do all the simple operations in order to get a good rating. But the difficulty of the procedures could be figured into the rating system.

Until such a system is established, patients may not be able to get such information, even from a cooperative surgeon. The fact is, the system doesn't encourage surgeons to keep records of the *results of their operations.* After the operation and postoperative checks, the patient is back in the care of the primary care physician — his family doctor, internist or general practitioner. And even if complications or death occurred while the surgical patient was still in the surgeon's care, the surgeon may not have kept records showing his rate in specific procedures.

William Nolen, M.D., the respected author of *Making of a Surgeon* (Random House, 1970) and *Surgeon Under the Knife* (Dell, 1976), told us candidly, "I don't keep records on mortality rates and success rates. Most doctors don't keep that kind of information. Some doctors might be offended that you asked, but most of all it just wouldn't be productive. If someone asked me what my mortality rate for gallbladder is, I wouldn't have the foggiest notion. Most patients wouldn't really understand if I did go into details and say, 'Well, I lost a gallbladder patient last month but she had already had three operations and it was an unusually complicated case.' I would just say, 'There can be problems, but given your case and your history, I don't anticipate any.' "

Until records in the operating room are made public, choosing a surgeon will be, in the words of Jonathan V. Wright, M.D., "very, very difficult." But Dr. Wright, a family practitioner in Kent, Washington, and a medical columnist for *Prevention* magazine, agrees with other physicians that choosing a surgeon still doesn't have to be hit or miss. Doing your own legwork can be time-consuming. But if you agree that "health is the first wealth," it's worth the investment.

Dr. Wright suggests that in the absence of a referral from a primary care physician he trusts, the patient could contact two general practitioners, internists or family practice physicians at opposite ends of town (decreasing the chance that they would be buddies and therefore be likely to "conspire") and ask for confidential recommendation, making appointments with each if necessary.

Your county medical society can probably give you information about where a certain surgeon received his degree and training, how long he has been in practice, what his specialty is and so on. It will not give you an outright recommendation, however, nor will it have information about a surgeon's record with a particular operation.

If the county medical society can give only minimal information, how might a newcomer to town find a surgeon? Say a patient is told by her primary care physician she probably needs gallbladder surgery. The patient is getting ready to move to another state and postpones a surgical consultation until she is settled in her new home. How would she, a stranger in town, find a surgeon? Posing as such a patient, one of the authors called the information number of a local hospital to ask whether Drs. X and Y (listed as general surgeons in the phone book) had operating privileges at the hospital, and if so, for how long. The courteous secretary told us both doctors did have privileges, one for 15 years and one for 20. We called a second hospital and were again transferred to administration, where a secretary told us how long the surgeons had been operating there. She would not tell us how often they performed gallbladder surgery—or whether they performed gallbladder surgery at all. That information, she said icily, would have to come from the physician himself.

Unable to get information from medical societies or surgeons themselves, some people rely on recommendations from other patients. Advice from a friend won't do you much good unless you can get a consensus from several people you respect. That's because patients look for different things in a doctor. Many patients judge a surgeon mainly by personality.

A surgeon may have infinite patience with querulous patients who telephone at midnight to ask why their bowels haven't moved. Yet he may not be a top-notch surgeon. A second surgeon may have a brilliant technique with the scalpel at the operating table but lack sensitivity in the examining room, forcing an icy speculum into a nervous patient while barking, "Relax!"

If you don't know a surgeon by reputation, your primary care physician's referral is a good place to start.

Relying on another doctor's referral has its drawbacks too, however, as the Boston Women's Health Collective points out in *Our Bodies, Ourselves* (Simon & Schuster, 1976).

> Doctors admit that even they are not sure how to find out how really competent another doctor is if they do not

> work with him every day. Asking a doctor's peers for an opinion, however, is like asking a blood relative for an objective opinion of a member of the family. Unless he is medically dangerous or behaving in a way that colleagues find politically threatening, the recommendations will usually be enthusiastic. In most cases doctors make referrals the way they give other kinds of nonmedical opinions; they select on the basis of friendship and their own experiences, or because an exchange of referrals has become profitable. . . . The competitiveness of big-city university-linked specialists should work in the consumer's favor, but most of the time it doesn't, because these doctors often behave like small boys on rival football teams.

The women's group makes a good case for the idea that one doctor's referral to another isn't always based on only medical considerations. If you know and trust your family doctor, this shouldn't be a problem.

If the surgeon who performs your operation does not know your primary care physician, however, your medical care might be fragmented. If the two of them have worked together before, or at least work in the same hospital, the chance that they'll consult closely on your case may be better.

That's why it's important that you have a good primary care physician, not just a surgeon as the need arises. A good primary care physician provides you with continuity of medical care. As Marvin Belsky, M.D., of New York, and Leonard Gross point out in their book, *How to Choose and Use Your Doctor* (Arbor House, 1975):

> A good primary care physician doesn't abandon you to a specialist or fragment your care. He does refer you if you have special, unusual problems beyond his ability, or if you simply want another medical opinion. He functions here as the integrator and synthesizer in the team concept of medical care. . . . It's in your own interest not to fragment your care by going to an orthopedist, allergist, or other specialist *at the outset.* If you have a problem of unknown origin, the best rule is to begin with your family practitioner or internist

> and then move on to the specialist if the situation warrants; in such cases the primary care physician can help determine the degree of specialization required, select a qualified specialist, and serve as your advocate during treatment.

Although Dr. Belsky isn't talking only about surgical specialists here, his advice applies as well to patients who need to consult them.

Obviously a specialist is trained in special solutions to problems, and through no fault of his own, he may lack the perspective to make a proper diagnosis. A gynecologist, an orthopedist and a psychiatrist might all suspect a different problem in a patient whose symptom is chronic low back pain. Better for the patient first to consult a primary care physician who knows him, his working conditions, his family situation and his physical problems well. Naturally, if you have no primary care physician and you suddenly develop a hernia, you don't have time to develop a solid relationship with a primary care physician before the surgery. But it's an opportune time to find a good family or general practitioner or internal medical doctor who can help you with this and future problems.

As Sylvia Porter wrote in her syndicated newspaper column, "Your Money" in 1977, seeking a good primary physician makes good sense financially as well as medically. Ms. Porter remarks:

> A properly trained family physician can treat 85 to 90 percent of all medical complaints. In the other one out of 10 cases, he (or she) will know to which specialist to refer you and he will stay on the case interpreting the specialist's findings for you, the patient. He looks at you, the whole person, not part of you. More than that, he considers your whole family and interactions among the various members which may affect the health of any one of you.

If the only trusted sympathetic family doctors you know of are the ones on television dramas, you can still make a judgment about your surgeon's technical competence on your own. You can do so with a combination of letters, telephone calls and library research. Probably no one has the time and energy to check *all* aspects of a surgeon's competence. A spot check, however, can be reassuring. Here's how:

See that your surgeon has a medical degree (and where he got it). Anybody can call himself a doctor or specialist, even with a degree from a mail order correspondence course. Just because he's listed in the Yellow Pages doesn't prove that a person is indeed a medical doctor. Call the surgeon's office to find out from what medical school he was graduated. Or go to the library and look him up in the AMA's *Directory of Physicians,* which lists all of the nation's legally qualified M.D.'s. *Directory of Physicians* comes in several volumes, including an alphabetical and geographical index. Look up your state and city to find a list of doctors that practice there. Read the code explanation in the front of the book and then see what year the doctor was born, when and where he received his medical degree, when he became licensed in the state in which he is now practicing, what, if any, specialty he is certified in and what memberships he holds in special societies.

Generally, the reputation of a medical school is closely linked to the reputation of the undergraduate school with which it is affiliated. If you don't know how to judge the school's quality, call the chief of staff at a nearby hospital or a college pre-med counselor.

Some American doctors attended or were graduated from foreign medical schools, often because their grades kept them out of medical schools in the U.S. All foreign-trained doctors, however, have to take a test, the National Board Examination, before they are allowed to apply for a license to practice in the U.S.

The reputation of the hospital where your surgeon took his residency might help you evaluate him. If you don't know how to judge the hospitals, ask a doctor, nurse, health insurance representative or medical student. The AMA puts out a *Directory of Residency Training Programs,* which will tell you if the doctor's training was at a medical school-affiliated hospital and if it was AMA approved. If the doctor trained many years ago, however, the standing of the training and of the hospital may have changed. You can find out where your surgeon trained by reading the certificates on his office wall, by asking him or his nurse or by looking him up in the *Directory of Physicians.*

If the prospective surgeon is a specialist, you can look him up in the *Directory of Medical Specialists.* Besides telling you in what specialty he is board-certified, it will tell what medical schools he has attended, the degrees he has received, what post-graduate education he has had, past and present teaching positions he has filled and the memberships he holds in scientific societies.

See if your surgeon is board-certified. In the absence of other information, surgical patients should consult only surgeons who are board-certified. Although board certification guarantees that your surgeon has achieved a minimum level of competence, it won't necessarily prove that he's a good surgeon.

Physicians don't have to be board-certified to describe themselves as surgeons. The general practitioner who delivers an occasional baby at the community hospital or removes warts and moles in his office may list himself as a surgeon in the Yellow Pages.

Recognition of the importance of board certification is growing; some hospitals allow only board-certified surgeons to operate.

Certifying boards exist for general surgery and for surgical specialties such as otolaryngology (ear and throat), anesthesiology, orthopedics (bone and joint), urology (genital or urinary tract), and so forth. Some surgeons are certified in more than one specialty.

To be board-certified, a surgeon must have been graduated from an approved school of medicine in the U.S. or Canada (strict standards apply to graduates of foreign medical schools). He must have taken courses in the basic sciences, and had clinical training and major operative experience. After medical school, he must train in general surgery and his specialty for several years. Then he takes a written qualifying exam followed by an oral certifying exam. A surprisingly high number of applicants fail the board exams, but they are able to try again after more study. You may learn that a surgeon is "board-*qualified*"—that means he has spent the required number of years in training but has not taken the written and the oral exams.

In telephone interviews, two board-certified surgeons commented on the pros and cons of board certification. Dr. Richard Egdahl (the Boston endocrinologist) said, "I would say for complicated surgery, the surgeon should be board-certified. If you're just going to have a routine D and C, it may not be necessary. You have to look at how often he does surgery. Some people are board-certified but only do one operation a year of a given sort—that's not good."

James O. Stallings, M.D., a plastic surgeon and director of the Plastic Surgery Institute in Des Moines, Iowa, told us, "From the standpoint of the consumer, the advantage of board certification is that you know that surgeon has taken a standard educational course—medical school, internship, x years of residency and two grueling examinations. It is not, however, a guarantee of a good result. Of course, no reputable surgeon can or would guarantee anything. There are two sides to the body, and complications can occur. Patients should beware of a surgeon who guarantees everything, or even anything.

"I know people who are board-certified surgeons who are not, in my opinion, very good," added Dr. Stallings. "I know people who are *not* board-certified as surgeons who are, in my opinion, better surgeons than board-certified surgeons. But again you're taking a chance. I would say that from the standpoint of a consumer, your chances of success are greater with a board-certified surgeon of whatever specialty.

"I think the best recommendation a surgeon can get is by word of mouth from satisfied persons," Dr. Stallings concluded. "Obviously you could go to your family doctor or county or state medical society, but usually all they do is give you a list of doctors in the area."

If you follow some of these steps in assessing your surgeon's technical competence, you're off to a good start. *These criteria are intended to be used only as a supplement to your judgment about the surgeon.*

Valuable as it is in making an evaluation, technical competence isn't everything you need to know about the surgeon. Notice if he listens to you and see if he takes *your* priorities into consideration as well as his own. If he thinks you need gallbladder surgery but the tests have been inconclusive, he may suggest putting you in the hospital for a few days for a full work-up of tests. How does he respond if you say you are uninsured and can't afford x days of hospitalization at x dollars a day?

It may sound from the advice in this chapter so far that your surgeon has to be a soulmate. He doesn't. You can't trail from office to office in quest of the perfect surgeon, while your symptoms persist and worsen. Unless your case is very difficult or your recovery protracted, you probably won't see the surgeon more than a few times.

Realistically, you won't want to take him to task because you don't like the rough way he palpates your kidneys or because he calls you by your first name while expecting you to call him "doctor." Save your breath for the important issues.

Does he fail to take a blood test, even though your medical record (to which he has access) shows you had borderline anemia the last time your blood was tested a year ago? Does he tell you the name, risk and purpose of a test that points your nether portions toward heaven while he surveys the convolutions of your rectum with what looks like a miniature Boy Scout flashlight? Does he ask if you are allergic to shellfish before scheduling you to have iodine shot into your veins for a test?

Remember also that the doctor's office workers, nurses and assistants are his representatives. If they do something that truly concerns you, say so. Did the nurse fail to put your call through to the doctor when you experienced severe worsening of symptoms? Tell the doctor. He'll probably thank you for it.

Don't be afraid to insist that something be done about a problem that is bothering you. A patient interviewed for this book said a doctor was willing to let a suture needle which was revealed by an x-ray, remain in her body because he could not pinpoint its exact location. The patient elaborates:

> I had a hysterectomy for endometriosis (a pelvic disease) and felt fine after the operation. About 7 years later, I had a

bad fall and went in for x-rays. I had broken my coccyx bone, and they saw a suture needle in the print after they took the x-ray. I was completely unaware of it.

I consulted a surgeon—not the one who did the hysterectomy, of course. Naturally, the surgeon didn't want to go in to take the needle out until he knew exactly where it was. He took so many x-rays, and still couldn't find out exactly where it was. He said, "Since it's been in for 7 years and it hasn't given you any trouble, why don't we just leave it there?"

I wasn't satisfied with that, so he agreed to try one more x-ray, and that time he did find it. I had a very minor operation—it was in the wall between the vagina and the rectum, and it was easily removed.

A less assertive patient might have agreed with the surgeon's suggestion to ignore the problem, and acquiesced because "Doctor knows best." Probably such a patient would continue to have nagging worries over problems the needle could cause.

Your questions shouldn't stop with the operation. If you can handle the possible bad news, ask the doctor to show you the pathologist's report on the tissue removed and to explain it to you afterwards. Some patients leave the hospital in astonishing ignorance about their conditions.

Edward Harrison (not his real name) confessed he has never known whether a bladder tumor he had removed 20 years ago was cancerous. A well-educated professional, the patient had no explanation for his lack of information. Perhaps the doctor sensed that he didn't really want to know. Harrison told us:

"I don't know exactly what they did when they went up there. I don't know if it was anything or not."

"But didn't the doctor tell you? Didn't you ask?" we wondered aloud.

"Well, he explained in a vague way, but I really didn't understand and he was busy, so I let it go."

Mr. Harrison's wife put in, "I think they said it was a low-grade malignancy, but nothing too bad because it was encapsulated—it hadn't spread."

Mr. Harrison shrugged uncomfortably and replied, "Well, maybe that was it, then. I don't know."

If you are going to ask the doctor to let you see your medical record or to give you the unvarnished facts about your prognosis, make sure you have tried to gauge your own psychological reaction to possible bad news. It isn't fair to the doctor to demand the whole truth and then resent him for being the bearer of bad tidings if he has found something serious and you can't handle it emotionally.

One elderly woman, hospitalized after her husband came home and found her unconscious, grilled her young doctor as soon as she recovered.

"I want you to tell me what happened. Don't sugar-coat," she commanded when he came into her hospital room.

"Very well," said the doctor as he shifted his feet and looked away. "One of the arteries leading to your brain is clogged. When it was clogged so much that oxygen couldn't reach your brain, you lost consciousness."

By the time the hapless doctor looked back up at his tough-talking patient, his straightforward explanation had caused her to pass out.

The other side of the coin is the patient who insists that the doctor remain unflaggingly optimistic, even when the evidence doesn't bear out such optimism.

A desperately cheerful woman didn't want to hear the prognosis after her husband's terminal cancer symptoms had been greatly relieved by chemotherapy and radiation. She became quite angry when the doctor reminded her that the remission was temporary and that the patient would die—quite probably in a year or two.

"But he's better," she shouted angrily. "Anyone can see he's not dying."

When the doctor tried to reason with her, she literally refused to listen.

The chances for misunderstandings like these are far slimmer if you welcome the information the surgeon shares and ask questions as they occur to you, jotting them down if you get too flustered to remember what you want to say during exams and treatment.

Doctors, as their hurried manner will sometimes remind you, are busy people. An excellent surgeon may forget to ask pertinent questions at times. Take some responsibility for your own health and tell him about things he may have overlooked when he took your medical history. Are you on birth control pills? They could have predisposed you to gallbladder disease. Does your mother have high blood pressure? Are your allergic to penicillin? Did you have a bad fall 6 months ago? Are you on any medication—even aspirin, laxatives or diuretics? All of these things can be important.

What to Ask Your Surgeon Before the Operation

Surgical patients can save themselves much anxiety and second-guessing by asking the same sort of questions the surgeon would want answered before he let himself or a member of his family be operated on. The following list might help you. No patient would be interested in the answers to all of them, but you might want to use a few that are pertinent to your case:

What are the surgical complications?
What are the chances that my problem will recur after surgery?
What would happen if I didn't have the operation?
Will you let me see my medical record throughout my hospitalization?
Who will be responsible for coordinating my care while I'm in the hospital?
If all goes as expected, what will your fees be?

Will you bill me for my preoperative and postoperative consultations and the operation in a lump sum, or separately?
Will you visit me before the operation?
What tissue will be removed?
What organs are involved?
Exactly where will you make the incision and how big will it be?
Will it show when I wear a bikini (swimming trunks, low-cut dress)?
Can you make the incision through the old scar I have in the same area from my previous operation?
What time am I scheduled to be operated on?
How often have you done this operation?
How often is it successful?
How long should it be before I feel perfectly normal again?
How soon after the operation can I resume sexual relations? Jogging? Skiing?
How soon after I get home may I stop taking the medications? Sitz baths? Temperature readings?
Will you refer me to one of your patients who has already undergone this procedure?
How will the results of the operation affect my life-style?
Would you recommend this operation to a member of your family in my physical condition?
How long would it be safe for me to postpone this procedure?
Where would it be best for me to have this done—at a large university hospital, community hospital, outpatient clinic?
Will you prescribe drugs I need by generic name instead of by brand name?
How long will I be in the hospital if the operation and recovery go smoothly?
How long will I be recovering at home if my case is typical?
How long is the operation likely to take?
How will the anesthetic be administered?
Who else will be in the operating room?
Will anyone but you examine me while I'm in the hospital?

Will anyone but you actually be operating on me and if so, what will he or she do?
Will you be in the operating room the whole time?
What medicine will I be taking?
Will there be any tubes in me after the operation?
Am I likely to have bleeding, pain, swelling or other symptoms postoperatively?
How long will my bandages stay in place?
How much lifting can I do? Could I lift a 3-year-old, grocery bags, a laundry basket?
Will there be stitches to remove?
Is it OK to get the incision wet? If not, how can I protect it?
Can my hospital records be sent to my family doctor?
Will my children be allowed to visit me in the hospital?
How soon will I be able to eat after the operation?
Will I need to change my diet after the operation?
Is there anything I can do to prepare myself physically for the operation?
May I take my nutritional supplements along to the hospital?
Will there be any permanent changes in me afterwards?
Will I limp? Have a swollen arm?
May I see a copy of the consent slip I will be expected to sign?

Ask this last question on the first visit and remember the consent slip is yours—you can cross out any parts you don't like. Beware of any consent slip that gives the surgeon carte blanche to operate however and wherever he deems necessary. Give your consent only for the procedure you expect to undergo, unless the surgeon has discussed the possibility of more extensive surgery with you. Perhaps if he finds any unpleasant surprises, you will want to be fully conscious to make a decision for subsequent surgery.

Your management of the consent slip depends partly on your temperament. For example, some women undergoing a breast biopsy (removal of a lump for cancer testing) want only a biopsy done, even if the breast is cancerous and will soon require more drastic surgery. Other women might want a mastectomy done should it be necessary, at the same time as the biopsy, without waking up in between the two procedures.

Other questions might arise from what the surgeon has to say about your particular case. Pin him down when he makes a generalization. If, for example, he says you will need to lose weight before he can operate, ask him how many pounds, how fast and on what kind of diet. If he says you need to cut down on smoking, at least while you're recovering, ask him how much. If he prescribes pain pills and says to take two a day, ask what time of day you should take them. If he says your kidney is diseased, ask him the name(s) of the disease. That way you can look it up in a good medical dictionary and understand your condition better. If he tells you to rest after the operation or not to work too hard, find out what that means in terms of your normal activities. Could you go back to work half-days? Must you rest in bed or could you rest around the house? If he tells you exercise can be resumed, ask what kind. Walks around the block, your daily 1-mile jog, jumping rope in the living room? If he tells you he will be doing a prostatectomy on you, find out exactly what that means. Varying amounts of the prostate gland and surrounding nerves are removed in different prostate operations. Some procedures impair sexual function but most don't. Find out ahead of time what to expect.

If questions like this offend or amuse the surgeon, find another surgeon. Take the time to make sure that the surgeon who operates on you is a person you can understand, trust and respect.

As Dr. Egdahl said, "It really shouldn't be hard to find a good surgeon. A very few have sometimes tarnished the reputation of the whole profession."

3
Getting a Second Opinion

How many times have you heard a relative say with a touch of pride, "The doctor told me on Tuesday that it had to come out and on Wednesday morning they were wheeling me into the operating room"?

Probably your relative's gallbladder, hernia or hemorrhoids did need removal or repair. But it's possible that a second doctor would have recommended treating him medically with less risk and results that would be equally acceptable. Even if the second doctor agreed with the first, the patient would only have delayed the surgery a few days by making sure. Possibly, his health insurer would have paid for the consultation in full.

Many public health researchers, health insurers and surgeons agree that seeking a second opinion is well worth a few days' delay in elective surgery.

Studies show that second opinion consultations have the potential to save money, discomfort and lives. In testimony before a Congressional committee, Eugene G. McCarthy, M.D., M.P.H., a clinical professor at Cornell University Medical College, reported the findings of a second opinion program he coordinated in the greater New York City area.

"To date, a total of 4,700 individuals have participated in the second opinion program. One-third of the total (30 percent) were not confirmed for surgery," he said ("Second Opinion Elective Surgery Consultation Program: Prepared Testimony," submitted to the Subcommittee on Oversight and Investigations, of the Committee on Interstate and Foreign Commerce, U.S. House of Representatives, May 2, 1977).

The American Federation of State, County and Municipal

Employees allows second consultations for employees in the Health Security Plan of District Council 37 in New York City.

One of the members who benefitted was Mrs. Mary Barber, who had been advised to have a hysterectomy to stop profuse bleeding and occasional pain when she menstruated. She took advantage of the union's willingness to pay for a second opinion. The consultant suggested a medical alternative to major surgery. She became one of 594 union members who decided against an operation ("Cost and Quality of Health Care: Unnecessary Surgery," report to the same Congressional Subcommittee, January, 1976).

Although there is a growing trend toward seeking second opinions, many patients don't seek them because:

- they don't want to bother;
- they trust the doctor so implicitly that they are certain his recommendation is correct;
- they want relief so badly they are eager to be operated on.

Not wanting to bother is understandable. Who wants to flip through 3-year-old copies of *Time* for 2 hours, waiting to answer the same questions the first doctor asked a few days before? Still, if the need for surgery is not confirmed, a frustrating afternoon in a doctor's office is better than a painful week in the hospital and 2 uncomfortable weeks at home.

Most patients who notice disturbing symptoms go first to a family doctor or general practitioner. You should be cautious if your doctor who isn't a surgical specialist suggests performing a major operation himself. Doctors who have not specialized in surgery should perform minor operations only. Board-certified surgeons say physicians who have not trained as surgeons should not operate at all, although those surgeons have a vested interest in keeping competitors out of the operating room. *Unless the surgical procedure in question is exceedingly minor and routine, the first nonsurgical doctor consulted should not perform the surgery.*

If your doctor thinks surgery may be needed, he will probably recommend a specialist. Should you need to find a specialist on your own, either because your doctor hasn't recommended anyone or because you don't want to go to the doctor he does recommend, use the approach outlined in the chapter, "Choosing and Communicating with Your Surgeon."

The first opinion then is rendered by that surgeon you are meeting for the first time, either by your own choice or on your doctor's recommendation. The second opinion is rendered by yet another surgeon, who will not be asked to do the surgery.

It is unlikely that either your family doctor or the first surgeon will resent your desire for a second opinion. Dr. McCarthy says, "The argument that seeking a second opinion will destroy the trust between a family doctor and a patient has no validity whatsoever. If surgery is a possibility, the family doctor or general practitioner will almost always refer the patient to a surgeon, who makes the recommendation for or against surgery. The surgeon sees the patient once, and the same is true of the second consultant, if one is sought."

The GP or family doctor's opinion is valuable because he knows the patient's history; equally valuable is the opinion of the surgeon who has seen and treated hundreds of diseased organs. Opinions of 2 surgeons, consulting with the family doctor, should give you confidence in your decision.

"Any doctor who gets angry when his patient wants a second opinion before going through elective surgery is stupid. If the doctor was on solid ground when making the diagnosis and recommendation, he has no reason to object. In fact, I encourage patients to seek a second opinion. Then if the patient does go through with the surgery, he'll feel more comfortable and confident about it," is the assessment of David Seitzman, M.D.

Dr. Seitzman, a urologist and director of the Center for Ambulatory Surgery, Inc., Washington, D.C., renders both first and second opinions for surgery. Like many other doctors who want patients to take an active role in maintaining their health, he believes the trend toward seeking second opinions is good.

Yet many patients fear that the family doctor or general practitioner will be angry at their presumed lack of trust in the specialist to whom he has sent them.

Ruth Haase, assistant vice-president of Blue Cross and Blue

Shield of Greater New York (which has had a second surgical opinion referral center since January, 1976), agrees that some patients are reluctant to seek a second opinion.

"They have implicit trust in their internist or the referring physician and transfer that trust to the first surgeon who sees them. They often intuitively like and respond positively to the first surgeon they see and feel it unnecessary to obtain a second opinion. In addition, the whole psychosocial issue of never questioning a physician's opinion or of incurring his disfavor also remains a factor for some patients who will not seek a second opinion.

"There are some physicians, highly respected practitioners, and diagnosticians who feel that where appropriate diagnostic work-up has been done and/or where medical regimen has failed that second opinion is not required.

"The Blue Cross and Blue Shield of Greater New York program has 2,000 cooperating physicians who are board-certified in various surgical specialties and who render second surgical opinions. It is important to bear in mind that in roughly one-fourth of the cases in which the second opinion is a nonconfirmation, the first surgeon did not necessarily make an incorrect diagnosis or incorrect surgical judgment. It must be remembered that medicine is still an art as much as it is a science. Criteria for surgery are not always precise and diagnoses may depend upon the individual physician's clinical acumen and the patient's subjective perception of discomfort and psychosocial factors, as well as objective signs and symptoms.

"Of those cases which were not confirmed, in a Blue Cross and Blue Shield study of patients who went through its referral center, only 15 percent showed no pathology [disease]. The other cases which were not confirmed were deferred for further tests or for medical management."

Eleanor Tilson, who administers health insurance benefits to members of the United Storeworkers Union in New York City, agrees with Ms. Haase that some patients are afraid to seek second opinions. Members of her union, however, can present the doctor with a ready-made excuse. The United Storeworkers will not pay benefits for surgery unless a second opinion has been sought.

Mrs. Tilson comments, "I think there are still many problems attached to questioning a doctor and asking the questions so you really get the proper information. But people do not think of doctors as God anymore. I think, though, that people are still afraid of doctors. In the ultimate analysis, they do control the situation in terms of your health — and that's sobering, especially when it's a case of life and death. But I must say the image of doctors is a changing one, and I think unfortunately and sadly to a great degree it's because of their greed."

Surgery is drastic, expensive and dangerous, no matter how good your doctor is. A second opinion won't always protect you. An unscrupulous doctor could remove your perfectly healthy spleen in an operation followed by a fast, routine recovery; a conscientious doctor could remove a diseased spleen in an operation followed by recovery prolonged by wound infection or blood clots.

A second opinion merely increases your chances that the operation is necessary. While seeking a second opinion in financial, legal and other matters has long been the mark of a wise consumer, few patients have traditionally used the same self-protection in medicine.

If a plumber told you all the pipes in your house would have to be torn out and replaced in order for you to have greater water pressure, would you agree to a steep fee and give him the go-ahead? Or would you ask yourself how bothersome weak water pressure really is? Would you fear offending your plumber by seeking a second estimate? Or would you check with another plumber — maybe 2 more plumbers — to see if less drastic and expensive repair might be in order?

The comparison between your body and your household plumbing system is not a frivolous one. In fact, a case could be made for the idea that most people take at least as good care of their houses and cars as they do of their bodies. While the miles and miles of arteries and millions of cells in your body are far more delicate than your household plumbing, both systems are vulnerable to aging, accident and malfunction.

Most doctors are honest people who want to get you back in working condition. Sometimes, there is a genuine difference of opinion on how to achieve that goal between two experts, neither of whom is greedy or callous. If the experts you have consulted do disagree, it's up to you, after weighing costs (both physical and financial), risks and benefits, to make the decision.

A few doctors speak disparagingly of patients who seek second consultations as "shoppers." But an intelligent shopper is not out to buy cheap goods that will cost more in the long run. He merely wants quality at a reasonable price. The wise patient approaches surgery the same way, not hunting for "bargains" with hidden costs but for quality care.

For decades, a few of the millions of Americans whose doctors recommended elective surgery have sought second or even third opinions before being strapped onto the operating table; usually, however, they were rich. With cost-conscious health insurers beginning to pick up the tab, that option is becoming available to patients of every income.

Esther Levitt, fund director for the Distributive Workers of America, says of the second opinion program offered by the union she represents, "We approach it in this manner and we did from the beginning. 'Rich people have second opinions, why shouldn't you?' And as soon as you say that, they agree. If Rockefeller needs a second opinion, then everybody else does."

The advantages of second opinions are that they:

- thwart the few doctors who, "when in doubt, cut it out";
- reassure the patient that surgery is the right course of action;
- weed out ailments for which alternative medical treatment, or even the passage of time, is a better healer;
- save money;
- save lives.

Disadvantages are that:

- some healthy patients may go from doctor to doctor until they find one who agrees to surgery;
- some patients who genuinely need surgery may try to find a doctor who recommends against it;

- repeated appointments can be inconvenient;
- a patient in severe discomfort may not want to delay treatment until a second opinion can be rendered.

A growing number of patients ask surgeons to perform operations for imagined physical ailments, Michael Curtis, M.D., formerly of Tufts University, told the Western Hemisphere Congress of the International College of Surgeons in 1975. Dr. Curtis warned surgeons to be wary of the "polysurgical" patient with a history of unsuccessful operations for pain relief. In such patients, he said, chronic pain is often located in the back or abdomen (*Clinical Psychiatry News*, August, 1975).

So far, only a minority of the subscribers to Blue Cross and Blue Shield of Greater New York who have gone through the Second Opinion Referral Center either persistently seek unnecessary surgery or fearfully avoid necessary surgery, according to Ms. Haase.

"We are aware that there are a few patients who need surgery but will go from physician to physician until someone says no. There are also those who are polysurgical addicts and will doctor-hunt until they get a 'yes.' We hope to be able to identify some of these patterns in our study to follow up the approximately 1,500 subscribers who used the Second Opinion Referral Center in the first 20 months of its operation."

Both Ms. Tilson and Ms. Levitt agreed that in their experience with union members, the number of psychosomatic patients seeking surgery is very small indeed.

When asked if many union members still wanted surgery even after the second doctor did not confirm a need for it, Ms. Levitt exclaimed, "That's like asking if I had 50 acquaintances, are 49 anxious to jump out of the window? Patients who learn they do not need surgery are as happy as anybody could be."

Ms. Tilson showed that mailings to those in her union's program who got a second opinion which did not confirm a need for surgery responded positively. "How marvelous!" and "Thank God I don't have to go through that trauma," were 2 typical replies.

Some patients seek surgery not because they are neurotic but because they dislike pain and want to get on with living a pain-free, normal life. Dr. James Graham and Donald Cooley addressed such patients in the book, *So You're Going to Have Surgery* (Hawthorn Books, 1970).

> People differ. There are those whose nervous systems make it extremely difficult for them to wait and see the results of medical treatment. There are patients who want to get things over and done without delay. If there is a choice between medicine and surgery and the risk of surgery is minimal, they'll take surgery. This is especially true when it has been suggested that medical treatment be used first on a trial basis. In some situations, the physician or surgeon, with good judgment, may ask the patient to make a choice. When the physician and surgeon both insist on medical treatment first, it's better to go along with them.

Just as dangerous as proceeding with surgery when it isn't warranted is deferring it when it is. At a meeting in Dallas, July 1, 1976, some members of the American Medical Association's House of Delegates protested second opinion programs because of the dangerous possibility that surgery might not be performed in cases where it is really necessary.

If symptoms worsen after surgery is deferred, a life-threatening emergency could result. The patient must be aware of that possibility when he chooses not to have surgery. But the AMA's argument perhaps overlooks the fact that if symptoms persist, the patient can have surgery later. Second opinion programs are so new (1972 or later) that long-term studies aren't available. But preliminary data show that most who have opted against surgery on the basis of a second opinion, don't need it in the future.

Of 4,514 people who participated in a second opinion program from February, 1972 through October, 1977, 27.9 percent were not confirmed for surgery by a board-certified consultant. Dr. McCarthy of Cornell University Medical College conducted the study of a program started in New York by the college and financed by several Taft-Hartley security union welfare funds.

On the basis of telephone interviews with 80 percent of the

participants, 6 months after their consultations with second opinion consultants, 82 percent had not yet had the surgery performed. Of those patients, 60.5 percent had had no medical treatment either. Continued follow-up will analyze how many of the patients did not jeopardize their health by deferring surgery.

In a study of surgical procedures most frequently screened, Dr. McCarthy and a research associate, Madelon Lubic Finkel, M.P.A., found that among patients who voluntarily sought second opinions, 12.2 percent were not confirmed for gallbladder surgery; 28.7 percent were not confirmed for breast surgery; 30.1 percent were not confirmed for cataract removal; and 40.3 percent were not confirmed for prostatectomy (Presentation of Health Care Financing Administration Conference on Research Results from Physician Reimbursement Studies, Washington, D.C., February 22, 1978).

After becoming aware of evidence like this, most patients recommended for elective surgery would want to seek a second opinion. The only exception might be a patient who already has tried more conservative methods of treatment and whose pain or discomfort is so debilitating that he welcomes surgery for relief. Even then, he should carefully consider the risk of complications or an operation which might prove unsuccessful in alleviating symptoms.

For the purposes of most health insurers, the first surgeon consulted (not the family doctor or GP) renders the first opinion. The pediatrician who thinks a child might need a tonsillectomy may send him to an ear, nose and throat specialist. A woman complaining of heavy menstrual bleeding may be told by the general practitioner that she has a fibroid tumor, but be sent to the gynecologist to see if surgery is required.

In the past, patients seeking a second opinion generally had to share the cost of the second or third opinion with the insurer, but that's changing. Since testimony before Congress in 1974 drew public attention to high rates of allegedly unnecessary surgery in the U.S., health insurers began instituting programs that pay the second or third consultant's fee. Some union welfare funds have found second opinions so effective in containing costs that they require patients to seek them.

Although the primary goal of second opinion programs is to assure quality while containing costs, Ms. Haase and other insurance administrators caution against making simplistic conclusions about costs saved by not operating. They point out that other patients may fill hospital beds left empty by those who decide against surgery. Alternate treatment can be expensive for patients who decide against surgery, some of whom may still have to undergo surgery later. Costs mount in paying second consultants and administering programs, too.

As a general rule, however, fewer operations performed means less money spent. For example, John Hancock Mutual Life Insurance Company saved $41,000 in estimated surgical costs in a 3-year period while insuring an East Coast trucking firm. Of 88 who requested second opinions, 43 had operations and 30 did not. Another 15 cases were still in limbo when the study was made. Administrative costs were $2,500, resulting in a net savings of $38,500.

In a study that covered about 1,500 subscribers who requested second opinions from January, 1976 through August, 1977, Blue Cross and Blue Shield of Greater New York demonstrated a savings of about $600,000. Administrative costs were about $300,000, resulting in a net savings of $300,000. In more than a quarter of the approximately 1,500 cases, the outcome was a second opinion against surgery. Those patients in the study group will be followed for approximately 5 years to determine how many of those both confirmed and nonconfirmed ultimately had surgery.

The mandatory second opinion requirement can pose problems for frightened patients who don't want to wait for a second opinion before having a possibly cancerous tumor removed. If the tumor is cancerous, a few days' time ordinarily makes little difference. The patient can use those days to fill out hospital and medical insurance forms, prepare himself psychologically and arrange for child care or absence from work. The program may waive a second opinion requirement for a frightening condition, even if the surgery is technically elective.

Patients who don't check with their unions can get stuck with large bills. Sometimes this happens when a surgeon frightens patients into believing they need surgery even more immediately than is necessary, according to Ms. Tilson.

"I think some of the problems that exist are problems of the surgeon, who leans hard on the member and uses scare tactics about the time span of getting a second opinion. Specifically in a hysterectomy case of a D and C (dilation and curettage) situation, a surgeon will say, 'Well, I think it's important and necessary you go in right away.'

"After that we talk to the member. We say, 'Look, we don't want to question Dr. So-and-so, but this is the program and we may not be able to pay anything if you don't get a second opinion.' The minute you use the word 'pay,' it's magic. A second opinion is sought."

Jack Thomas (not his real name) went to an internist because he was coughing up blood. The internist called a surgeon who came immediately to her office and checked a spot on Jack's lung.

Both doctors agreed Jack needed surgery and quickly admitted him to the hospital. The frightened patient, who later learned he had a malignancy, was so shaken that he forgot entirely about his union's mandatory second opinion program. When a bill of $4,500 came several weeks later, Jack went to his union for reimbursement. Because he hadn't followed regulations, the union technically didn't have to reimburse him at all. A sympathetic benefits counselor arranged for the union to reimburse the surgeon its maximum $800 surgical fee. That left Jack with a bill for $3,700, a little less than half of what he earns in a year. If Jack had contacted the union before undergoing surgery, the second opinion would probably have been waived and the surgery performed as soon as possible by a surgeon who cooperates with the union's plan. The cooperating surgeon's fee would have been less than a fourth of what Jack was finally assessed, and he would have paid no out-of-pocket fees. Jack says:

> I'm grateful to be alive, and I'm not angry at the surgeon. The surgeon did a good job on me. $4,500 is his fee. I think it's exorbitant, but in a life and death matter, I don't

> argue. I wasn't about to ask how much it costs and say, "Well, I'll look around" when I had cancer. I'm paying $50 a month and his office doesn't bother me. Eventually, the surgeon will have to make a settlement. I make $9,000 a year and I'm paying for chemotherapy and radiation, too.

Second opinion consultations are now mandatory for Medicaid recipients in Massachusetts and New York State for certain elective procedures. Most insurers who offer second and third opinion programs do not require them, however. Among such insurers are some of the groups covered by Blue Cross and Blue Shield, Aetna Life and Casualty and Connecticut General. In 1976, the New York State Insurance Department required that all health insurance contracts provide coverage for second surgical opinions.

The first step in seeking a second opinion is to check with a benefits counselor from your health insurer. Details of plans are difficult to remember. Furthermore, requirements may have changed since you signed up for the policy, and you may have ignored or forgotten brochures notifying you of changes. It's *your* responsibility to find out what your policy covers, not the insurer's to tell you.

Generally, the second opinion programs work this way:

1. The primary care physician thinks the patient might need surgery and sends him to a specialist. The specialist does not have to be one of the insurer's cooperating physicians, although the insurer may be able to help you find a good specialist if the primary care physician doesn't.

2. After hearing the specialist's recommendation, the patient contacts the health insurer. The insurer gives the patient names of several surgeons in his area who cooperate with the insurer. The patient chooses one and makes an appointment.

3. Although arrangements can usually be made to keep the second consultation secret, most patients fill out a form which is sent to the primary care physician or the doctor who gave the first opinion. It is sent, along with the patient's history and lab test results, to the doctor who will render the second opinion, saving

the patient the inconvenience, expense and hazards of repeated tests. Some doctors' offices forward the records to the consultant; sometimes the patient is expected to bring the materials along. Find out from the insurer and doctor's office what you should do.

4. Through agreement with the insurer, the doctor who renders the second opinion will usually not be allowed to perform the operation, even if the patient wants him to. This provision removes the consulting surgeon's financial incentive for recommending surgery.

5. After the second opinion is rendered, the patient decides whether to have an operation. Some insurers reimburse for a third consultation, but few patients seek it, according to Dr. McCarthy. Under all the plans we've investigated, the final decision is left up to the patient regardless of what the second doctor has recommended.

6. If the patient decides to have surgery, some insurers will reimburse any surgeon whose fees are reasonable and customary. Other insurers will only reimburse surgeons who cooperate with their plan. (See the chapter on Surgical Costs and Insurance Coverage.)

Now the decision is yours to make because only you know how you feel.

Perhaps the first doctor said your gallbladder should come out and the second suggested you try a different diet and some medicine for a few months. How frequent are the attacks? How painful? How valuable is the time the surgeon estimates it will take a person in your condition to recuperate? What conditions (obesity, diabetes, heart disease) do you have that would make you a greater than average operative risk? In what percentage of cases does surgery relieve gallbladder symptoms? How well can you afford the baby sitter and cleaning person you may need while in the hospital and recuperating?

If you are not insured or your insurance company will not pay for a second opinion, you might still want to seek one.

Be sure to tell the second surgeon that you are consulting him only for his opinion, and that he will not perform the operation. In 1977, surgeons' fees for a second opinion ranged from $50 to $200 without laboratory and test fees. If you seek a second opinion on your own, find out beforehand how much it will cost. If the doctor replies that it depends on the number of tests he needs to make a thorough diagnosis, assure him you will bring your medical history and previous test results when you come. If he says he needs to conduct more tests, ask for the costs and reasons, but don't be too suspicious. Most doctors are busy and stand little to gain financially from unnecessary testing, because lab fees are predetermined. Do be skeptical, however, if he will not accept the results of tests already conducted on you by a reputable doctor and an approved lab.

If you have trouble finding a doctor, try contacting the hospital outpatient clinic, neighborhood health center, public health clinic, disease-oriented private organization or county medical society near you for advice.

One consumer who could have benefitted from a second consultation is Mrs. Marie Valenzuela from Woodland, California. At the same Congressional hearing in which Dr. McCarthy testified, Mrs. Valenzuela and her daughter Linda testified about a routine but unnecessary operation that resulted in severe complications. According to the report:

> In the winter of 1969, Mrs. Valenzuela brought her youngest child, who had been running a high temperature, to a physician who informed her that the child would need a tonsillectomy.
>
> On a return visit, following treatment of the daughter with penicillin, Mrs. Valenzuela brought her other three children, at the doctor's request, so that he could examine their previously healthy throats. The physician determined that all the children needed their tonsils removed. Mrs. Valenzuela had brought along a young niece who had been experiencing nosebleeds on occasion. After a brief examination, the physician indicated that this child would need her tonsils removed as well.
>
> The surgeries began and one of Mrs. Valenzuela's children experienced brief respiratory difficulty but had no serious complications. Linda Valenzuela did not fare as well.

> Six days after being discharged from the hospital she began bleeding profusely from the neck and required 3 different surgical procedures. The operations left Linda with half the normal cerebral blood circulation. She was very near death from the bleeding, developed pneumonia, required a tracheotomy, and subsequently became anemic and contracted hepatitis. The loss of carotid circulation on one side increases the likelihood that sometime in the future Linda might experience brain damage. Laboratory tests determined that the operating physician had removed healthy tissue from each of the 5 children (Congressional report, "Costs and Quality of Health Care: Unnecessary Surgery," January, 1976).

Although Mrs. Valenzuela's unfortunate example shows venality on the part of the doctor, a doctor doesn't have to be greedy to recommend unnecessary surgery.

Reasons a doctor would remove healthy tissue or recommend surgery when medical indications are questionable might be: to decrease vulnerability to malpractice suits, to relieve the complaining patient's symptoms as finally and quickly as possible, or to solve a problem which was honestly misdiagnosed.

More than a little of the blame must be shared by patients who sue when an emergency condition results because surgery has been delayed in favor of more conservative medical treatment. A general surgeon in La Jolla, California, Clifford Graves, M.D., illustrates this problem with an example from his own experience:

> The other day I was asked to see a 70-year-old woman with a nontoxic thyroid adenoma of moderate size. In England, this patient would have been told to forget about the problem and come back in a year. But in this country, a surgeon can't afford to send the patient home. Suppose the adenoma turns malignant while you wait. A lawyer would make mincemeat out of you. So, out it comes (*Medical World News,* October 20, 1975).

Some gynecological surgery deals with health problems that are more annoying than dangerous. A surgeon might recommend hysterectomy to a woman who has completed her family and undergone multiple dilation and curettage (D and C) operations for bouts of heavy uterine bleeding. For such reasons (and there is debate among gynecologists about whether such a problem is a good reason to operate) health statisticians often name hysterectomy the most frequently performed surgery in the U.S. after tonsillectomy. If hysterectomies continue to be performed at the current rate of increase, according to the National Center for Health Statistics, more than 50 percent of American women will have had their uteruses removed by their 65th birthdays. Various authorities estimate from 30 to 40 percent of hysterectomies performed are unnecessary, according to W. Gifford-Jones, M.D., in *What Every Woman Should Know about Hysterectomy* (Funk and Wagnalls, 1977). (For more information, see the chapter on Hysterectomy.)

Reviews of surgical cases by a doctor's peers provide a safeguard against unnecessary surgery, according to the medical establishment. A study in Vermont showed doctors performed far fewer tonsillectomies after a review committee published reports of their soaring and regionally varying rates — but that didn't help the children who had already undergone them unnecessarily (*Pediatrics,* June, 1977).

When a second opinion program was instituted by the Distributive Workers of America, Ms. Levitt says, a few of the union's cooperating doctors were angry. They objected to the idea of recommending a union member for surgery only to have him sent to another doctor.

Ms. Levitt comments, "You have to be careful with doctors as you are with other professionals, not to step on their toes and to take care of them.

"They said, 'If we're cooperating with you, why do you send the people elsewhere?'

"And we said frankly, 'Wouldn't you send someone in your own family for a second opinion?'

"And the answer was invariably, 'Yes.' "

4
Choosing a Hospital

While most Americans wouldn't reserve vacation lodging without learning about its price and quality, they don't apply the same common sense when it comes to choosing a hospital.

Persons who are emergency or urgent cases, of course, don't have much choice: they go where the ambulance takes them. Since your surgery is elective, you do have a choice. Finding an appropriate hospital for your treatment should take less time and energy than choosing a surgeon. But first, a look at the picture nationwide will show you your choices.

The 7,000 hospitals in the United States, offering over 1½ million beds, are attended to or staffed by hundreds of thousands of physicians. With so many institutions available, the room for differences in quality is tremendous.

Although many patients still believe that the big, medical school-affiliated hospitals provide the best care, no significant relationship has been found between the outcome of surgery and the hospital's size, percentage of board-certified doctors or medical school affiliation.

More important in determining the outcome of the cases is the proportion of registered nurses (R.N.'s) on the staff and the care the hospital takes in screening attending doctors.

To evaluate these aspects of the hospital, you might want to ask the hospital administration office what its criteria are for allowing doctors to perform operations and what the ratio of registered nurses to patients is. In his book, *Talk Back to Your Doctor* (Doubleday, 1975), Arthur Levin, M.D., warns patients to beware of hospitals where there is not at least one R.N. on each floor or where there are more than 10 patients to each R.N.

A 1974 study of differences in outcomes of surgical cases among 17 hospitals reinforced previous studies showing a great variety in care from hospital to hospital. Conducted by the Stanford University Center for Health Care Research, the study concluded that a patient having an operation can be 2½ times more likely to die or suffer serious complications in Hospital A than in Hospital B.

Influenced by studies like this one, many patients say they worry about the general quality of health care in this country. It seems paradoxical then, that an overwhelming majority say they are personally satisfied with the care they receive. Does this show they feel superior about their abilities to make wise health care choices? Or are they whistling in the dark?

A pair of University of Chicago Public Health Department researchers suspected the latter when their 1978 study showed 61 percent of Americans think there is a crisis in health care. Only 12 percent, however, said they are dissatisfied with their own health care!

"Why this paradox exists is a mystery. . . . It could be a product of the human propensity to seek reassurance and support when in need," they speculated.

The best way to get reassurance and support when in need (and anyone about to undergo surgery is certainly in need!) is to know that you can expect good care at a reputable institution.

In a national poll by Louis Harris, respondents ranked hospitals second and the medical profession third in a list of 28 industries needing attention from the consumer movement. Only food manufacturers were rated more in need of attention, with hospitals and the medical profession ranked more in need than the oil industry, used car dealers, nuclear power plants and the advertising industry.

Despite that healthy skepticism, however, many consumers automatically go to the hospitals their doctors recommend or to those nearest their homes. While both of these sound reasons need to be considered, they should be supplemented by knowledge about the institution where you will have your operation.

A study of the history of hospitals in this country shows that from the turn of the century until the Depression, one-fourth of the hospitals were privately owned. Economic woes closed them down in the 30s. Later, voluntary nonprofit organizations or municipal and county government took over hospital administration with the help of federal Hill-Burton funds.

There are 3 types of hospitals today: proprietary hospitals, operated for profit and run by physicians, investors or both; voluntary nonprofit hospitals; and government hospitals. Patients should find out which type of hospital it is where they are to be admitted.

Proprietary hospitals do not generally offer internship or residency programs for training young doctors. They usually have fewer full-time staff members than the other 2 types, with part-timers taking up the slack.

Since about 1970, investor-owned chains, operated by hospital management companies, have been growing faster than any other segment of the hospital industry. Despite an old and frequently inaccurate image of being money-grubbing at the expense of patients' health, they have been welcomed in rural or suburban communities where voluntary groups have had trouble getting federal hospital funds. Often they replace older, dilapidated structures and offer basic, but not ultraspecialized care. This makes them less than ideal for the patient who requires sophisticated treatment for a rare disease.

For most elective surgery cases, though, a proprietary hospital should be fine if it measures up to standards of quality detailed later in this chapter. As a plus, commercial proprietary hospitals often compete with nonprofit ones by offering inducements such as food that is unusually tasty by hospital standards.

Government or other nonprofit hospitals, which outnumber proprietary ones, may be medical school-affiliated or teaching institutions. Although there are more in the Northeast than elsewhere, large teaching hospitals are located throughout the country. A teaching institution is affiliated with a medical school and offers training to residents and other health personnel. A smaller hospital in a small town, suburb or rural area is often called a community hospital; a few community hospitals also have less extensive teaching programs.

Many doctors and health care experts say that if you are very sick, you are probably better off in a hospital that is affiliated with a medical school. That's because patients in such hospitals are seen by a variety of doctors: anyone from a medical student or an intern to the chief of surgery.

To prevent your care from being fragmented, of course, you should find out who is in charge of coordinating your care while you are in the hospital by asking your surgeon or your family doctor. As long as you manage to keep in touch with the doctor in charge throughout your hospitalization, being observed, examined and questioned by several physicians in a research and teaching-oriented environment could enhance the quality of your care. A student nurse may ask the question about your medical history that throws light on your case; a resident may notice an important symptom you thought was too minor to report; a medical student may correctly suspect that an allergy to the fabric in the hospital gown is causing your eyes to swell, and so on. Some doctors say patients should try to go to surgeons who have operating privileges at a medical school-affiliated hospital, even if they plan to be operated on in a community hospital. Working in an environment oriented toward education, they say, helps keep surgeons' knowledge current. Furthermore, medical school-affiliated hospitals have the reputation of adhering to strict standards for their attending surgeons.

If there is no medical school-affiliated hospital near you, you may want to travel to one if your surgery is very complicated. Of course, you will have to find a surgeon in the city where that hospital is located. You will have to weigh being away from friends, family and home against the seriousness of your illness. Unless money is no object and travel is possible, follow-up on your case will be difficult. See what your family doctor and surgeon say about the idea.

For the same reasons that medical school-affiliated hospitals are good for the very sick or the patient with a rare disease, they aren't necessarily the best environment for someone whose case and treatment is simpler and more straightforward.

Probably a smaller community hospital would be just as good, if it is accredited and if you have a good surgeon. Your uncomplicated hemorrhoids aren't very likely to intrigue the staff of a medical school hospital. If you know what your problem is and how the doctor hopes to solve it, being examined by several doctors a day is likely to inconvenience you.

Because interns and residents generally stay only 1 to 7 years, there is a high rate of turnover in teaching institutions. Young doctors on the house staff (doctors who work for the institution as opposed to attending doctors, who send patients from their private practices to the hospital) may not be as familiar with the hospital routines as older doctors. Confusion about exams performed or tests ordered can increase as more staff members — some new to the hospital — work on your case.

If you go to a teaching institution for surgery, try not to schedule it near July 1, traditionally the day when new interns and residents arrive at the hospital to begin training.

Attorney George Annas, a Boston University medical school professor and author of *The Rights of Hospital Patients* (the Basic American Civil Liberties Union Guide to Hospital Patients' Rights, Avon, 1975), gives this advice:

> I would say if you're going to have some ordinary surgery, go to a community hospital. If it's going to be a complicated operation, go to a medical school-affiliated hospital. You'll have many more people looking at you. However, most people there are not going to be too interested in a tonsillectomy. They've probably seen more of those than they ever wanted to see. If you're an uninteresting case, you won't get any special treatment.

Whether it's a teaching institution or a small community hospital, finding the perfect hospital won't do you any good until you become a patient of a surgeon who attends there.

Elective surgical patients must be referred to a hospital by a surgeon. Some surgeons operate at more than one hospital. Either ask the surgeon where he operates or call the hospitals where you want to seek treatment and ask if the surgeons you plan to consult operate there.

Once the need for surgery is confirmed, a hospital's accreditation or the lack of it could be a deciding factor in your choice. Of the 7,000 hospitals in the U.S., 4,900 are accredited by the Joint Commission on Accreditation of Hospitals (JCAH). Accreditation is voluntary—a hospital must request the JCAH to send its evaluation team consisting of a physician, hospital administrator and registered nurse for an on-site survey. Proprietary hospitals are not eligible for JCAH evaluation — you will have to judge them by other criteria.

The JCAH, sponsored by the American College of Physicians, the American College of Surgeons, the American Hospital Association and the American Medical Association, is not a profit-making or government institution. Some insurance companies have recognized JCAH accreditation as a criterion in payment for claimants.

Most accredited hospitals will display their JCAH certificates prominently in the lobby. Probably your surgeon or county medical society could tell you if the hospital where you will seek admission is accredited. Or you can call or write the Public and Professional Relations Department of the Joint Commission on Accreditation of Hospitals, 875 N. Michigan Avenue, Chicago, Illinois 60611.

If you are interested in an unaccredited hospital, you may be able to make some judgments about it by contacting the licensing bureau of your state's Department of Health. There you could see accounts of government inspections of the institution as well as follow-up inspections to evaluate areas in need of improvement. They are a matter of public record.

Once you know how the hospital selects attending doctors; what the ratio of R.N.'s to patients is; whether the hospital is proprietary, government or voluntary nonprofit; whether it is a teaching institution; whether it is accredited; and whether it has fared well during licensing inspections, you may want to ask a few more questions. Of course, you might not always get answers.

To what hospital(s) has my surgeon or members of his family been admitted for surgery in the past?

Does the hospital have a patient representative to whom I can turn if I have problems?
Will the hospital allow me to view my chart?
What hospital does my surgeon and/or family doctor recommend?
Will my insurance policy cover surgery performed at the hospital?
What were my experiences other times I was admitted to the hospital?
What do former patients of the hospital have to say about it?
Does the hospital have a pastor, rabbi or priest?
How near is it to my family, friends and home?
Does it have services I might require, such as physical therapy and dietary departments, blood bank and intensive care unit? (Your need for these services would, of course, depend largely on the surgery you undergo.)
How much is my visit likely to cost? (See the chapter on Surgical Costs and Insurance Coverage.)

Once you have made your decision, take a tip from many mothers-to-be and visit the hospital before the surgery. If you want a tour, contact the public relations officer. If not, go on your own and informally familiarize yourself with the layout of the building.

Know Your Hospital Rights

Many hospitals print public information about the institution which you can request before or upon admission. Some hospitals have adopted *Hospital Patients' Bill of Rights,* published by the American Hospital Association.

Although the rights guarantee little more than courteous treatment of patients by staff and outline only patients' legal rights that have already been established in court, many hospitals are leery of them. The bill does not even include the patient's right to view his own medical record. He must get a subpoena for the record in court if his doctor will not show it to him.

In a study undertaken 3 years after the association adopted the rights and made them available for hospitals to post or distribute to patients, only about 500 of the 7,000 hospitals surveyed were giving patients a copy.

Reasons for the caution ranged from fear of an increased number of malpractice suits to a reluctance of the hospital officials to appear to be stepping in between doctor and patient.

As hospital patients begin to behave more like consumers than frightened children, though, the move toward spelling out rights is increasing. Minnesota and Pennsylvania both require their hospitals to post bills of rights for patients.

Even if the hospital you select makes no bill of rights available (a situation you should view advisedly), the AHA's bill applies to you. We don't believe it's strong enough, but it is a good start. The rights include:

1. The patient has the right to considerate and respectful care by competent personnel.

2. The patient has the right to obtain from his physician complete current information concerning his diagnosis, treatment, and prognosis in terms the patient can be reasonably expected to understand. When it is not medically advisable to give such information to the patient, the information should be made available to an appropriate person in his behalf. He has the right to know, by name, the physician responsible for coordinating his care.

3. The patient has the right to receive from his physician information necessary to give informed consent prior to the start of any procedure and/or treatment. Except in emergencies, such information for informed consent should include but not necessarily be limited to the specific procedure and/or treatment, the medically significant risks involved, and the probable duration of incapacitation. Where medically significant alternatives for care or treatment exist, or when the patient requests information concerning medical alternatives, the patient has the right to such

information. The patient also has the right to know the name of the person responsible for the procedures and/or treatment.

4. The patient has the right to refuse treatment to the extent permitted by law, and to be informed of the medical consequences of his action.

5. The patient has the right to every consideration of his privacy concerning his own medical care program. Case discussion, consultation, examination and treatment are confidential and should be conducted discreetly. Those not directly involved in his care must have the permission of the patient to be present.

6. The patient has the right to expect that all communications and records pertaining to his care should be treated as confidential.

7. The patient has the right to expect that within its capacity a hospital must make reasonable response to the request of a patient for services. The hospital must provide evaluation, service, and/or referral as indicated by the urgency of the case. When medically permissible a patient may be transferred to another facility only after he has received complete information and explanation concerning the needs for and alternatives to such a transfer. The institution to which the patient is to be transferred must first have accepted the patient for transfer.

8. The patient has the right to obtain information as to any relationship of his hospital to other health care and educational institutions insofar as his care is concerned. The patient has the right to obtain information as to the existence of any professional relationships among individuals, by name, who are treating him.

9. The patient has the right to be advised if the hospital proposes to engage in or perform human experimentation affecting his care or treatment. The patient has the right to refuse to participate in such research projects.

10. The patient has the right to expect reasonable continuity of care. He has the right to know in advance what appointment times and physicians are available and where. The patient has the right to expect that the hospital will provide a mechanism whereby he is informed by his physician or a delegate of the

physician of the patient's continuing health care requirements following discharge.

11. The patient has the right to examine and receive an explanation of his bill regardless of source of payment.

12. The patient has the right to know what hospital rules and regulations apply to his conduct as a patient.

5
Walk-In Surgery: The New Ambulatory Centers

A pregnant mother learns that her 6-year-old son needs minor surgery. A 2- or 3-day stay in the hospital would be not only traumatic for him but exhausting for her. She learns that the procedure can be done as safely at an ambulatory surgery facility for less money, in less time. Her insurance policy will reimburse in full for the procedure. Within an hour after the surgery, the boy is at home, begging to ride his bike. . . .

An uninsured foreigner working in an American city develops an inguinal hernia. He cannot possibly pay surgeon's fees of $450 in addition to the $1,000 normally charged in the city for 2 nights' hospitalization. His doctor recommends the surgery be done in an ambulatory surgery facility. His hernia is repaired and he is on his way home 4 hours after admission. The ease of his recovery is matched by the ease with which he pays the facility's bills — $230, excluding surgeon's fees. . . .

An executive needs a dilation and curettage (D and C) which her doctor hopes will help diagnose excessive uterine bleeding. She is eager for the bleeding to stop, but she does not want to postpone a business trip scheduled the next week. The doctors posts her case on Friday at an ambulatory surgery facility. Monday morning she is on the plane, the bleeding staunched and its cause diagnosed. . . .

These are true stories of patients who were well served by ambulatory surgery facilities. Born in the 70s, the centers are for the basically healthy patient who needs minor surgery. Ambulatory surgery can be performed in either a free-standing center designed solely for the ambulatory surgical patient, or in an outpatient surgery unit of a hospital. Hospital outpatient units existed before ambulatory surgery facilities, but were not widespread.

Wallace Reed, M.D., and John Ford, M.D. (who is no longer with the facility), founded the first ambulatory surgery facility under the registered name Surgicenter®, in Phoenix in 1970. Why? Dr. Reed says, "Starting the Surgicenter® was an attempt to respond to criticism about doctors not being interested in the rising cost of medical care. I wanted to show that there are doctors who are interested. I put my reputation and money on the line to show it.

"We do not practice defensively [as protection against malpractice suits] — that's one of the ways we save money. We don't do extra x-rays — we accept them from other places. We do our own simple tests, but we don't charge extra for them, they are included in our lump fee. We've given ourselves a ceiling, in other words. We don't add on an extra charge for IVs, drugs, oxygen and other items."

David Seitzman, M.D., a Washington, D.C., urologist and the executive director of the Center for Ambulatory Surgery, Inc. (CASI), performs surgery on both an inpatient and outpatient basis. He described the need for ambulatory surgery this way: "There is tremendous emphasis today in the cost of medical care. One way that medical costs can be contained is in the use of alternative methods and one alternative to surgery in a hospital is surgery on an outpatient basis.

"It's been estimated that in the U.S. 20 to 40 percent of surgical procedures can be done on an outpatient basis," Dr. Seitzman told us. "At the present time only 5 percent are done on an outpatient basis. Now that outpatient basis need not necessarily be in a free-standing ambulatory surgery facility. It can be in an ambulatory setting in a hospital."

Currently, a battle about the merits of the 2 types of ambulatory facilities — hospital-affiliated and privately funded — is being waged between their administrators. Yet, not one of the free-standing or hospital unit proponents interviewed for this chapter argued that actual medical care is better in his type of facility.

As long as your doctor approves and you feel satisfied with the facility's reputation and credentials, *which of the 2 types of facilities you choose will probably make little difference in the medical outcome of your case.* Prices are comparable, and although some hospital-affiliated Blue Cross and Blue Shield Plans resist reimbursing the free-standing centers, most private insurance carriers encourage their members to go to either.

Going under trade names like Surgicenter® and Minor Surgery Center®, the free-standing clinics are privately funded and not affiliated with a hospital, regardless of the hospital affiliations of the surgeons who treat some of their patients in them. In this chapter, they will be called "free-standing ambulatory surgery centers." The term will refer to centers where a variety of minor surgical operations are performed, as opposed to a single-procedure facility like an abortion clinic.

Generally hospital-based, and always hospital-affiliated, some hospital ambulatory facilities operate as separate cost centers and some are subsidized by the hospital. In this chapter they will be called "outpatient surgery units." The term "ambulatory facility" will refer to either type of facility.

An ambulatory facility is particularly appropriate for:

- patients undergoing diagnostic techniques;
- patients who can't afford the time away from work or from home that a hospital stay would require;
- patients who are uninsured; and
- children or other patients who would be emotionally traumatized by being away from home overnight.

Examples of procedures commonly done in the ambulatory setting are: diagnostic procedures such as cystoscopy (examination of the bladder), dilation and curettage, abbreviated as D and C (stretching of cervix and removal of material or growths from uterus), breast biopsy (removal and examination of breast tissue for diagnostic purposes), laparoscopy (visual examination of the interior abdomen); or such simple procedures as minor oral surgery, tooth extraction, wiring the jaw, fracture correction, for example, minor orthopedic procedures such as removal of bunions, sterilization procedures, such as tubal ligation in women (severing or pinching of uterine tubes), and vasectomy in men (removal of the ductus of the vas deferens).

Ambulatory surgery is not for every patient. It is emphatically not for those who are dangerously sick and it is normally not for those who are high operative risks because of diabetes, hypertension, old age, obesity, cardiac conditions and other problems. An accredited facility will not allow a patient to be operated on without a referral from a doctor who serves the ambulatory facility. In order to remove the financial incentive for performing operations, physicians (except possibly a staff anesthesiologist) are not employed by the facility on a full-time basis.

If you know, for example, that you want a growth on your foot removed in an ambulatory facility but your podiatrist does not operate at such a facility in your community, your county medical society can provide names of other local podiatrists, whom you can ask about ambulatory surgery. (The ambulatory facility cannot directly refer you to physicians who use their facility.)

Any licensed surgeon may apply for operating privileges at an ambulatory facility. Patients, however, are very carefully screened by the doctor who is to perform the surgery and the anesthesiologist before acceptance by the facility, in order to weed out high-risk patients.

Marian Kennedy, R.N., director of nursing at CASI in Washington, D.C., explained her facility's policy: "The patients that are posted are generally in good health. Every one of them has some impediment to their health or well-being, or they wouldn't be coming to us. But we don't do anyone who is acutely ill.

"Now that does not mean we will not do people that have problems," she added. "But they are people that have known problems and they are monitored by internal medicine specialists who consult closely with the surgeon.

"For example, we operated on a diabetic under general anesthesia. And we operated on one gentleman who was 88 years old, chronologically, but he was a very healthy individual and recuperated beautifully."

She added that such patients are painstakingly monitored and that backup systems, required by the accrediting society (described later in the chapter) exist for their protection.

Advantages of ambulatory surgery are that it saves time and money and provides the individual with streamlined, often personal care. Because the facility will assess you a lump sun regardless of your need for "extras" like intravenous feeding, fruit juice, phone calls and bandages, you know in advance exactly what the procedure will cost. That lump sum will not include your surgeon's fee or the diagnostic procedures you undergo before admission to the facility. As you learned in the chapter on choosing a surgeon, you should find out from the surgeon what his fee will be ahead of time. Administrators at the facilities expect their doctors to charge reasonable and customary rates, but they exert no direct control over the surgeon's fee and won't be able to tell you how much he will charge. The surgeon's fee is strictly between you and the surgeon.

In addition to the actual dollar savings you gain from ambulatory surgery over hospital surgery, you save time. Although this concern is less compelling for the elderly and children, for some patients, the old saying that "time is money" holds true.

A study, conducted by the National Bureau of Economic Research in Stanford, California, on what kinds of people used surgery in 1963 and 1970, showed some interesting income and educational differences. The people in the high-income brackets generally underwent more operations than the less affluent. But highly educated, prosperous men, aged 20 to 64, were less likely to undergo surgery than were the less educated in their income group (*New England Journal of Medicine,* September 29, 1977).

The researchers of the study speculated that doctors may recommend surgery less often for members of the high-education, high-income group because they think these patients will comply with alternative treatments in home conditions conducive to successful outpatient care. The researchers added, however, that the patients themselves may avoid surgery because their time is too valuable to spend in the hospital.

Lost time, surgeon's fees and hospitalization charges are not the only costs of surgery in the traditional hospital setting. Indirectly, utilization of surgery drives insurance premiums up.

More directly, it can cause the patient to spend money for child care during the time away from home. Often a spouse will leave work for a few days to take care of the home or be with the patient at the hospital. This can use up the spouse's vacation or sick leave.

These costs are minimized by ambulatory surgery.

John I. Smith, a photographic manufacturer in Washington, D.C., is a case in point. Mr. Smith who is self-employed, uninsured and committed to the care of his invalid mother, avoided hospitalization for personal, financial and business reasons. In a telephone interview, he told about problems caused by his need for surgery and how he solved them:

> I stepped off my bike very hard into some guttering on the street. I felt some warmth in my groin right afterwards. It wasn't discomfort, really, just a peculiar feeling of localized warmth. I felt it a couple more times and noticed a pouch on my groin. So I went to my surgeon. He said surgery would have to be done.
>
> Going into the hospital just wasn't feasible for me. For one thing, I'm self-employed so I don't have Blue Cross. But more than the money, it was a time problem. My mother is terminally ill with atherosclerosis and I take care of her. It just wasn't possible for me to go to the hospital for the 6 days it would normally take for the surgery. Time was the overriding consideration. So my doctor suggested I go to a man downtown who ran a clinic and did surgery on a walk-in, walk-out basis. He thought I would find the doctor and the clinic attractive.
>
> I wasn't really concerned about what would happen if there were complications. I felt the clinic was adequately equipped and I knew there were hospitals 2 blocks away. I

was concerned, though, that I might have considerable discomfort.

When I went to the clinic, I thought it was more like an airline office or a good restaurant than a clinic, which was good. I liked the color scheme very much. The colors are really nice and the recovery room's design is well calculated to make you want to get up and feel like living again. I guess it's maybe a little futuristic, a little 2001, but I like that. Most of these damn hospitals, even the new ones, have such an institutional aura, if not odor!

Everything was explained to me and I felt I was getting a lot of attention. I needed a lot of attention to be operated on and released in that amount of time. I was under general anesthesia for 40 minutes and on my way home in 2 hours. I also felt I had adequate postoperative instructions. I was told not to drink alcohol for 24 hours. I did and was consequently very sick the next day, but that was my own indiscretion.

I had been told that I was to go back in for a postoperative check in 4 days, but I misunderstood and thought they said a week. So in 4 days they called me and said, 'Where were you?'

After 3 weeks I was back on my ordinary schedule, which I worked up to gradually. I had to wear support garments for a while, but eventually I was able to discard them.

When I got home after the surgery, mother and I had nurses 8 hours a day, but I took care of us the rest of the time. I was able to handle us both the first night after the surgery. The first night I slept in a chair. I had to half-carry mother to the bathroom every hour or so — actually, my mother is ambulatory but very unsteady on her feet. I had discussed this with the doctor who did the surgery, and he thought I would be able to manage it, which I was.

I would have surgery done there again if I needed an elective operation, and I would certainly recommend it to other people.

Part of the reason that Mr. Smith was handled so rapidly is that ambulatory surgery facilities are open only during regular business hours, and every effort is made to discharge patients by the end of the afternoon. That doesn't mean that you will be kicked out into the street still woozy if you're physically not able to leave by 5 o'clock or your ride is late. It does mean that if the operation goes smoothly and your recovery is routine, you will be on your way home in at least a few hours.

For children and their parents, the time saved by ambulatory surgery may not be as important as the emotional trauma they are spared.

In a 5-year study of over 5,000 children undergoing surgery on an outpatient basis at Children's Hospital in Jamaica, West Indies, there were no deaths or major complications.

According to Mohammed El-Shafie, M.D., and Robert P. Shapiro, M.D., of the Medical College of Ohio who reviewed the results of the surgery, "The incidence of complications was 2.7 percent for 2,662 general surgical procedures [as opposed to specialty surgery]. The most common complication, superficial wound infection, was seen in 1.58 percent of the patients and none required admission [to the hospital]."

The researchers also noted that "Parent cooperation played an important role in the program. Due to the shortage of qualified nurses, parents were encouraged to participate actively in looking after their children in the preoperative and postoperative period, and did so with enthusiasm and competence" (*Pediatrics,* October, 1977).

Even when nurses are plentiful, most parents are happy to be involved. Jo Anne Burka of Potomac, Maryland, was only too glad to help in preoperative and postoperative care when her 6-year-old son underwent ambulatory surgery for a minor urological problem. Mrs. Burka and her physician husband were allowed to stay with the child in both the preoperative holding area immediately before surgery and in the recovery room immediately after. Dr. Burka was in the operating room during the procedure. Mrs. Burka described her experiences in a free-standing ambulatory surgery center this way during a telephone interview:

> My son needed the type of surgery that could be performed in an ambulatory setting — enlargement of the

opening of the penis. He had undergone surgery for an undescended testicle in a hospital when he was 3. He was hospitalized again for a tonsillectomy and adenoidectomy when he was 5. His surgery at age 3 was especially traumatic because he was so young. He had to be hospitalized the night before, although he wasn't really ill. Of course, the nurses had to spend some of the night looking after him. I was pregnant and afterward I was exhausted from lost sleep while he was in the hospital. There were no facilities for parents who stay overnight. It was a 2½-day ordeal.

I know from experiences as a surgical patient in hospitals that the staff is often understaffed and overworked. When you are not critically ill but not able to care for yourself independently, you hesitate to make extra demands.

If the type of surgery needed can be performed in an ambulatory surgical unit, it is less traumatic for the patient. The family is better able to handle postoperative care. Having my son's surgery done on an ambulatory basis made everything much easier. Because of the large picture window in the postoperative room, you are able to see the child as soon as he is wheeled out of the operating room. As soon as they have him ready, you can go in and see him. The first thing the child sees when he wakes up is his mother. In fact, the parent is able to assist the nurse during recovery.

I thought the ambulatory center was just fantastic. There was so much obvious concern for both the patient and the family. The staff works regular hours, they aren't exhausted from overwork, and their only job is to take care of people like you.

Robert C. Brownlee Jr., M.D., at Children's Hospital of Philadelphia, writes that much more pediatric surgery can be performed on an ambulatory basis, in an editorial in the same issue of *Pediatrics* cited for the Jamaica study. His opinion:

Various authors including El-Shafie and Shapiro indicate that approximately one-third to one-half of all surgery cases in children can be done appropriately as outpatients. Perhaps after more experience with this approach, we can

> look forward to an even greater percentage falling into the day-care category.
>
> There are obvious advantages, but they warrant emphasis. In this time of accountability for all that is done, of cost consciousness and increased concern for people as individuals, it is imperative that we consider all of these factors. Estimates of saving for outpatient surgery versus in-house surgery vary from place to place and range from $100 to $500 per case, depending upon the institution and type of surgery. . . .
>
> While this [cost containment] is very important, it likely is not as important as the savings in emotional costs to the young child. The trauma of separation from home and parents brought about by hospitalization and surgery is tremendous and has long-range implications that we cannot overlook. The potential for long-lasting emotional trauma must diminish tremendously when a child scheduled for surgery in a day-care situation can have his parents by his side until the actual surgery is done, can recover under mother's and father's ministrations and can return home to a familiar bed and room and siblings (if any).
>
> Other factors such as lessened postoperative infection, savings of bed space and freeing of nurses and other personnel for higher priority work should also be remembered.

Part of the reason that children (and other patients) are not retained overnight is that they are not as heavily anesthetized in an ambulatory surgery facility as they might be in a hospital.

Dr. Reed (founder of the Phoenix Surgicenter®) said just enough anesthesia to keep the patient pain-free and provide suitable operating conditions for the surgeon is administered during surgery at his facility, thereby saving the patient time and money.

As past hospital surgical patients can testify, some hospitals administer enough anesthesia to keep the patient hazy for hours after he reaches the recovery room. Using minimal anesthesia can backfire, however, according to one patient operated on at an East Coast facility. On an anonymous card returned to the institution after recovery at home the patient wrote: "As for the pain, the doctor said I absorbed the anesthetic very rapidly, so he had to inject more before the surgery was complete. So I was in great pain before I could get home and take medication."

Even so, the patient rated the service at the facility excellent, and added that she would return should she need a minor elective procedure again. Her postscript: "It was the first time I ever had surgery and had delicious chicken broth afterward. And I do so love chicken broth!"

If the idea of being whisked in and out of surgery makes you anxious, ask to be posted early in the morning at a free-standing ambulatory surgery center or go to a hospital outpatient surgery unit so you can be admitted to the adjoining hospital should a problem arise. (Patients from free-standing centers can be admitted to hospitals, too, of course, though they will have farther to travel.)

The only other patients at an ambulatory facility will be ambulatory surgery candidates like yourself. That means that you will not be bumped off the schedule by an emergency case, as you might be from the traditionally crowded hospital operating room schedule.

Administrators at the ambulatory facilities admit that the doctors who perform surgery there could be detained at the office or hospital, but they say such a situation would only delay your operation, and only very rarely postpone it to the next day.

Even a basically healthy person undergoing minor surgery at 8:00 A.M. in a hospital would probably have been admitted the night before and be discharged the day after surgery, resulting in a 2-night stay. Patients undergoing diagnostic procedures, such as breast biopsies, are particularly inconvenienced by this overnight hospitalization. If the test result is negative, they want to hurry home; if it's positive, they need to make arrangements for child care or sick leave for their upcoming days in the hospital.

Some hospitals retain patients for a standard amount of time after surgery regardless of the speed with which they recover. Sometimes standard stays are as much a matter of habit as of medical imperative. As any mother of a 25-year-old can tell you, women used to be hospitalized twice as long after delivery a generation ago as they are now.

Even in the traditional hospital setting, doctors are beginning to realize the logic behind releasing patients after "right stay" rather than "standard stay."

A study of patients who underwent routine abdominal surgery in a British hospital showed that the 47 who were evaluated and discharged on a right-stay basis were hospitalized an average of 2 days less than those discharged after the standard 10 days (*British Medical Journal,* June 11, 1977).

A follow-up report showed that the medical progress of the 2 groups was comparable. The time before they returned to work did not differ significantly. The main differences were that patients in the right-stay group complained less often about the length of time they spent in the hospital. They were also slightly freer of minor postoperative symptoms, such as disturbed sleep, than the fixed-stay patients, who reported more symptoms during recovery at home.

The report concluded that the shorter stay, though often overlooked, can reduce the demand for bed-space and better serve the patient, who usually wants to get back home as soon as possible.

After free-standing surgery centers came into being, hospitals were quick to follow suit with their own outpatient surgery units, built with the encouragement of the American Hospital Association.

Since the Minor Surgery Center® of Wichita opened in Kansas in 1974, for example, 3 Wichita hospitals have begun to offer ambulatory surgery.

M. Robert Knapp, M.D., president of the Wichita facility, welcomes the proliferation of units for outpatient care. He said that in every instance he knows of where a free-standing center was built, a hospital in the same area created or enlarged an outpatient surgical service soon afterwards.

"We do have evidence in Wichita that more outpatient surgery starts to be done at the hospital when the free-standing center is introduced," said Dr. Knapp. "We don't compete with the traditional system as much as complement it. I do think, however, that the ambulatory center offers advantages over the hospital outpatient facility.

"For one, the cost is less. That doesn't mean that the charges are lower to the patient. Sometimes the outpatient facility of a hospital charges the patient less than a free-standing center. But the overall cost of operating the free-standing center is less, and ultimately the hospital is going to pass on that extra cost to the consumer.

"The most important difference between the 2 is intangible. The ambulatory centers offer personal care to each patient and the staff deeply feels its responsibility for the patient. We're concerned with the individual — he's not just another number coming down the line," Dr. Knapp said.

Douglas Hawthorne, assistant administrator of the Presbyterian Hospital of Dallas is quick to agree that "hospitals have been somewhat lax in not initiating this kind of care in their own environment."

He maintains, however, that in today's climate of medical cost containment, hospitals should start providing this service; that fashioning an outpatient unit from an existing portion of the hospital makes good sense, and that the units are cost-effective if operated as a separate cost center of the hospital. In Dallas, the Presbyterian Hospital's Day Surgery Unit was created *before* a free-standing ambulatory surgery center that eventually folded. Mr. Hawthorne said, "The hospitals that establish ambulatory surgical units are not duplicating existing facilities that are already available. The significant difference between the hospital outpatient facility and the free-standing is that we have all the emergency backup services of the hospital at hand. There is emergency service and hospital admission available when somebody wants it. This happens in about 3 percent of the cases. A complication develops in the operating room or recovery room, usually excessive nausea or bleeding. It isn't always a medical complication. It may be a case of patient apprehension. For example, parents might decide that they would feel more comfortable with their child hospitalized overnight rather than taking him home. That's fine with us."

Hospitalization won't necessarily expedite recovery, though, according to Dr. Seitzman (Washington, D.C., urologist and CASI director). Based on surgery experiences in both the hospital and ambulatory setting, he said, "Some of my patients in the hospital tend to spend extra time because they're confined. They have a tendency to feel ill because of this. Whereas if you go home, although you may have the same degree of pain, you're at home. If you're home, you are ambulatory and you may not feel as sick. You have a little closer relationship with your surgeon because he's the only person you're dealing with. You're not dealing with nurses, hospital staff, residents and others. If you have a problem, you contact your surgeon. And then it becomes a different, if not a better, rapport between the surgeon and his patient."

Only one patient in CASI's first 10 months of operation subsequently required hospitalization, Dr. Seitzman said. The patient suffered chest pains from gas.

Responding to arguments that hospital units aren't cost-effective, hospital administrator Mr. Hawthorne conceded, "When you incorporate a same-day surgery unit, you reduce the overall length of stay in the hospital. Now that does cut into the revenue. In our instance, the same-day surgery unit is a separate cost center. With our daily service charge and revenue from x-ray, we are able to finance the unit independently of the hospital. Even if we weren't, you have to ask the question: Which is more important, losing a few days of occupancy or providing a service that the patient needs and wants?"

If better service is the goal, then why did hospitals jump on the ambulatory surgery bandwagon only after the privately funded facilities were open, asks Robert Williams. Mr. Williams, who is executive director for the accrediting body, Freestanding Ambulatory Surgical Association (FASA), says, "Hospitals have had 50 years to do what free-standing ambulatory surgical facilities are doing, but they just became interested in providing this service in the last 5 to 7 years. There is more money to be made on the hospital inpatient as opposed to the hospital outpatient. With this being the case, how can a hospital, from a financial standpoint, be totally committed to a program which empties inpatient beds?

"When attempting to develop an outpatient surgery program," Mr. Williams explained, "frequently the hospital administration will look for a service of the hospital which is underutilized. Such an area may be the Obstetrics unit, since in many areas the annual birth rate is decreasing, or the emergency room. There is certainly nothing wrong with this approach except the commitment usually isn't taken far enough. These ambulatory surgical units are frequently expected to share services with other departments within the hospital. As an example, when such a unit is incorporated into an existing emergency room area the equipment and personnel already present in that area may be called upon to function in the outpatient surgery unit as well. On the surface such an arrangement appears to reflect sound economic planning. However, when demand for emergency treatment is high, both personnel and equipment may be pulled from the outpatient surgical function and pressed into use to satisfy the emergency needs at hand. This either causes postponements or cancellations of scheduled outpatient surgery. The net result is that rather than risk such inconveniences physicians tend to schedule what are really outpatient surgical candidates as inpatients in order to insure that their patient is considered as a first priority."

Thomas O'Donovan, Ph.D., author of *Ambulatory Surgical Centers: Development and Management* (Aspen Systems Corporation, 1976), and administrator of Mount Carmel Mercy Hospital in Detroit, agrees that costs are higher for hospitals operating outpatient surgery units than for the privately funded facilities. That's still not a good argument against them though, he said. "The reason that argument doesn't make sense is that most hospitals are reimbursed for costs they incur, not just for what they charge the patient."

An American Hospital Association staff specialist in ambulatory care, Eugene Wood, flatly dismissed the arguments over the relative merits of the 2 types of facilities. "The difference is that the free-standing centers are not under the auspices of a hospital. Surgery is surgery. It doesn't matter where you have it," he said.

When asked how a patient can safeguard himself against facilities that are not up to par, Mr. Wood said, "I would go where my physician sent me. I trust him to make that decision in my best interests."

According to Dr. Seitzman, doctors try to send people where they need to go, financially as well as medically. "If a patient doesn't have insurance, physicians — the ones that I know — will try to perform whatever is required in the most expeditious and the most economically feasible way. If the patient has the best insurance — whatever that may be — then there is no requirement for him to worry about the cost. And if the patient has insurance where the first dollar is covered, there is no concern, from the patient's or the physician's viewpoint, because 100 percent is covered.

"Patients have the mistaken idea that if they have insurance they can avail themselves of anything, and insurance will pay for it," Dr. Seitzman pointed out. "If you tell a patient that you can do something equally as well, equally as safely, but cheaper, the answer that you frequently will get is 'But I pay my insurance, let them pay for it. I have insurance coverage why should I bother or care?' And you try to get across to the patient that he has to pay for his premiums and he's concerned when next year's premiums go up. But that's a watered-down thing because people do not think about this on an individual basis.

"Physicians are also paid by the third party carrier. And they don't necessarily concern themselves with the specific hospital costs. A patient may go to one hospital or another depending upon the physician's preference — not by the cost of one hospital or another," explained Dr. Seitzman. "Even if he has the choice of one or the other, it isn't done on a cost basis. It's done on 'Where am I going to be that day?' or who referred the patient.

While patients may be oblivious to costs covered by insurance, the insurance carriers naturally are not. Mr. Hawthorne (the Dallas hospital administrator) said insurance companies have not reduced premiums even though costs to patients are less because of shorter overnight stays. Ambulatory surgery, he said, saves insurance companies more money than it saves hospitals.

Joseph Clune, manager of the group claims division of Metropolitan Life Insurance, was enthusiastic about the savings involved for the patient, as well as beneficial psychological effects.

"We've found that the patient saves 43 to 52 percent by having surgery done in a free-standing center," he said.

Having personally visited 127 facilities for ambulatory surgery and accepting only 48 of them for reimbursement, Mr. Clune admitted some facilities are substandard but said the consumer can protect himself against them. When the facilities became popular, Mr. Clune said, Metropolitan Life had to arrange a way for the privately funded centers to be approved because contracts between the company and the groups it covers mention only hospital reimbursement.

"Use of the centers depends in part on surgeons' awareness of them and whether their patients are aware of them as an option.

"Of course, I've seen a couple of promoters out on a scheme to get rich and I've seen some cases where you wouldn't put a sick cat in the damn place.

"The centers we reimburse in full have to be accepted by us. If a patient would have surgery done in a center we don't work with, he would only be reimbursed for 80 percent of the balance after a $100 deductible," he said.

The criteria Metropolitan Life uses in accepting a facility for full reimbursement are similar to those used by FASA, the accrediting body for the free-standing centers. The Joint Commission on Accreditation of Hospitals (JCAH) has not yet established specific guidelines for hospital outpatient surgery units, but each unit is reviewed along with the hospital as a whole in accredited institutions.

Unfortunately, persons who learn they need surgery aren't always in a position to research what the most economical alternative might be. They are more interested in finding safe, convenient facilities reimbursed by their insurance carriers. Always call the insurance carrier *before* your case is posted, not after you receive the bill. Since emergency surgery is not performed at ambulatory centers, lack of time is not a reason for failing to make this call.

Patients who are going to have ambulatory surgery should be sure that the free-standing ambulatory surgery center they go to is either accredited by FASA or is at least a member of it and has applied for accreditation, according to Dr. Reed. Patients undergoing outpatient surgery in hospital units should make sure that the hospital is accredited by JCAH. (See the chapter on Choosing a Hospital.)

To locate ambulatory surgery facilities of either type within your community, call the county or regional health center, ask a knowledgeable doctor or check at nearby hospitals. FASA claimed 65 member facilities in 1978. Marian Kessler from the AHA's Office of Research Affairs said in June, 1978, that to their knowledge, no accurate tally of hospital outpatient surgery units exists, although such a study (by AHA) is underway.

After you have found an attending doctor, checked with an insurance carrier, established that the facility is up to standard (by checking accreditation and licensure, asking the doctor, touring it), given your medical history, undergone the appropriate lab work for admission, ascertained what you will be charged by *both* the facility and the surgeon, and decided that ambulatory surgery is right for you temperamentally, you should be ready for the procedure.

It is important that you have an adult pick you up and drive you home and perhaps stay with you a few hours or all night. You should ask for postoperative instructions concerning food, drink, activity, return to work and follow-up visits. Know how to contact the surgeon should a problem arise.

With this preparation, a good surgeon, a basically healthy body, an eagerness to get well and no unexpected complications, your reaction to ambulatory surgery might be as enthusiastic as that of the patient who raved about his visit to an ambulatory facility: "Excellent service, convenient location, pleasant surroundings, economical cost, and enthusiastic staff — an exciting concept whose time has come."

6
Preparing for Admission — And the Operation

Lying uncomfortably in bed, the hospital patient thinks it's wonderful that doctors are sawing open a man's chest, recirculating his blood and fixing his heart — just one floor below him. But if they can do that, he keeps asking himself, why can't he get a bedpan or a pain pill sooner than half an hour after he has rung his bell?

Threatened by strikes, high prices for equipment, fuel shortages and increasing government regulation and consumer skepticism, the hospital is caught between technological advancements and patients' increasing if reasonable expectations.

The doctors, nurses, social workers, dietitians and other health care team members we consulted agree that in *most* American hospitals, medical care is adequate if not superlative. Americans who have had the misfortune to have been hurt or fallen ill in underdeveloped countries abroad would quickly concur. But what often bothers hospital personnel — and patients — is the sometimes depersonalized manner in which health care is delivered.

Of more than 10,000 nurses who answered a questionnaire in the professional journal *Nursing 77,* the vast majority said both nurses' and doctors' skills were good to excellent. But 77 percent said the level of psychological support given the sick was fair to poor. Results were published in the journal in December, 1976 and January, 1977. (It should be noted that readers volunteered their answers and were not randomly polled.)

The most commonly offered weapon against dehumanization in hospitals (itself the topic of hundreds of conferences, books and articles) is better communication between patients and staff.

Your stay will be much more pleasant if you know what to expect in the hospital and how to communicate with the staff. Not knowing what is going to happen may make you feel more anxious. If you have questions, ask to see the surgeon or anesthesiologist working on your case.

Patients who were visited by an anesthetist before surgery had less preoperative anxiety than those who were not visited in a study at a Surrey, England, hospital.

Researchers noted that those who were able to meet the anesthetist personally and ask questions were also less anxious than those given a 10-page booklet explaining anesthesia. Both groups were less anxious than those given no preoperative information about anesthesia (*British Medical Journal,* October 15, 1977).

If you feel as if hospital staff members are speaking Greek when they answer your questions, you have plenty of company. You have every right to the same sort of clear explanation you would ask for if a car mechanic answered questions about repairs on your Chevy in hopelessly technical jargon.

This is what happened when Jonathan M. Silver of Albert Einstein College interviewed hospital patients:

> To determine the deficiencies in patients' understanding of their physicians' explanations, I interviewed 109 patients at a public and voluntary hospital. On questioning their use of medical terms, I found some striking misconceptions. For example, a woman knew that her eyes and skin were yellow and that her liver was enlarged, but did not realize that these signs were related to her being 'jaundiced.' Similarly, when explaining a paracentesis to a patient, I used the terms 'anesthetic' and 'antiseptic.' Talking with the patient afterward, I discovered that he did not know what these words meant. A virtuous attempt at explanation failed because medical terms had been used instead of the lay words 'pain-killer' and 'germ-killer.'
>
> Patients often do not understand common medical procedures. Six patients undergoing intravenous treatment at the time of the interview had no idea why the needles were

> in their arms. Another enigmatic procedure is electrocardiography. For instance, the first time one patient had an electrocardiogram coincided with the same office visit during which his diabetes was diagnosed. He came to the conclusion that the electrocardiogram was the diagnostic procedure for his diabetes. Another patient believed that the electrocardiograph pumped her heart. . . .
>
> In conclusion, physicians should not assume that patients understand their illnesses and treatments. Narrowing of this communication gap is challenging, but achievable. After an explanation of the situation, the physician should solicit questions from the patient and provide the opportunity to correct any misconceptions. The patient should be asked to explain his or her understanding of the illness and therapy. Through these logical steps many of the problems of noncompliance or unnecessary patient anxiety can be avoided" (*New England Journal of Medicine,* May 18, 1978).

Middle-aged or elderly patients who haven't been hospitalized since their own births or the deliveries of their children are probably in for a shock when they go to the hospital today. The corridors are labyrinthian, the machinery sophisticated, the tests bewildering. They might find themselves wondering, "Doesn't anybody care?"

But even in the most imposing institution, your own small human voice can be heard and respected. *The trick is neither to whisper nor shout, but to state your own needs as often as you have to in a firm, polite voice.*

Many hospitals are rightfully criticized for failing to provide nonsmoking waiting and patient rooms, dispensing only junk food from their vending machines, allowing accidents to happen, lacking follow-up after patient discharge, and being noisy.

Sensitive from his own discomfort or put off by an exasperated tone of voice from a busy nurse, a patient easily forgets that most hospital staff members literally wish him well. Surrounded by death, trouble, odors, tears and complaints, it isn't always easy for them to show it.

"The medical profession," remarked one blunt East Coast

hospital social worker, who asked not to be named, "has a poor public image. Americans are woefully ignorant about health, and the whole system reinforces them for being passive. The patient who has a thousand questions shouldn't be punished, even if a busy nurse or doctor would really like to have a nice, quiet, compliant patient. Patients are partly to blame for making doctors godlike. They burden doctors and nurses with total dependence. Even if they're not aware of it, it's a dreadful weight of responsibility for the staff to carry."

In an attempt to alleviate the problems the social worker described, many hospitals are making changes. Some have adopted the American Hospital Association's Bill of Rights (see the chapter on Choosing a Hospital) or a document similar to it. Over a fifth, or 1,420 hospitals, have a patient representative or patient advocate, an ombudsman who trouble-shoots between patients and staff. Some have hired translators for their patients who don't speak English. Others stretch the rules on visiting hours and other matters in selected instances. Colorado, Minnesota and New York have state laws requiring patient grievance mechanisms within health institutions. Patients get some protection from Professional Standards Review Organizations (PSRO) which are federally financed but doctor controlled. Although often criticized for not being tough enough, PSRO doctors do monitor each other's patient care in matters such as length of stay, medication orders and so forth.

Although abuses still exist, such programs for improvement make optimism possible. In a speech before the Medical Society of the State of New York in New York City, in November, 1976, David M. Thompson, M.D., the director of New York Hospital in New York City, concluded:

> The hospital edifice may seem austere and inhuman, but the interior can be just the opposite. Specialty units are structured and geared to the needs of individual patients as they are affected by their disease. Treatments and routines must be carried out, but at the same time, a person's right to privacy and to accept or decline treatment must be recog-

nized as an integral part of the delivery of health care. Notice that I said person, not patient. If we remember that patients are people and we treat them as such, we will not lose sight of the humanism factor.

Are hospitals dehumanized? I think they might have been, and maybe in many instances still are, but I think they are trying. I believe all of us recognize that a large part of curing is caring and that only by caring will we be able to maintain a humanized hospital" (*New York State Journal of Medicine,* August, 1977).

Before Admission

Generally, elective surgical patients get a call from the admissions office a day or 2 before they are scheduled to enter. Jot down a list of any nonmedical questions you have and leave it by the phone. The caller will probably ask a few biographical questions and find out what, if any, insurance coverage you have. If you sound prosperous enough from your answers, you will probably be asked if you prefer a private or semi-private room. Find out the difference in costs, and recognize the risk of acquiring a noisy roommate with a gang of visiting relatives before you answer.

If you have questions and the admissions office hasn't called as your admission approaches, call it. Among questions you might want to ask are:

Will I be allowed to wear my own gown and robe?
What toiletries, if any, will you provide? (Many hospitals provide a "free" kit with items like toothpaste and mouthwash upon admission. The cost is reflected, indirectly anyway, in hospital bills.)
Do I need to bring any cash?
When are visiting hours?
What are visiting rules for children?
What is my admitting diagnosis?

When is my operation scheduled?
What floor is the admission office on, and which entrance should I go to?
May I leave my car in the lot while I'm in the hospital?
Where do my visitors park?

Many hospitals provide information booklets which help to answer many questions asked by patients on admission.

By the time you have been admitted, you should have asked your doctor whatever you wanted to know about your condition and the upcoming operation. If you would like to supplement the information he has given you, look up your condition in a good medical dictionary.

The American Cancer Society offers general information in laymen's terms to patients about specific diseases. Printed information is free while films and tapes can be borrowed. Every state has several chapters. Check the phone book for the one nearest you.

If you are going to undergo surgery that may have a profound emotional impact on you or change your life-style, ask the surgeon to put you in touch with a patient who has undergone the procedure. There are many self-help groups to encourage patients who undergo operations like mastectomies or colostomies. It may not be as helpful to contact friends or acquaintances who have been through similar surgery, as their actual operations and physical conditions could have been much different than yours will be.

Remember that you have a right to feel anxious — it's a rare surgical patient who doesn't. When psychiatrists Thomas H. Holmes and Richard H. Rahe compiled a list of 43 well-known commonly occurring life events that cause stress, personal injury or illness ranked sixth. It was assessed as causing more stress than being fired, retiring or changing financial states. Your relatives and friends may also feel anxious when you are hospitalized — change in health of a family member was ranked eleventh among the 43 factors.

C. Eugene Walker, Ph.D., a clinical psychologist who wrote the book *Learn to Relax* (Prentice-Hall, 1975), suggests that anxiety isn't always a bad thing. He wrote:

> Anxiety is a lot like pain. We prefer to experience as little of it as possible, but it serves a very useful purpose in alerting us and activating our defenses in times of danger. Moderate amounts of anxiety motivate us to plan to for future events and increase our ability to cope with situations as they occur.

Use your anxiety. A healthy amount of it may be constructive if it makes you double-check your insurance policy, find out as much as you can about your condition, prepare yourself nutritionally or make arrangements for your absence from home or work.

Maureen Gilligan, supervisor of the Visiting Nurse Association in Brooklyn, New York, works with many elderly patients both before and after hospitalization for surgery. She told us, "Very often, patients can reduce their worries by throwing themselves into the busy work of going into the hospital — leaving the house clean, stocking up on groceries, buying a new nightgown or pajamas, stopping the newspaper, finding someone to water the plants and so on."

Ms. Gilligan also suggests that patients try whatever customarily relaxes them, noting that some young patients seemed to have been helped by techniques like transcendental meditation.

Several postoperative patients told us what worked for them. One man's family sensed his anxiety and gave him a preoperative party — complete with new p.j.'s and a cake that said, "Happy Operation." A woman entertained guests the night before her admission to keep her mind off the upcoming operation. Other people have used self-hypnosis, exercise, soothing herb teas like camomile and peppermint, meditation and hobbies to relax.

Perhaps a book on relaxation will help. One of the most popular is Dr. Herbert Benson's *The Relaxation Response* (William Morrow, 1975).

Basically, meditation for relaxation involves concentration on thinking about nothing, nothing at all. By following a few simple instructions, practicing deliberate relaxation once or twice a day for 20 minutes or so can effectively reduce tension and anxiety.

First, select a quiet room and sit in a comfortable chair. Adjust yourself so that you are as relaxed as possible. You should probably slouch forward a bit, resting your hands on your thighs, and keeping your feet flat on the ground, somewhat in front of the position of your knees.

Close your eyes. Now, consciously relax all your muscles, beginning with your feet. Move up through your legs, your stomach, your chest, your arms, your neck and even your face, jaws and mouth. When your jaw muscles are really relaxed, your lower teeth will probably not be touching your upper teeth.

Breathe through your nose, and draw the breath into your belly, which should be rising and falling. Become aware of your breathing, but don't make a big deal out of taking deep breaths. They aren't necessary. Breathe normally and naturally.

Now, as you breathe out, say the word "one" to yourself. Inhale. Exhale and again repeat the word "one."

Keep the muscles of your body relaxed and continue breathing rhythmically and easily, in and out, repeating the word "one" with every exhalation.

It's only natural — stray throughts are going to pop into your head. They won't interfere with the exercise. Just think, "Oh, well," and let the thought drift out of your mind. If it returns, don't worry about it and don't try to fight it. Just keep repeating to yourself the word "one," breathing easily and rhythmically and keeping your muscles relaxed.

Continue for up to 20 minutes. When you finish, sit quietly for a while and then gradually open your eyes.

Anxiety may make you feel like turning to coffee, cocoa or leaf tea for its warmth and reassuring aroma. But don't suddenly increase your intake or you may experience unpleasant symptoms.

As too much caffeine can interfere with sleep, raise blood

pressure, cause heart irregularities and gastrointestinal disturbances, and a myriad of other symptoms, it's probably wise not to drink much caffeine-containing coffee or tea in the hospital. Too much may even cause your vital signs (such as pulse and blood pressure) to be misread. You might want to take some herb tea or other favorite noncaffeinated beverage with you and ask for hot water when you want it. Most hospital kitchens offer decaffeinated coffee on their patient menus.

Several nurses and dietitians we spoke to said patients complain more frequently about food than about anything else in the hospital. Patients say they complain because the food is genuinely poor; hospital staff members suspect it's because the food is the easiest target for the general dissatisfaction brought on by illness and discomfort in alien surroundings.

At any rate, it may comfort you to have a familiar snack at your bedside. Unless you will be on a special diet in the hospital, consider bringing along favorite foods that don't need to be refrigerated. Also, bring any nutritional supplements you customarily take (as long as you have told your surgeon about them). You will probably need to check these items in when you're admitted. You will also need toiletries, sleepwear and slippers and a small amount of cash for magazines and other small purchases. Since you will spend some time waiting for tests or treatments in even the most efficient hospitals, it's best to bring something to read or do with your hands. The period of hospitalization could be a good time to catch up on correspondence or a book you've been meaning to read.

Clear up last minute doubts before admission. If you come down with a severe cold or sore throat during the week or 2 before surgery, call your physician. Colds increase the possibility of postop respiratory complications, and elective surgery may have to be postponed until the infection clears up.

Be sure to alert the staff to any food or drug allergies you may have, to avoid reactions during tests or the operation. One woman we spoke to broke out in a rash after a TB skin test, which involves a small injection right under the skin. Instead of TB, more tests revealed she was merely allergic to the adhesive bandage that was put on the injection site. You should also tell the staff about any medication you regularly take — it could interact with drugs given in the hospital or produce misleading test results. Cortisone, for example, can cause an elevation in blood sugar level, which might make doctors suspect diabetes.

Before the Operation

Let's follow a patient through a routine operation.

Carl is feeling draggy toward the end of the day. His stomach is often vaguely upset and he needs more cigarettes and coffee than ever to face the feisty geometry students he teaches in a junior high school. Among the other teachers, he has a reputation for possessing the patience of Job in his classroom. But lately, he snaps at students and refers to them mentally as "snotty brats." At the insistence of his concerned wife, Alice, he visits his family doctor in October.

"Well, Carl," Dr. Marcos responds to the schoolteacher's vague complaints, "you smoke too much, you don't exercise and 190 pounds is just too much to carry, even on a 6-foot frame. That could be why you don't feel any better than you do."

When Carl tells him about the recent attacks of pain in his upper right abdomen, though, the doctor begins to ask questions. Tests bear out the doctor's suspicion of a diseased gallbladder. The doctor tells Carl to have the surgery at his convenience, preferably within a year. He advises him to stay away from fried, fatty and gas-forming foods, but doesn't specify which ones. Carl thinks of a ditty he heard one of his least favorite students singing about beans, the musical fruit, that day in the school cafeteria.

"No more beans for me," he tells Alice that night. She agrees with his idea to schedule surgery when school is out in May.

Except for a few mild attacks of indigestion, Carl is fine until March. When his 2 daughters come home from college for a weekend, Alice celebrates by fixing stuffed cabbage, a

> favorite family dish. By 10:00 P.M., the mild-mannered Carl amazes his daughters and wife by literally howling in pain. A surgeon is consulted the next day, and Carl quickly agrees to have the gallbladder out in a week.
>
> On the scheduled day, Alice drives Carl to Clark City General, an older community hospital where both of their children were born. After paperwork is taken care of in the admissions office, Carl goes to his assigned room to unpack and is then summoned back down to the laboratory for tests.

If the hospital is crowded, you may have no choice of room. Actually, Carl did, but didn't know it. If cigarette smoke and noise bother you, you can request a nonsmoking roommate and a location away from the nurses' station and elevators. Some hospitals have attempted to set up nonsmoking areas and patients' rooms, with mixed success.

Contrary to the old stereotype of nurses tiptoeing along silent corridors, hospitals are very noisy places. The whirs of machinery, conversations of staff, visitors and patients, ding of call bells and clank of trays all contribute to the bedlam. Once you are admitted, with any luck, to a quiet room, it's time for any necessary tests that weren't done on an outpatient basis.

Testing procedures vary from hospital to hospital. Besides diagnostic tests done in the doctor's office, outpatient clinic or hospital before surgery (Carl had a gallbladder series, for example), all patients are required to take certain general tests upon admission for surgery.

Blood and urine specimens will be taken and your chest will be x-rayed. Electrocardiograms (abbreviated either EKG and ECG) are usually administered to all patients over 40. Other tests you may have are a skin test for tuberculosis and a kidney function test.

A common method of evaluating kidney function is to test the blood urea nitrogen (BUN) level. This test screens kidney efficiency. If your kidneys weren't working as well as they should, a sudden drop of blood pressure from anesthesia and surgery could temporarily shut them down. If that were the case, surgery would be postponed and you would be given intravenous fluids to correct the condition.

You may have tests as an outpatient a day or 2 before admission. Possibly you will be asked to bring a urine sample from home. Or you may be admitted to the hospital before the testing begins. Some hospitals have you proceed directly from the admissions office to the lab. Others send you to your room first, take the urine and blood samples there and schedule EKG and chest x-rays for later in the day. If the hospital has portable equipment, all or most of the tests could be taken in the room. If you are asked to fast from midnight on the day before admission, you are probably going to have a fasting blood sugar test, which will rule out diabetes.

Ask when your tests will be if you are ushered to your room without a word about testing. If you are directed immediately to the lab, perhaps an accompanying family member or friend can drop your things off in the room.

The EKG will study heart patterns and rule out previous heart attack while the chest x-ray rules out various pulmonary diseases. When your chest is x-rayed, you may be asked to don a heavy lead shield that will protect your reproductive organs and a fetus, if you are carrying one, from possible harm. Tell the technician if there is any chance you are pregnant.

Your blood will probably be checked in the several tests that comprise a complete blood count (CBC). This includes a hematocrit, which measures the volume of red blood cells in comparison to your total blood volume, and a hemoglobin test, which measures in grams the red blood cell pigment in your blood. Both are used in the diagnosis of anemia. Evaluation of the shape and size of red blood cells would help determine the type of anemia if you are anemic. White blood cell count measures the number of white blood cells in the blood and helps determine the presence of infection. In a differential white blood cell count, 100 of your white blood cells are examined by microscope to determine the proportionate amounts of the various types of white blood cells. This test helps determine the type of infection if you have any infection. A microscopic exam of the number of platelets in your blood helps diagnose any clotting abnormalities. The results of all these blood tests should be ready for the doctor within 24 hours of when the specimens were taken.

Your blood may be typed and blood from a blood bank reserved for you in case a need for transfusion arises. The need would be determined not only by your blood count but also during surgery by the pressure measurement in the great veins of the chest. If you have already lost a considerable amount of blood, you may be given a preoperative transfusion to offset the loss and boost your supply for the operation.

Some surgical patients, especially those who are undernourished because of vomiting or lack of appetite, will also be checked for the blood mineral levels, including potassium, sodium, chloride, calcium, phosphorus and magnesium. The results of all these blood tests should also be ready for the doctor within 24 hours of when the samples were taken.

Being in awe of doctors and nurses, Carl doesn't ask what his blood tests are for, although he winces a little when the nurse sticks the needle in the crook of his elbow and draws the blood into 4 rubber-topped tubes. Because he is a heavy smoker with a mild case of emphysema and chronic cough, Carl's surgeon had ordered Carl to go to the hospital for a chest x-ray a few days before. Three days before the surgery, the surgeon also had Carl come in for inhalation therapy, so that ultrasonic humidifiers and mist vaporizers could liquefy the mucus in his bronchial tubes.

After Carl has the blood tests, he waits in the lab for half an hour, until his name is called by the EKG technician.

"I just had an EKG in the doctor's office a few months ago," Carl tells the technician.

"We need a current EKG, Mr. Johnson," the technician replies.

Although he has been having EKGs with his routine check-ups for the last 10 of his 55 years, Carl always feels like an actor in a science fiction movie when he has to lie prone on a cot in a soundproofed room, stripped to the waist with his chest dotted with grease-smeared electrodes. The technician also straps 4 electrodes to his wrists and ankles. The electrodes are attached by wire to an electrocardiograph, a machine about the size of a small TV mounted on a stand. The technician moves a fifth electrode over Carl's chest to specified positions, just as a doctor would with a stethoscope.

The wires, which sense the electrical current that courses through Carl's heart with every beat, lead to a mechanism that records the beat. The impulse of the beat from the upper to the lower heart chamber appears as vertical peaks and horizontal valleys on graph paper in the EKG machine. Later, a doctor interprets the tracings, which show that Carl's heart is working normally. The EKG doesn't take long, and the voltage of the electrical current is so low that Carl feels no pain or discomfort.

Before he goes back up to his room, a nurse leads Carl to a bathroom and presents him with what looks like a transparent Dixie cup.

"Can you pass water for us, Mr. Johnson?" she asks euphemistically. Carl's urine will be checked for specific gravity, which is the degree of concentration of the urine, to rule out urinary tract obstruction, kidney damage and dehydration.

Determination of the urine's pH, or degree of acidity, would help show if Carl has kidney, lung or other conditions which might lead to too much or too little acid in the body. Carl's urine is also tested for protein, which would help diagnose kidney damage if there were any. The amount of sugar in his urine is meaured to help rule out diabetes and hypoglycemia; the urine is also checked for the amount of ketone bodies (a chemical compound) in it, to help rule out metabolic disorders. His centrifuged urine is checked in a urine sediment exam for indications of kidney damage, urinary tract infection and gout. The results can be analyzed in a few minutes.

Your surgeon will visit you some time before the operation to review the planned surgical procedure, its probable results and relative risks. If you haven't already signed a consent form, authorizing the specific procedure, he may ask you to do so at this time. Take this opportunity to be sure you clearly understand the surgeon's explanation of the nature and purpose of your coming operation.

> Except for the emphysema, Carl's test results are normal, and the surgeon tells him when he visits that afternoon that smoking is the only factor that might make for an uncomfortable recovery.
>
> "No more smoking now until after the operation," the surgeon warns him on his way out of the room. "See you tomorrow."
>
> During the afternoon, Carl stays in bed and reads an Ian Fleming book. Except when the nurse interrupts to take a short medical history and check his pulse and blood pressure, he pictures himself as James Bond instead of a geometry teacher awaiting gallbladder excision.

You will probably be admitted in the afternoon of the day before surgery. Since hospitals have only minimal staff on weekends, the earlier in the week you are scheduled, the better. Although you will probably not be in discomfort the day before an elective operation, the hospital atmosphere may encourage you to take to your bed. While patients aren't usually allowed in the main part of the hospital, you can probably roam around your floor or visit with other patients in the recreation room the day before the surgery. Lying in bed may encourage you to feel sicker and dwell on the upcoming operation.

To prevent confusion, however, tell a nurse when you leave your room. Nurses will appear periodically to check your vital signs, establishing a record of your normal readings and assuring that whatever condition you've been hospitalized for hasn't become worse.

> Around dinnertime, Alice comes in to bring Carl the evening paper and the day's mail.
>
> "Better for you to read this than your tacky spy novels," she sniffs. There is also a get-well card from Carl's first pe-

riod class, with a picture of an outraged rabbit getting a shot in the behind.

Usually a hearty eater, Carl is hungry by the time his dinner tray arrives.

"Enjoy your dinner, Mr. Johnson," says the nurse. "You won't be eating again until after the surgery."

Carl doesn't know it, but a sign on his door warns kitchen personnel "n.p.o." That means he can be given nothing per mouth ("os" is "mouth" in Latin), not even water. Scared by the attack he had a few days before, Carl didn't gorge before he went into the hospital.

Some patients have a gargantuan "last supper" before surgery, like prisoners taking a last fling with freedom — not wise, especially if you will have general anesthesia. The less in your stomach the day of the surgery, the better.

Since the time Carl has entered the hospital, half a dozen different nurses have already been in and out of his room. Part of the reason is that the day shift has gone home and the night shift has come in. Years ago, registered nurses could be identified by the white caps they wore. That's no longer true, but you can still tell them from other hospital personnel by what's on their name badges. Registered nurses (R.N.'s) have the most training and handle administration and the more complex aspects of nursing care; licensed practical nurses (L.P.N's) handle routine patient care, while nurses' aides perform the chores. The head nurse on the floor is a registered nurse. If you have a complaint about a floor nurse, ask to see the head nurse. But before you complain, discuss your problem with the floor nurse and make sure it isn't a matter of flawed communication. Some patients worry that a nurse will retaliate in ways such as withholding pain pills if they complain. Nurses we talked to said this is highly unlikely if the supervisor has been informed.

A former nurse who is now a patient representative in a Pennsylvania hospital said some of the bitter complaints patients make arise from their failure to speak up.

"Some patients almost expect nurses to read their minds.

You have to speak up when you need something," she stressed. "Many people in the hospital become docile — and although I hate to say the word, almost childlike. They don't want to make trouble. They just want you to make them better so they can go home. Having been in the hospital as a patient myself, I can understand that. In fact, I said when I got home I'd like to write a book about what it's like on the other side.

"One woman told me she had undergone surgery 2 days before and had never been offered anything for pain. What had happened is that the doctor had written on her chart an order for pain medication as necessary, or p.r.n. A very busy nurse might forget to ask the patient if he or she needs anything for pain if the patient doesn't ask."

Carl Johnson is a passive patient throughout his hospitalization. He doesn't like to make trouble. Only pain or hunger prompt him to complain, and then quietly. When he's cold, it's his visiting wife Alice who rummages through the drawers in the hospital room and finds a blanket. When the noise from the nearby elevators interrupts his sleep and the nurses say the door must remain open, Alice brings him cotton balls from home to put in his ears.

Although Carl is in a semi-private room, the bed next to him is empty. He's glad, because tonight he doesn't feel like talking to anybody, even Alice. He's a little relieved when she kisses him goodnight and goes home. He tells himself he isn't really alarmed about the surgery, but he keeps thinking he and Alice are the right age to make a will. This thought is interrupted by the arrival of Dr. Anders, the anesthesiologist.

She explains that Carl will have general anesthesia and suggests putting him to sleep by the combination of an injection and inhaled gases. Then she asks a few questions about drugs Carl takes, his previous reactions to anesthesia, family history and so on.

"First you'll get a shot to make you drowsy and comfortable, before you leave the room. Then throughout the operation," she concludes, "I'll be continually testing your vital signs to see how you're tolerating the anesthesia. You're in pretty good shape — though you ought to stop smoking — so I don't foresee any problems. Everything sound OK with you? Do you have any questions?"

"No." Carl smiles and shakes the doctor's hand. Actually, he's curious about when he'll be "put under" and how soon after the operation his head will clear, but he feels silly asking. He has an uneasy memory of his elderly father, who died several years before, being thoroughly disoriented for several days after undergoing surgery for lung cancer. Was that because of the anesthesia, he wonders?

According to Ms. Gilligan (from the Brooklyn Visiting Nurse's Association), elderly patients may want to ask if their surgery could be done under local anesthesia. She said, "Older people who are perfectly able to cope at home do become disoriented in the hospital. Their senses are overloaded. If they have some hearing and sight deprivation and some slowing of their mental reflexes, general anesthesia will exaggerate this. They may feel disoriented for several days."

The terms anesthetist and anesthesiologist are often used interchangeably, but they have different meanings. An anesthetist is anybody who administers anesthesia — a nurse, for example, can be an anesthetist. An anesthesiologist is a medical doctor who has specialized in studying and administering anesthesia. Carl's anesthesiologist, Dr. Anders, is a woman. Because anesthesiologists keep rather more regular hours than most doctors, it is an especially appealing field for women with family obligations.

You should tell the anesthesiologist about any drugs you take or disease you have, even if you feel you've already been through the same thing ad infinitum with your family doctor, the surgeon and possibly the registered nurse who welcomed you to your room. If any blood relatives have had unexpected reactions to anesthesia, such as high fever, say so. This tendency can run in families.

After Dr. Anders leaves, Carl watches his favorite detective drama on TV and puts the light out at 10:00 P.M. When he is almost asleep, he feels a touch on his forearm. The white-suited young man towering over him looks familiar in the dim light from the hall. When the orderly turns the light on, he and the older one recognize each other — he's one of Carl's former students. While the orderly goes through his preoperative routine with Carl, the two of them reminisce. The orderly doesn't tell Carl why he is scrubbing him from the breast to groin. Carl doesn't ask.

Later on, though, he worries about the size of the shaved area — is the incision going to be *that* long? He feels like an offering about to be sacrified.

Not knowing Carl is worried, the orderly doesn't say that the size of the area cleansed and shaved bears little relationship to the length of the incision. Although both scrubbing and shaving (to facilitate making the incision and prevent infection) are usually done, the hair in the operative area may merely be trimmed short instead. It depends partly on the procedure and partly on the surgeon's thinking. Some surgeons still believe hair carries contaminants into the operating room that can pose a threat to the patient; others think shaving causes tiny nicks and scratches that serve as a breeding ground for bacteria. Although Carl didn't think to take a shower — he had had one in the morning before being admitted — it wouldn't have been a bad idea. Showering the night before surgery would help guard against infection, particularly if he scrubbed the entire area where the surgeon will be working.

"Just one more thing, Mr. Johnson."

"School's out. Call me Carl."

"OK Carl. Want to roll over now?"

Only Carl's pride is hurt when the enema is administered, but afterward, advised to hold it for 10 minutes, he is extremely uncomfortable. Usually one who follows directions to the letter, he cheats a little and dashes to the bathroom in 8 minutes, just in time.

Until early morning, Carl is left in peace. Only once does a nurse come in to check his blood pressure, and she steals in so gently, using a flashlight, that he barely awakens.

At 7:00 A.M., when Carl has long been awake with hunger pangs, an ample nurse marches in and hands him a hospital gown and 2 yellow pills.

"Take these. Change into this," she barks. Carl thinks fleetingly of his days in the Marines. Once he is back in bed in his breezie nightie, she fits him with white elastic knee-high socks (which will help support his leg veins) and asks him to remove his wedding band, both to prevent it from being stolen and to keep one more foreign object out of the operating room. Just before he is taken to the operating room, his hair is covered with a disposable cap, which will keep hair-borne germs out of the operating room.

Just as the nurse leaves the room, Alice arrives.

"Excuse me, nurse. Could you or someone else let me know when Carl comes out of the operating room?" Alice asks on her way in.

"Yes. Stay in the waiting room and someone will come and tell you when he goes to recovery," the nurse replies.

"Where is the waiting room?"

"First floor."

Although Carl wonders about when his operation is scheduled, what tubes will be inserted in him afterward and if he will be returned to the same room, he doesn't ask.

Patients can save themselves worry by finding out these details before the operation. Afterward, fear exaggerated by pain could make them panic and jump to conclusions. Even to relatives, patients who have routine postop equipment attached to them can look much sicker than they are.

Jewelry cannot be worn to the operating room. Leave it with a visiting friend or relative until after the operation or give it to a nurse to put in the hospital safe. You should scrub off any make-up and nail polish so the anesthesiologist can check the color of your face and nail beds. Dentures should be removed so that anesthesia can be easily administered. If they are not removed, they can be broken by the anesthesiologist's apparatus or come loose and block the passage of air.

If, like Carl, you have anxious relatives waiting to hear how the surgery has gone, assign just one of them as the family envoy

— communications break down if several family members ask doctors and nurses for progress reports. The envoy can call the others who are waiting to hear about you. If no one can come to the hospital, write a note of explanation with the phone number of a close friend or relative who expects the call and give it to the nurse to clip on your chart. That way, the surgeon will know whom to call. If the friend or relative will be in the hospital, ask him or her to stay in the waiting room or the room you will be returned to after the surgery so he or she can be easily contacted. You should also ask the surgeon how long the procedure will probably take, so that relatives or friends won't worry as time passes. Length of a procedure isn't always an indication of its gravity. Furthermore, an emergency operation on a different patient can delay yours or you can be kept in recovery a long time without your family or friends knowing it.

> Alice and Carl joke a few minutes to ease their mutual nervousness. Then the ample nurse returns with a formidable assortment of equipment. Carl reads her name tag as she looms over him and learns she is B. Maldor, R.N.
>
> "Are you his wife?" she asks Alice before baring Carl's genitals and inserting a rubber catheter in the tip of his penis.

The catheter is inserted in the urethra (urinary passage) because if Carl's bladder were to fill up with urine during the operation, it could get in the surgeon's way. A catheter, which drains into a clear plastic bedside bag called a Foley bag, is used with many different kinds of surgery. It isn't painful, although it can be uncomfortable.

Urinary catheters can be inserted before, during or after surgery. It is easier to insert them in women, because the urethra is shorter in women than in men. If you are a woman with a tendency to get urinary tract infections, you may want to ask for a sterile funnel which fits into the urethra with the catheter passing through it. Since the catheter will then touch only the sides of the funnel instead of the skin around the urethra's opening, you'll be much less likely to become infected.

There are several reasons for catheterization. One is to measure the hourly output of urine (which shows how well the circulation of blood is working). Another is to empty the bladder to avoid distention; if the bladder is distended, its muscles could be weakened. Also, a distended bladder can get in the way during surgery; it could be a particular problem in prostate surgery. The surgeon has to be able to distinguish the bladder from other organs by feel. Another reason for catherization is to relieve bedridden patients who cannot relieve themselves.

After the catheterization, Carl thinks he is ready at last for surgery. He is surprised when Nurse Maldor approaches him with another tube, this time for his nose. The tube is to prevent Carl from vomiting and then aspirating, or breathing in the contents of his stomach. Inserting the n-g or nasogastric tube is a little more difficult than inserting the catheter. Well lubricated, it is inserted through the nose and into the back of the throat.

"Keep swallowing," orders Nurse Maldor as Carl's gag reflex rebels. She brings him a few chips of ice to suck on, and then the tube slides easily down Carl's throat. Its presence bothers him, making his throat ticklish and rather sore, just like it feels when he has a bad head cold.

A piece of tape is used to secure the tube across Carl's nose and upper lip.

"Now one last tube and we'll be on our way," the nurse tells Carl. The insertion of the intravenous tube into the inside bend of Carl's elbow isn't nearly as uncomfortable as the last procedure. He feels only a prick from the steel needle that is inserted. The needle is at the end of a clear tube which the nurse tapes to his wrist. The tube is attached to a glass bottle of fluid hanging upside down from a bracket on the top of a pole. The pole rests on casters. The bottle is filled with a combination of saline and dextrose, the clear fluid which will nourish Carl until he is able to eat again.

Doctors say the IV also serves the purpose of keeping one of Carl's veins open while he is in the operating room, giving access to his circulatory system so that drugs he may need can be easily administered.

If the tender membranes in your nose are scraped when an n-g tube is inserted, you may have a nosebleed. That is nothing to worry about, nor is the fluid you may see draining from that tube. The tube may be connected to a container, which, when plugged into the wall, provides a low level of intermittent suction that will keep your belly from distending.

Nasogastric tubes can be used for different purposes. They can be used to prevent vomiting, as Carl's was; for stomach-pumping; for drawing off gas or seepage from the patient; and for keeping the stomach and upper intestine from distending. Sometimes the tube is inserted by the anesthesiologist after you are unconscious. After surgery, your mouth and nose may be sore from the tube. Request ice chips or an anesthetic jelly for relief.

In abdominal operations, the tube will probably remain in place until the bowels function, probably 2 to 4 days. In other types of operations, if it's used at all, it can come out much sooner. Sometimes the tube is just used periodically for suctioning excess fluid.

The use of the intravenous tube is more universal. At worst, an IV will make your arm sore — moist compresses will help relieve that discomfort. In the fluid administered by IVs, there may be salt, minerals, glucose, vitamins and antibiotics. Just water may be used if an IV is inserted only for the duration of the operation. Although IVs are generally inserted into the inside bend of the elbow, they can also be put in a prominent vein, such as one that runs across the forearm or the back of the hand.

To keep the needle from coming out of the vein, you should keep your arm flat and motionless. Your arm may be strapped to flat pieces of padded wood to help you do so. If you have an IV for several days you may want to ask the doctor or nurse if you can have some antiseptic salve to put on the vein where the needle enters it. This may relieve the soreness, and will guard against vein inflammation and infection. If you speak up as soon as you feel ready to take food by mouth, the staff may be persuaded to detach the IV from you sooner. (See the chapter on Nutrition for Surgery Patients.)

Not all surgical patients undergo all these procedures. You may undergo some or all of them after you are in the operating room, either anesthetized or so premedicated you are only dimly aware of them. If you should awake with a catheter, IV, n-g tube or small tube protruding from the surgical incision to drain it, don't be alarmed and don't yank on the tube. The use of any of these tubes is a perfectly normal procedure. None of the tubes will be acutely painful, but they may make you uncomfortable and sore. You'll be rid of them as soon as it is possible.

> With the IV in place, Carl has only one more indignity to submit to before he is wheeled to the operating suite.
>
> "Roll over, now," the nurse commands, after checking Carl's identification tag. Carl winces as he feels an injection in his right buttock. The nurse is administering "premedication" — usually a combination of drugs — which will relax him, dull his pain, and dry his saliva and mucus.
>
> Whistling "I Left My Heart in San Francisco," a bearded orderly wheels a mattress mounted on a cart alongside Carl's bed.
>
> "Time's up," he remarks jovially, hoisting Carl and his network of equipment onto the bed.
>
> "See you soon, dear," Alice calls from the door as Carl is whizzed along the corridor; the orderly shouts greetings to his friends from behind Carl's head. After a trip down to the first floor in an elevator, Carl is pushed through formidable double doors labeled with a large sign in huge red letters. He is too confused to read the words, "Surgical Suite — Authorized Personnel Only." Along with several other patients stretched out on rigs like his, Carl is pushed lengthwise against the wall. Three other patients precede him in the line leading to the operating room. Masked workers emerge and enter through its swinging doors, oblivious to the motionless patients lined up along the wall. Carl lifts his forefinger, which feels as heavy as a barbell, to trace a plaster patch in the shape of Cuba on the wall. Sometime later — his sense of time has vanished — he is wheeled into the operating room.

It's a rare elective surgical patient whose operation takes place promptly when it's scheduled. If you're such a patient, you may go directly into the operating room from your own room.

Otherwise, patients may be taken first to a preoperative holding area, to the recovery room (where they will also be returned after surgery) or to a corridor, as Carl was.

Writer Michael Clark shared with us a vivid account of waiting for orthopedic surgery in a small community hospital: "On Wednesday morning, about 9:30, I was given a shot of something to make me groggy. I was then wheeled down to the operating room. By the time I got down there, I was just about out. However, I was wheeled into the room on this little cart. My last conscious memory was this: There were approximately 4 or 5 operating room personnel standing around the operating table. They had green gowns on, caps over their hair and masks across their faces. Each of them held their paychecks in their hands. They were, to a person, all complaining about the amount of tax which had been taken out of their paychecks."

Like Michael and many of the other patients we talked to, your last impulse before being operated on might be to jump off the operating table and run to the nearest exit. You will be too groggy to do so. But if you know what to expect in the operating room, you may feel calmer.

7
What Happens in the Operating Room

The silent nurses scurry back and forth in a frenzy of grim activity, communicating only by nodding their heads or widening their Bambi eyes. A mysterious mask tied over his rough-hewn jaws, the surgeon performs with the tight-lipped concentration of a ballistics expert defusing an atomic bomb. The only sounds are the ominous blip of the electrocardiograph and the clink bloodied instruments make as they are tossed into metal trays.

Unless you work in a hospital, your idea of an operating room probably comes from the movie M.A.S.H. or soap operas. Even if you have had surgery before, you were probably so heavily anesthetized that you only recall being wheeled in. The operating room (OR) in a real hospital bears little relationship to the one described above.

Radios and cassette players may fill the room with the sound of the surgeon's favorite music; one nurse may massage the tired shoulders of another who stands holding a tray aloft; OR personnel may joke with each other and periodically leave or enter the room.

Although a few bloodied "sponges" — really 4-inch squares of thin gauge — will be dropped into buckets as the operation progresses, there is very little gore. Many people have the idea that the entire operation room is sterile or bacteria-free. While the entire room is *clean,* only the area around the table is actually sterile. Even the anesthesiologist at the head of the table is out of the sterile operative field.

Most operating rooms are not large — some are no bigger than a living room — and only a very few are equipped with the windowed amphitheaters you see in the movies. If observers are present, they are more likely to stand on portable steps outside the sterile operative field. In some hospitals, observers may watch the operation on a closed-circuit TV screen in a corner of the room.

Part of the OR mystique is the surgical garb. It lends an air of anonymity; nurses who have worked together more than once may not recognize each other outside the OR, without their masks. Everyone working in the room wears a cap, a mask and a cotton uniform — either pants and tunic, which men and some women wear, or a dress. Paper booties are worn over the shoes to reduce friction and prevent a buildup of static electricity — a spark could cause the combustible gases used in anesthesia to explode.

Only the surgeon(s) and scrub nurse(s) (called "scrubs") wear sterile gowns and latex gloves. They scrub their hands in antiseptic solution for about 10 minutes and move only in the sterile operating field, the area immediately surrounding the patient. The circulating nurse doesn't scrub, but when she brings materials to the surgical team she takes off the wrappings without touching the materials directly. Her job, basically, is to fetch and carry.

The strange costumes worn in the OR, incidentally, are no longer always green — they are sometimes cheerily flowered.

The OR's major distinguishing characteristics are the operating table and high-intensity light. The table can be broken into various positions to accommodate different types of surgery; some sections can be elevated or lowered when the patient is aboard. Special equipment, such as electrocardiographs and surgical instruments, rests on portable stands, stainless steel carts and shelves and tables along the wall.

> Carl, the patient we left waiting outside the operating room in the last chapter, won't remember much of this scene. After the scrub nurse checks Carl's identification bracelet against his chart, she and the circulating nurse roll his litter to the operating table and help him scoot onto the table. A modest man, Carl is still awake enough to be embarrassed when his gown rides up in the process and exposes him. To his relief, he is quickly covered.

The premedication he received in his room makes Carl feel cold. He is grateful to be enveloped in a blanket that feels deliciously warmed, like a sheet that has just come out of the dryer. Now Dr. Anders, the anesthesiologist, begins her work. First is the blood pressure cuff, which will be attached to Carl's arm throughout the surgery. Then the electrodes from the electrocardiograph machine are affixed to his chest, as they were the day before when he had his preoperative EKG. The anesthesiologist's EKG machine will monitor Carl's heart throughout the operation. Dr. Anders detaches the IV with the saline-dextrose combination from the inside bend of his elbow and replaces it in the same site with a slightly larger tube (see the chapter on Nutrition for Surgery Patients). It will be used first to administer the sodium pentathol which will initially put Carl to sleep, and later, a muscle relaxant. The smaller tube, which administers the saline-dextrose combination will be replaced in the recovery room.

The 3 types of anesthesia are: general, in which you are unconscious and feel nothing at all; spinal, in which you are awake but numb in a general area, usually the lower half of your body; and local, in which you are awake, and only the particular area to be operated on is numb. With either spinal or local anesthesia, drugs can be given to make you groggy or even as completely unaware of your surroundings as you are under general.

Before getting any of these types of anesthesia you will probably have premedication — pills or a shot — to make you drowsy and calm. The premedication may also dry your mouth, as some anesthetics increase the flow of saliva and the anesthetist needs to keep your windpipe clear. (If you drink heavily or take barbiturates, narcotics or tranquilizers, tell the anesthetist well in advance of surgery. More than the ordinary dosage of premedication may be needed to have the desired effect on you.)

Anesthesia works by blocking pain. General anesthesia acts on that part of the brain that recognizes pain, to make you unaware of it. Local anesthesia cuts off transmission of pain signals between the site it is administered and the brain.

If you have general anesthesia, it will be administered either by needle into a vein or by inhalation. If by inhalation, either a liquid form is dropped onto a mask covering your mouth and nose or more likely, a gaseous form is sent directly into your lungs via an endotracheal (throat) tube. Your anesthesiologist may combine techniques in your case, perhaps injecting you to put you to sleep, then administering inhalation anesthesia with a throat tube. This sounds more uncomfortable than it is — the only after-effect of it, if any, will be a mild sore throat. Although it could be hard for the doctor to insert the tube in a wakeful and tense patient, an anesthesiologist is able to guide a tracheal tube into a relaxed throat with the gracefulness of an expert seamstress threading a needle.

Spinal anesthesia is injected into the spinal canal by way of the membrane that covers the spinal cord. It is not injected into the cord itself, as you may have suspected or feared. You will get a local anesthetic first, just under the skin, to keep you from feeling pain when the deeper spinal anesthesia is administered by a different needle. When the needle is removed, you are then positioned for your particular surgery. You will be numb in the legs and pelvis and possibly even higher depending on the way you are positioned. If you haven't been put to sleep, the numbness may give you the eerie (and fortunately mistaken) feeling that you've been cut in half.

It may take longer to come out of spinal anesthesia than it does out of general — up to several hours. You may suffer a headache upon awakening which can last up to 2 weeks. This pain is not abnormal — it occurs in about 1 out of 20 patients — and results from tiny losses of spinal fluid. You can lessen it by lying flat, following the hospital staff's directions and requesting pills or injections for pain.

Caudal and epidural anesthesia are also injected into the spinal area, but differ from spinal anesthesia in that they are injected outside the spinal canal and do not cause postoperative headaches. Caudal anesthesia, often associated with childbirth, is injected between the lining membranes at the lower end of the spinal column, just above the rectum. Epidural anesthesia is injected into the epidural sac to block the nerves in a large area of the body, such as the legs.

Local anesthesia can be administered several ways. A surface or topical anesthetic can be applied as a solution or jelly to the skin or mucous membranes to block pain from nerve endings. A nerve block can be achieved by injecting around a peripheral nerve at a distance from the area to be operated on, blocking pain impulses at the trunk of the nerve rather than at its branches.

Carl, you remember, is having general anesthesia. Because of the premedication, Carl's ability to feel, see, smell and taste has been considerably dulled. (To some patients it may seem they are tasting the anesthetic rather than smelling it.) Hearing, however, is the last sense to desert him and the first to return. That's part of the reason that it is considered unprofessional for the OR team to discuss the patient in anything but relevant medical terms. In Carl's case, they are discussing the exacting expectations of one of the hospital's attending surgeons.

"He wants you to kiss his feet," whispers a spiteful voice.

"I'll say," another voice agrees.

Before Carl was wheeled into the operating room, Dr. Anders and the nurses cleaned up from the last operation and prepared for his. Equipment was checked, supplies such as gauze and towels were laid out, antiseptic solutions were measured, record forms were readied and the operating table was draped with sterile cloths. Electrical switches were all double-checked to make sure they were turned on, again to prevent an explosion. Dr. Anders checked her console, a big box containing devices by which she can continually monitor Carl's condition. She measured drugs into syringes to inject, when necessary, into Carl's veins.

After he is on the table and the equipment is ready, Carl hears someone tell Dr. Anders that the surgeon, Dr. Morris, is almost through scrubbing.

Dr. Anders injects the fast-acting barbiturate, sodium pentathol into Carl's arm. As it sometimes does, the pentathol triggers a few hiccups; then Carl falls deeply asleep. From this point until he is wheeled to the recovery room, he will remember nothing about the operation. Varying doses of the sodium pentathol which put Carl to sleep can be administered throughout the operation.

The surgical team swings into high gear. Dr. Morris, who entered the room quietly before Carl was asked to start counting backward from 100 (while the anesthesia took effect), sets up a screen, a foot-and-a-half square, at Carl's chest. This "ether screen" (so named in the days when ether was a frequently used anesthetic) separates Carl's head and shoulders from the part of his body to undergo surgery. It helps the surgeon's visual concentration and separates the anesthesiologist from the action of the sterile operative field. Then the surgeon washes Carl with soap and water and paints an area of skin from just under his nipples to his pubis with a bright red antiseptic.

The area of your body that will be washed and painted depends on the operation. Just as the size of the territory covered by the scrubbing and shaving you have the night before the surgery has no relation to the size of the scar, neither does the surface painted. Some of the red solution may wind up on the tabletop. To keep the procedure sterile, the surgeon paints Carl with a piece of gauze clamped in a forceps, the surgical equivalent of a paint brush.

In abdominal surgery like Carl's, the solution is worked into the navel. If you were having vaginal or rectal surgery, it would be worked into these areas.

While Dr. Morris paints Carl, Dr. Anders continues working. She checks the endotracheal tube continually to see that it is functioning properly — otherwise, Carl's lungs could collapse. Carl is hooked up to a ventilator, or rebreathing machine that records the amount of gas being administered. The gas is recirculated through the machine, where wastes such as carbon dioxide are removed from it. Then it returns to Carl freshly supplied with oxygen. This system saves money — because the anesthesia is reused — and prevents the gases from escaping into the OR room, where, over a long period, they could affect the health of OR personnel.

Carl is by now a human porcupine, bristling with tubes. Besides the IV, catheter, ventilator and tracheal tubes, a mechanical airway is placed over his tongue to keep him from swallowing it.

Sometimes this airway, which reaches to the back of the tongue but not down the throat, will be left in place until you reach the recovery room. It will be removed when the staff decides you are no longer in any danger of choking on your tongue. You may feel it upon awakening.

The anesthesiologist's job does not stop with these preparations. The vital signs must be recorded on a chart every 10 minutes. Your temperature may even be monitored through the ear via a probe, which rests against the eardrum and alerts the anesthesiologist immediately if the body overheats; measures for cooling can be administered right away should they be necessary. If you have a mild postoperative earache, that could be why.

Anesthetic drugs depress nerve-cell activity. They render you not only unconscious, but also pain-free. Upon awakening, you will not even have a memory of pain.

But even combinations of drugs to make you sleep and depress your nerve activity do not sufficiently relax your muscles for surgery. A muscle relaxant will be injected into your veins, without which your surgeon would have to use force to budge your internal organs in order to operate. When your muscles are relaxed, gentle pressure with delicate instruments will do the trick. The step greatly reduces postoperative pain.

Since even your tongue is a muscle, it may be so relaxed after the operation that you will be able to communicate verbally by groans only. All these things — tongue relaxation, combined with premedication, the mechanical airway and the fact that you will be asleep almost instantaneously — should eliminate any worries you may have about ranting and raving while in a mental twilight zone from drugs.

> When the muscle relaxant is administered, Carl's body looks almost as if he is having a seizure. It twitches, quivers and then dramatically relaxes. After this, he is immobile throughout the operation. He coughs (or "bucks" in OR lingo) once or twice and Dr. Anders quickly responds to a command from Dr. Morris: "Take him deeper."

Overweight people require more anesthesia because fat absorbs anesthetic very readily. After the operation, the anesthesia leaves the body, filtered by the liver and kidneys. This is why your liver and kidney function should be tested preoperatively. If they were not up to par, the anesthesia could build up in the organs to a toxic level.

After you go to sleep and the anesthesiologist is sure your vital signs are stable, your body will be positioned. Since you are relaxed to the point of flaccidity, you will be strapped to the table. Positions vary with the surgery — during hand surgery, for example, you lie on your back with your arm upraised; during kidney surgery, you lie on your side; and during hemorrhoidectomy, you lie on your stomach. Some of these necessary positions are so unnatural that you wake up with unexpected aches. If it's going to be a long operation the anesthesiologist may suggest that your limbs be given a rest or that your position be changed slightly from time to time.

> Once Carl is anesthetized, positioned, washed and painted, Dr. Morris pulls Carl's gown back over the ether screen and the scrub nurse frames the operative field with sterile towels.
>
> Dr. Morris then drapes the patient. The drape is a sterile sheet, with a slit down the middle. Some drapes are disposable, and many are made of polyester. (If you are allergic to polyester, tell your doctor before surgery is scheduled. One woman told us she woke up with mysterious welts after an operation. Her allergist later concluded she was allergic to the drape. Once an operation was delayed 20 minutes with the patient fully anesthesized because she was allergic to polyester and the all-cotton drapes were late in arriving from supply.) Such drapes are used in all surgical cases. You don't need to worry about being vulnerably nude while you are under anesthesia. Carl is completely covered by the drape except for his head, the arm in which the IV is inserted and the abdominal area where the operation is to be carried out.

When patients think of being cut, they may think of emergency room victims of stabbings and car wrecks, blood gushing from torn flesh. That is hardly the case in elective surgery. Surgery does produce a wound, of course, and it is traumatic to the body. The surgeon, however, will cut so methodically and gradually that the process is neater than you would expect. Because sterile instruments are used and organs have neither ruptured nor perforated, the procedure is considered "clean" rather than "contaminated." Elective patients therefore stand much less risk of infection than emergency ones.

Before he starts to cut, the surgeon will ask if the anesthesiologist — and you by implication — are ready. If so, he doesn't just take a knife and plunge right down to the organ he wants to examine. The human body is composed of layers, filled in by connective tissue. First there is the skin, then the underlying fat, then the fascia (a band of fibrous tissue). The organs lie beneath all these layers encased in protective membranes. A cross section might remind you of a diagram of the layers of the earth.

In some operations, the surgeon will operate through existing openings; for example, he operates through the mouth in tonsillectomies, the vagina in dilation and curettage and some hysterectomies, the tip of the penis in some prostatectomies, the rectum in hemorrhoidectomies. In other operations, the only way to reach the diseased area is to cut the skin. Since Carl's surgery is abdominal, that is the case with him.

Starting with the skin, the surgeon cuts through the layers a bit at a time, using the blunt handle of the scalpel to push and pull, as well as the blade to cut. The surgeon or his assistant will sponge up any blood, which is more likely to bead unobtrusively than spurt dramatically. Occasionally, a small blood vessel will stretch and break. The vessel will be cauterized electrically (burnt at the end) or closed off with a small clamp called a hemostat. Then it is ligated (tied) with a tiny suture. (The word "suture" means stitch and is used both as noun and verb, e.g., the surgeon can suture you with a suture.) The clamp is removed once the vessel is tied. The work of the tied-off vessels is done by new ones that grow in, as well as by collateral circulation, one of the body's natural backup systems. If you start to bleed too much — which isn't likely in routine elective surgery — the surgeon will use suction equipment to draw off the blood. If it is necessary, he will order a transfusion of blood which has been matched against yours and kept on hand. If your blood was not tested and typed before the operation, you could be given blood from a universal donor, with a calculated but small risk of having a bad reaction.

Surprisingly, fat bleeds more heavily than any other layer because it is so heavily infiltrated by blood vessels. That is only one reason why overweight people are advised to lose weight before elective surgery. Fat also makes the surgeon's gloves very slippery, thus prolonging the operation. If you've ever handled the fat on a cooked ham, you'll know why surgeons are loath to operate on fat people.

After you are opened, the surgeon will do what's necessary to correct your problem and observe by sight and feel the organs and tissues not known to be diseased. If he encounters anything abnormal — a sore, a hard spot, a reddened area — he'll take a specimen of it to have it tested for malignancy. A tiny specimen is removed and frozen, then clamped on to a slicing machine in the pathologist's lab. A paper-thin slice is taken from the sample and transferred to a slide. After it is stained with dye, the pathologist examines it by microscope and reports back to the operating room within 15 minutes. Lab reports on specimens other than frozen sections take longer to complete, but are more accurate. The surgeon will also take a specimen for a follow-up report by the more time-consuming procedure.

Anything removed from your body — hemorrhoids, a tumor, an appendix, a gallbladder, a bit of tissue — is taken to the pathologist's lab where it is analyzed; the test results are recorded on your chart. Your surgeon should be able to give you a report soon after the operation. If he forgets, ask him.

In some cases, an x-ray will be taken during the operation. An x-ray tube mounted on a wall of the OR or even a tube built into the table has a built-in film carrier. X-rays are taken while the wound is open, and instant prints can be developed on instant film a few feet from the operating table. For example, the surgeon operating on a hip replacement case could quickly be sure that the bones were correctly positioned before driving in a screw.

> Dr. Morris takes a plastic tube, the thickness of a pencil lead, and threads it into Carl's main bile duct to see if there are stones. Then he takes pictures. The x-ray prints from this procedure (x-ray of the bile ducts and gallbladder), which is done with the x-ray pointing straight down into the wound, are called cholangiograms.

Before you are closed, sponges and surgical instruments will be tallied. If anything is missing, the portable x-ray machine will be used to make sure nothing has been left in your body. Every sponge has had a thread sewn into it that will show up on the x-ray machine. When all equipment is accounted for, suturing begins. You will be closed, layer by layer, as meticulously as you were opened.

The surgeon will use various suture methods depending on your case and the layer he is closing. He may use a surgical stapler, which is faster and considered just as safe as a needle and thread. Fat will not hold stitches, so it must be spread between muscle and skin like the filling in an Oreo. If you are obese, you will probably heal more slowly and painfully than people of normal weight. Extremely obese people may even be returned to their rooms with the wound still open, a dressing and powder or ointment their only protection against infection.

Both the opening and closing of the body are considered the most routine parts of the operation; they are the times when the surgeon is most likely to ask a resident to take over. Having a resident or other doctor assist with the operation is not considered unethical "ghost surgery" as long as the surgeon remains in the room and closely supervises the assistant.

Before the skin is closed, any drainage tubes you will need to help wounds heal uniformly will be inserted. In Carl's case a small hole is made under the skin in his flank and the drain is threaded through to the outside of his body. Drains are not threaded back out through the wound. Most common is the Penrose drain, a quarter-inch rubber tube lined with absorbent gauze. A safety pin is put on the end of the drain to keep it from going back inside the body. Don't worry if you see a drain protruding from you after surgery. They slide out easily and comfortably in a few days and shouldn't bother you if the bandage over them is changed frequently.

Finally, your skin is sutured with a thread, either the kind that is absorbed or the kind that can be removed when the wound is healed. Sponge-backed buttons or small plastic bridges may be placed on the skin to maintain proper tension of the sutures. A bandage is placed over your wound. Heavy, bulky bandages aren't used much in surgery anymore. Of course the bandage size depends on the surgery, but you may be surprised at how small it is. An excessively bulky bandage could hamper your breathing if it were used on your chest or abdomen. It could also prolong wound healing by blocking air from your skin and the wound edges. Blisters and ulcerations are less likely to develop if the bandage is kept simple. Some incisions are not bandaged at all, but sprayed with a substance that creates a plastic covering. Or you may have only a simple gauze pad with ointment on it.

> Once Carl is closed, drained and bandaged, all the drugs — anesthetic gas, muscle relaxant and barbiturate — are cut off in the reverse order in which they were introduced. Only the oxygen is continued as he is coaxed back to consciousness. Dr. Anders replaces the IV tube containing saline-dextrose in his arm.
>
> While the other attendants tidy up and Dr. Morris dashes off to take a phone call, Dr. Anders and the circulating nurse stay with Carl. He is conscious but so groggy that he is not aware of being awake. He is soon able to obey simple commands such as "Wiggle your toes."
>
> Dr. Anders slides the tracheal tube out as easily as she slid it in. The airway remains in place over Carl's tongue.
>
> "He's reactive now," the circulating nurse observes.
>
> "Yes. We'll wheel him out," Dr. Anders replies.
>
> The motion of the cart to which Carl with his tickling tubes is gently transferred makes him as wildly nauseated as he's been since his daughters persuaded him to take them on a roller coaster ride after a Chinese dinner. His instinct is to grip the side of the cart, but his hand is heavy and remote.

In his drugged confusion he thinks about Dr. Christian Barnaard transplanting apes' hearts into humans. He is stricken by the panicky conviction that his hand has been replaced by an animal paw. He opens his mouth to protest, but his tongue feels thick, dry and foreign, as though a wad of terry cloth has been stuffed into his mouth.

His communicating mechanisms refuse to be activated by orders from his brain, and Carl feels so helpless that he is ready to cry. Curiously, that is the one way he can communicate. Anesthesia may keep a patient from speaking, making a face or moving his limbs, but it can't paralyze his tear ducts. Finally, Dr. Anders notices Carl's flickering eyelids.

"You're OK now, Mr. Johnson. We're in the recovery room," Dr. Anders whispers. Only seconds have elapsed since they left the operating room.

Reassured, Carl's irrational fears vanish as quickly as they materialized — in fact, he is frustrated by his inability to maintain a thought. He drifts into a sleep as dark and cool as a night in a forest.

8
How to Get Back on Your Feet Faster

When you are in the process of spring cleaning, all your paraphernalia is strewn around the house. It looks like a cyclone's hit. But it has to look worse before it looks better. Surgery is the same way. In elective cases, you'll probably feel worse immediately after the operation than you did before it.

You can expect a slightly elevated temperature, slightly higher pulse rate, slightly faster breathing, a loss of weight and reduction of energy — all of which means that your body is doing its job of first-stage healing. The medical staff becomes concerned, however, if these deviations from your normal state are more than slight. That's why your blood pressure, temperature and pulse will be checked so frequently after surgery — to make sure that your vital signs are gradually returning to normal.

In most operations, *complications are more likely to occur during recovery than during surgery.* That is why the "success" rates of certain operations can be misleading — if the surgeon computes the rates on the basis of deaths or complications occurring on the operating table rather than on the basis of those occurring soon after surgery.

A good number of postsurgery deaths are preventable, Charles G. Child, M.D., of the University of Michigan, told a U.S. House subcommittee on April 25, 1977. In a 1973–75 study Dr. Child directed, 796 of 1,695 complications following 1,493 operations were preventable. So were 85 deaths.

If you have carefully chosen your surgeon and hospital and prepared yourself for surgery, you've already considerably decreased your chances of having postsurgical complications. Some complications can't be helped, and no amount of foresight or vigilance on your part or your surgeon's can prevent them. But alertness and *willingness to participate in your recovery* will decrease your chances of having preventable complications even more.

After surgery, the patient is taken to the recovery room before he is returned to his room. Ideally, the recovery room is staffed by at least one registered nurse for every 2 patients, one anesthesiologist and one respiratory therapist. The purpose of the recovery room is to keep postop patients near sophisticated equipment such as a machine to administer external cardiac stimulation in case of heart problems. Transfusions and respiratory help are also available until the danger of immediate postoperative complication is past.

In the recovery room, you and the other patients will be lined up on stretchers with your heads toward the wall and your feet pointing to the center of the room like recruits sleeping in boot camp. The staff, which operates from a station in the center of the room, can easily watch for signs of trouble in any patient in the room. Depending on the type of surgery you had, you may be hooked up to heart and respiratory monitors that ring an alarm when a pulse is too slow or a breath takes too long coming. Recovery rooms are notoriously noisy; phones ring, patients moan and stretchers clank against the wall as the patient is wheeled into position.

In the last chapter, we left our patient Carl in a deep and peaceful sleep as he was wheeled into the recovery room by his anesthesiologist, Dr. Anders.

When Carl begins to blink, an R.N. hurries to his bed, which is equipped with side rails to keep him from rolling out.

"How are you doing, Mr. Johnson?"

He nods sluggishly and she takes his blood pressure. Anesthesia and premedication can lower blood pressure slightly, as they have done in Carl's case. Were it to dip too low, the nurse would be alert to the possibility that Carl might be going into postoperative shock. Until he leaves the recovery room, his vital signs are checked at least every 20 minutes.

"Can you wiggle your toes for me now, Mr. Johnson?" she asks. "That's good."

Dealing with Problems and Discomforts

Coming out of anesthesia, Carl is discovering, is a little like being born again. After the black oblivion he went into when he inhaled the anesthesia, the recovery room seems unbearably bright. His limbs are heavy, the air feels cold and the blips and beeps of machines seem deafening.

Because Carl is a heavy smoker who has undergone abdominal surgery, his nasogastric suction tube is reinserted after the operation to remove his secretions, clear his bronchial "tree" and stimulate his cough reflex.

Tubes aren't automatically used with all patients — if you are able to cough on your own, the equipment may not be necessary. Many abdominal operations do require the tubes, however, partly because they keep the upper intestine from distending. Normally, they are removed 2 or 3 days after the operation, as soon as the bowels start to function.

After coming out of general anesthesia, you may be given oxygen by a mask or catheters in one or both nostrils. These would probably be connected to a wall tank, not a tent like the ones you see in medical dramas on television. Oxygen helps to disperse the anesthetic and get the patient over the shivering and disorientation he may be experiencing.

The nasogastric tube, IV and catheter all tug a little when Carl moves, making him uncomfortable. You may even yank instinctively at these tubes when still fuzzy from the medication. Doing so will only earn you the discomfort of having them inserted again. If you have asked beforehand what tubes will be attached to you, perhaps their presence won't alarm you and you won't be as likely to grab at them.

Because he has a tube in his nose, Carl has been breathing through his mouth. The combined effect of the premedication he had been given to dry up his secretions and the mechanical airway to keep him from swallowing his tongue makes his mouth feel like a cornfield in an August drought. He is able to bring the nurse back to his side by moaning. He points feebly to his mouth and silently forms the word "water" with his lips.

"No water yet, Mr. Johnson. You might throw it up, I'm afraid. But we can get rid of this contraption for you," she offers, slipping the plastic airway out of his mouth, "and I'll bring you a chip or two of ice to suck on."

The ice chips bring Carl enough relief to allow him to fall back to sleep. He wakes fitfully during the periodic checks of his blood pressure, pulse and temperature. At one point, the nurse asks him to roll over and gives him an intramuscular injection of a pain-killer in the hip. He hasn't begun to feel pain yet — in fact, he doesn't even feel that his body is occupying space — but the doctor has ordered that the medication should be started in the recovery room so that Carl will be pain-free throughout the first postoperative day.

Intramuscular injections are usually given rather than pills by mouth during the day of surgery because they are faster-acting and less likely to trigger nausea. Starting with the second postoperative day, pills are more likely to be given.

After Carl has spent 2 hours in the recovery room, Dr. Anders reappears. She asks him to cough, turn over and wiggle his toes. These actions stimulate his blood flow, help keep fluid from collecting in his lungs, and demonstrate that he is able to react to suggestions. Satisfied that his color is good and his vital signs stabilized, she tells the R.N. that an orderly can take him back to his room.

If Carl had undergone more serious surgery, such as a coronary bypass operation, or if there were reason to think his general condition was precarious, he would be taken to the Intensive Care Unit (ICU) instead of to his room. In very small hospitals, the recovery room and ICU could be one and the same, or intensive care could be administered with special equipment in a regular hospital room. Large hospitals, however, generally have several intensive care units: one for pediatric patients, one for medical patients, one for surgical patients, and even, in some cases, separate units for coronary, respiratory, kidney, burn or premature infant intensive care.

As in the recovery room, monitors are available and there is a high ratio of staff members to patients. Visiting hours are limited and flowers are probably not allowed in the patient's room because of the possibility that germs in the vase could infect the vulnerable patient. Flowers also tend to get in the nurse's way as she maneuvers sophisticated equipment.

ICUs are for people who need to have vital signs, EKG and fluid balance monitored; who need respiratory support or who need to have problems such as shock, heart instability, hemorrhage, overwhelming infection, or similar serious conditions carefully managed.

Few elective surgical patients are taken to intensive care. Chances are you'll be returned to your room no longer than a few hours after surgery. You may have been so woozy throughout your stay in the recovery room that the first memory you will have after the operation is of waking up in your room. When you first wake up you may feel euphoric that you've survived — this feeling may later give way to the blues about anything from your inability to urinate to the tastelessness of the food you are given by mouth when the IV is removed. If you're like many patients, you may become obsessed with your body and its functionings during the first few days.

It may help to see a loved one at your side during those first few hours after surgery when you are drifting in and out of sleep. Some hospitals allow an adult visitor to sleep on a cot by the patient's side the first night or two, even in a semiprivate room.

Studies have shown, not too surprisingly, that touching can be comforting, both physically and emotionally, to the recuperating patient.

"Touch provides the critical human element to machine-oriented care," is the way one nurse put it. Others we interviewed commented that backrubs and baths can be especially comforting. That is something for your visitors to bear in mind if the nurses are busy. Besides cheering you, massages can stimulate the skin surface, which is good for you when you're immobile. Massages of the lower back can help stubborn bowels move again.

Pain. Discomfort is inevitably associated with surgery. But barring unusual circumstances, there is no reason for you to bear intense pain silently after elective surgery. Some patients don't know they can ask the nurses for pain medication. In many cases, the doctor orders pain medicine for your "p.r.n." or "as necessary." *It's your job to tell the nurse when you think it's necessary.* It's her job to give or withhold the medicine in accordance with the doctor's orders on your chart.

In a study on how patients cope with surgery, 2 researchers discovered that patients classified as "copers" requested and took more pain medication than did other patients (*Psychosomatic Medicine* September-October, 1973).

Remember, though, that the doctor must strike a balance between relieving your pain and coaxing your body back to normal. The after-effects of anesthesia and premedication plus a generous dose of pain-killer could knock you unconscious. If the doctor and nurses are aware of your discomfort but ask you to tolerate it, they probably are trying not to sedate you so much that your recovery is prolonged.

Pain can come from several sources besides the incision. In routine cases, incisional pain will be severe for only a day or 2 and will subside in 3 or 4 days.

Urinating. Especially if you have prostate trouble, are bedridden or have undergone a rectal or hernia operation, you may have trouble urinating after surgery. If you have an IV, part of the reason for the discomfort is that you have been taking nourishment in the form of liquid all day. When you ask to use the bedpan or bathroom, certain that you are about to flood the bed, you discover that your bladder won't release a drop. If you were not routinely catheterized during or before the operation and you are not able to urinate by the end of the day of surgery, you will probably be catheterized. Some patients dread catheterization so much that they tell the nurse they have urinated when they actually haven't, a bad idea since a bulging bladder can cause permanent urinary tract damage. Catheterization should be the last resort after you have tried running water in the sink or running a few drops of water over your vulva or the tip of your penis, tricks that sometimes help start your urine to flow.

If your condition permits, ask if you can have someone help you to the bathroom rather than use the bedpan. It's easier to urinate in the usual setting. Even so, you might be asked to use a bedpan that fits in the toilet bowl. The nurse will then have the unlovely task of measuring the results for your "intake and output" chart, which assures the staff that what you take in — fluids and later solid foods — is in proportion with what you put out — urine and later feces.

Although catheterization is often necessary when you really can't urinate, it has its hazards — especially if you are prone to urinary tract infection. Sometimes catheterization through the urethra can be avoided by draining the bladder with a tube that bypasses the urethra and goes directly into the bladder. The tube (which is less likely to cause infection than a catheter because the procedure is sterile from tube to collection bag) is inserted with a catheter needle into the lower abdomen. The clamp on this tube can be closed to see if your bladder is cooperating. If it is, the tube can be removed. If it isn't, open the clamp and try again later. That's its advantage over the catheter generally used, which has to be reinserted if you can't urinate when it's removed.

If you're unlucky enough to become infected from a catheter, the infection will develop within 48 hours after the catheter is removed. Your temperature could rise to as high as 104 degrees and your flanks could become tender. Treatment would include fluid intake, antibiotics or even another catheterization because of your continued inability to urinate.

Bowel movements. It takes awhile for your body to start functioning smoothly again after surgery, and your bowels may be even more stubborn than your bladder. Once you are graduated to a liquid, then a semisolid and finally a solid diet, stay away from foods that normally constipate you. Try to eat bran and drink fruit juices and plenty of fluids unless for some reason they are off limits for you. It helps to move around, even from side to side in bed. Walk as soon as you are allowed to. A massage of the lower back might also help get things going. Probably the nurses and the surgeon will be asking you about your bowel movements, especially if you have had abdominal surgery. And the surgeon will periodically listen to your bowel sounds. He'll use a stethoscope on your belly to detect "peristalsis" — the intestinal activity that occasionally makes your stomach growl. After surgery, peristalsis is so reduced that the normal sounds are reduced to a distant rumble that can't be heard by the unaided ear. As soon as he is able to detect bowel activity — probably in 48 to 72 hours — the surgeon will order your nasogastric tube removed. You are likely to feel momentary nausea as it slides painlessly out. It's to your advantage to admit it if you've passed gas — this is another sign the tube is due to come out and that you are ready to take food by mouth.

If you remain constipated, you may be offered a laxative, a suppository or an enema. Fecal impaction can occur in a patient whose colon or rectum wasn't emptied before surgery or who has not been able to take liquids by mouth. The symptoms are diarrhea or very small, hard stools, and straining. You may have lower abdominal cramps or feel an urgent need to move your bowels. You may not feel empty, even after you've had a bowel movement, and you may not be able to control your bowels.

Fecal impaction is relatively common in the bedridden elderly, and even in vigorous younger people confined to bed. It means just what it sounds like — a hard mass of feces is stuck in the rectum. Sometimes overnight oil enemas followed by soapy water enemas the next morning will take care of the problem. In other cases, the impaction will have to be broken up by the doctor's or nurse's gloved fingers. This can hurt, but you can ask for medicine to dull the pain (if it isn't automatically given to you). Only rarely does the mass have to be removed surgically.

Gas pains. Predictable as they are, gas pains are the nemesis of many a surgical patient who is otherwise recuperating beautifully. They are an especially common complication of abdominal surgery. The nurse isn't likely to get as excited about them as you are. You might even mistake them for heart attack symptoms. They usually disappear in 1 to 3 days, depending partly on how much gas was in your intestines before the operation. They come also from air you swallowed after surgery, from your intestines' lack of motion, and sometimes from the handling of your intestines during surgery.

Coughing, walking and passing gas will give you some relief, as will having a small enema to help you expel gas. Avoid carbonated drinks and gas-forming foods such as beans and peas if they appear on your tray. If you are given a straw to drink liquids, throw it away — it increases the amount of air you swallow. Raise the head of the bed and drink slowly from the rim of the cup. Remember not to gulp it, or you might vomit.

Other intestinal problems. Tell the nurse if the gas pains are still bothering you after 4 days. They could be signaling a more serious complication such as intestinal obstruction (when raw edges of internal wounds catch a loop of bowel between them and grow together or around it), or paralytic ileus (when the small intestine is uncharacteristically still and quiet), or intussusception (when a loop of bowel slips back into itself like a spring does when you sit on the bed).

Soreness. You may be sore or achy in areas other than the site of the surgery. This could be a result of your positioning during surgery or from lying in bed. If your heels get sore, ask for a rubber air ring to support them. If the tubes connected to you are uncomfortable, ask if you can have some anesthetic jelly. The jelly could prevent infections as well as relieve the discomfort.

Moving around. With incision hurting and tubes protruding from it like the legs of a centipede, it's little wonder that many a postsurgical patient is reluctant to walk, stand upright, or move in bed. He's afraid he'll make himself worse through strain or exhaustion, leave a trail of apparatus in his wake as he shuffles down the hall, or worse yet, faint, fall, or break a bone.

You shouldn't get out of bed until the nurse or surgeon gives you the green light, of course, but chances are they'll be hounding you before you think you're ready. The nurse — acting as the hospital equivalent of a disco dance teacher — will exhort you to cough, roll over, wiggle and walk through a postoperative routine. The regime will start as early as a few hours after surgery. Believe it or not, the exercise is good for you.

> Our friend Carl is typical in his attitude toward exercise. A lamb in the waiting room and doctor's office, an unquestioning patient who silently opens his mouth wide to receive his unidentified pills, he turns into a rebel when asked to cough.
>
> No sooner is he back in his room from recovery than the nurse is cranking up the foot of his bed to normalize his blood pressure and stimulate the flow of blood in his legs. She asks him to move to his other side each time she comes into his room hourly to check his temperature, overall appearance, blood pressure and pulse. In the evening she appears with an air of mission.
>
> "We're going to get you on your feet again tonight, Mr. Johnson."
>
> Carl looks down over the mound of his bandaged belly at his forlorn feet, motionless white stumps at the end of the bed.
>
> "Oh no we're not," he thinks.
>
> The nurse orders, "But first you're going to cough."
>
> Carl clears his throat delicately, like a church soprano.
>
> "That won't do. Cough," she insists.
>
> Carl closes his eyes and concentrates. When he coughs, this time with more gusto, his eyelids fly open. First he checks the ceiling, to see if his guts have splattered on it; then he peeks beneath his bandage to make sure the surgeon remembered to sew him up.
>
> "That was pretty good, but you're going to have to do better or we'll never be able to take that tube out of your

nose. The more you cough, incidentally, the less likely you are to have gas pains."

"Why?" Carl asks.

The nurse, obviously a graduate fresh out of nursing school, glories in her reply.

"Because coughing increases the pressure on your diaphragm and presses down on your intestines, where the gas is trapped. Smokers are especially prone to fluid collection in their lungs. Because you smoke — and you shouldn't — we're going to have you cough often. If we didn't make you move, you could wind up with pneumonia or something worse. That's another reason we're going to get you on your feet tonight. The upright position permits expansion of the base of your lungs."

Carl whimpers a little and grasps at his bile drainage tube as if it were a life preserver as the nurse helps him edge to the side of the bed, lets down the side rail and swings his legs over the side. She puts her arm around him, chirping "Up, Up and Away." Woozy but vertical, he can't believe he is on his feet so soon after surgery.

"That's enough for tonight," the nurse decides after he takes a few feeble steps, "but tomorrow we'll let you walk down the hall."

"Promise?" Carl growls.

"You bet," she crows, missing his sarcasm as she returns him to his bed. Carl, who had been feeling lonesome after his wife went home for the night, is relieved to see her go. He is only too glad to turn out the lights and commune with his sweet white pillow.

Besides bringing your energy back to its former level and restoring an appetite you may have mistakenly thought you'd be happy to lose, postoperative exercise restores muscle tone. It helps prevent bedsores, lung complications, blood clots, constipation and other intestinal problems.

You should ask if it's OK for you to get up before you dance down the hall with your IV pole clanking rhythmically along. But even confined to bed, you can breathe deeply (but not quickly), keeping the supply of oxygen going to your heart and brain; deep breathing strengthens your pulse and clears your head. Keeping your shoulders drawn back and expanding your chest as much as possible will help keep the air sacs in your lungs from sticking to each other thereby tempting pneumonia.

You can also bend and straighten your knees, flex your thighs, or ask the nurse or a visitor to help you "bicycle" in bed. Thigh muscles shrink quickly when you're confined to bed.

The importance of postoperative exercise was recognized during WW II when physical therapy programs sprang up in U.S. Air Force hospitals. If your hospital is understaffed, the nurses might not have time to cajole you to exercise. You'll recover faster if you do it yourself, always remembering to ask first if it's OK, then for help if you need it.

A physical therapist may be called in on your case if, for example, you've lost muscles as in a radical mastectomy, or if you have undergone bone surgery. Otherwise your exercise instruction will be informal. If you would like to see the physical therapist, mention it to the surgeon — the therapist can only visit patients if the doctor has asked him to.

Helping the wound to heal quickly. You may regard the surgical wound with some combination of revulsion and fascination. It probably won't be nearly as horrible as your imagination and the mysterious bandage lead you to expect. Seeing it for the first time is a little like confronting your first wrinkle or gray hair. Look at it squarely as soon as possible — which could be quite soon if the dressings are changed often. You earned it, after all. Before long that fiery red will subside to a lackluster pink and then a pale white.

Because many elective operations are "clean" (as opposed to "contaminated" operations where, for instance, an appendix has ruptured), elective patients have less chance of wound infection. Possible complications include suture abscesses, hematomas, seromas, streptococcal and staphylococcal infections, wound dehiscence, incisional hernias and suture failure.

Not all bodies absorb the sutures that are supposed to be absorbed. In such people, a tiny boil, or suture abscess, forms along the incision. Don't pick it — when it comes to a head and drains, a bit of suture may be found inside.

A hematoma is a collection of blood, or blood clot, that occurs in a tissue inside or outside the wound. It is usually accompanied by swelling and discomfort, and appears within 24 hours after surgery, although it may take longer if it is deep inside the body. If the blood is inside, the wound can be reopened and the blood evacuated. If the bleeding is superficial, removal of a suture or 2 and drainage of the blood may be enough.

A seroma is a collection of serum in a wound, and is most apt to occur in surgery involving large flaps of skin, like breast surgery. Sometimes the fluid can be drawn out by a needle. The wound may have to be explored in the operating room.

The better the supply of blood to the wound, the less chance you have of becoming infected. Wound infections usually appear about 5 days to a week after surgery. Some infections appear sooner, within a day or 2. Symptoms are redness of the skin and fever; treatment is administration of antibiotics.

Other infections produce collections of pus in the wound, which have to be opened and drained. Only rarely are the muscle and fascia (fibrous tissue beneath the muscle) layers involved — usually just the skin and subcutaneous tissue lying directly under it are infected.

Wound dehiscence is the opening of several layers of the wound. Occurring most commonly in obese patients, it isn't generally evident until the sutures are removed. Then, triggered by coughing or straining, a fluid of blood and serum is discharged. The patient may feel as though a giant kernel of corn has popped under his skin. Once the process starts, the wound spreads open like a zipper. Another operation must take place. Without treatment, the bowel or peritoneum can spill out into the open wound. Extremely obese or poor risk patients may be elaborately bandaged until they are ready for a second operation, but their problems can be compounded by an incisional hernia.

An incisional hernia occurs most often after abdominal cases. The fascial layer separates under the closed skin and organs can sometimes protrude through it. This condition also requires a second operation.

Broken sutures will cause the wound to gape like a hole in a garment. If this happens to you, you won't be sewn again but taped so that you can heal from the inside out. Resuturing doesn't "take" in a wound where stitches have broken.

Timing of suture removal depends on the operation. Abdominal sutures are removed in about a week and neck sutures after 2 or more days. You don't need to stay in the hospital to have the sutures removed. Painless and simple, it can be done in the doctor's office. Even so, the procedure may make you squeamish. It helps to divert your attention — think about a favorite person or place. The sutures aren't deep — remember that each of your layers was separately stitched, and you are sewn inside with sutures that won't be removed. The sutures will be cut and picked out from only the top layer, your skin. They are coming *off* more than coming *out*.

When the bandage is taken off, you might be surprised to see straps, sponge-backed buttons or small plastic bridges attached to your skin to distribute tension evenly on the sutures. Such devices keep the sutures from pulling on your skin.

Blood clots. Say the word "blood clot" and most people look appropriately grave. Blood clots or thrombi of the deep venous (vein) system are a dangerous postoperative complication. Blood clots of the superficial venous system (the blue lines visible just below your skin) are not dangerous, although they can look ugly and feel tender.

The blood systems of the arms and legs comprise 2 systems — the superficial venous system and the deep venous system, the bigger veins hidden deep in the body behind muscle tissue. The deep venous system is responsible for most of the blood return to the heart from the legs. That's why you can have varicose veins removed without impairing your circulation — they are part of the superficial venous system, which isn't doing much of the circulatory work anyway.

Blood clots in the deep venous system, which are composed mostly of red blood cells and fibrin (a fiberlike substance that forms in the blood during clotting), are most likely to appear in the legs. Their threat is that they can dislodge from the legs, travel by way of the bloodstream through the right side of the heart and then to the lung. There they block pulmonary arteries, preventing essential flow of blood. In the lung, they are called pulmonary emboli, and they kill 1 out of every 10 victims. Nobody knows quite why blood clots form, but several factors are known to make people more vulnerable to them. Among them are operations, especially on the hips or pelvis, malignancy, oral contraceptive use, varicose veins, lack of movement, previous history of blood clots, and age over 60. They are rare in patients with coagulating deficiencies.

Prevention consists of leg exercises, elevation of the leg either by the patient or by mechanical inclination of the foot of the bed, use of elastic support stockings, walking soon after surgery and certain drugs. Although walking is encouraged, sitting and standing are discouraged because they tend to make blood pool in the legs.

A German doctor has been able to reduce the incidence of thrombi in a trial of 600 patients from 38.5 percent to 7.7 percent. He used both stockings and a pedal-operated appliance. Patients who pedalled the "bed bicycle" for 5 minutes 3 times a day had far fewer clots than patients in the control group (*Medical Tribune,* January 25, 1978).

Large-scale trials have shown that heparin, a substance found in various tissues, is remarkably effective in preventing blood clots. Low dosages of it are injected just under the skin. You can be taught to inject it at home. When it is administered this way instead of by mouth, it can't be digested from the gastrointestinal system. In 1977, the American Heart Association predicted heparin could save 4,000 to 8,000 lives a year (*Circulation,* February, 1977).

Because heparin can cause minor bleeding during and after the operation, patients are screened by several blood tests and asked not to take aspirin or other platelet anti-aggregating agents for 5 days before the operation. It is not recommended for patients who will undergo prostate, brain, eye or major bone operations, but it is recommended for patients over 40 who will undergo major abdominal or chest surgery.

If you do get deep vein thrombosis in spite of preventive efforts, you might not know it. Symptoms are silent in about half the cases, and you could be unaware of any problem until the clot travels to the lung.

Symptoms can include aching, discomfort and tightness in the calf or thigh, pain aggravated by exercise, or pain behind the knee when the foot is bent backwards. Swelling might be so slight that it is undetectable unless the doctor measures the circumference of both your legs.

Several tests are used in the diagnosis of blood clots. Ascending phlebography and venography are considered highly accurate. In ascending phlebography, a contrast medium is injected into the foot and x-rays are taken. If the column of dye halts, doesn't fill the vein uniformly or is diverted in its flow, the patient has a blood clot. Venography is similar and uses radioisotopes instead of dye.

After a blood clot is diagnosed, the patient is treated by bed rest with his feet and legs in elastic stockings, elevated *15 to 20 degrees,* or about a foot, above his heart. Warm, moist dressings are applied to the affected leg. The treatment reduces swelling, pain and chance of forming new clots. After 7 or 8 days, or whenever the clots are thought to be safely adhered to the vein walls, you can gradually begin walking again. Sitting and standing are still banned and the wearing of elastic support stockings encouraged for 3 to 6 months. You might also be given anticoagulants or heparin. If heparin is given, your blood clotting time must be tested each day — otherwise there could be complications with bleeding. You should not take aspirin.

Several New York doctors have reported that they successfully treated patients with deep vein blood clots through an at-home program of self-administered heparin, elastic stockings and exercise. The patients walked, swam and took hot baths to increase blood flow and stimulate fibrinolysis. Heat stimulates fibrinolysis, a process in which enzymes dissolve fibrin, thus destroying the clot. Blood clots travelled from the legs to the lungs in only 7 of the 407 patients, none of whom died (*Surgery, Gynecology and Obstetrics,* August, 1977).

Answering Some Common Questions

Will you need a private nurse? Unless you are very, very sick, in an understaffed hospital or have no relatives or friends who visit often, you probably don't need a private nurse. If you can afford it, though, having one might make you feel more comfortable. Because you hire the private nurse on a day-to-day basis she has only you to care for. This gives her time for the amenities a busy floor nurse might skip — wiping brows, turning pillows, lending an arm during walks down the hall. Several nurses we talked to, however, mentioned that many private nurses are part-timers with family obligations. They work when they have the time or need the money. As a result, they aren't always up on the latest in hospital care, and may not know how to operate the equipment attached to you if it is new and sophisticated.

What do you need to know about the drugs you're taking? From drops in the ear to needles in the vein, your hospital stay will probably star a rainbow array of drugs, ranging from powders to tablets to liquids to capsules. The average hospitalized patient is usually given at least 8 drugs during his stay, according to a study conducted by the Colleges of Medicine and Pharmacology at the University of Florida (May et al., *Clinical Pharmacology and Therapeutics,* vol. 16, no. 5, 1974).

Many of them are lifesaving and pain preventing. It's a rare patient who would want to undergo even the simplest operation without some form of anesthesia. All the same, you have every right to know what you're taking, why you're taking it and what it could do to you. You have 5 rights when it comes to medicine — right time, right amount, right route of administration, right drug, and the right to refuse to take it. The surgeon, of course, has the right to refuse to treat you if you won't take the drugs he thinks you need to get well. When confronted with a myriad of sedatives, barbiturates and antibiotics, many patients think longingly of the good old days when Granny's bicarb was the strongest medicine around. But even without elaborate pharmaceuticals, our predecessors hoped their own special treatments would make them well.

Donald Gould borrows some historical examples to make this point in his essay "How Doctors Generate Disease" in the book *Equalities and Inequalities in Health Care* (Academic Press, London, 1976). Gould writes:

> The greatest damage doctors do to their patients involves the misuse of drugs. Excessive and overenthusiastic treatment is by no means a new phenomenon. Louis XIII is said to have suffered 212 enemas, 215 purgatives and 47 bleedings within the course of a single year, and a canon of Troyes was once sued for the cost of 2,190 enemas administered to him over a period of 2 years. However, the major virtue of the therapies of the past is that if few did those subjected to them any good, most did not do all that much damage either.
>
> Modern drugs have created an entirely different situation. Their very value depends upon the fact that they are capable of altering the biochemistry of cells and organs. It therefore follows that no effective drug can be innocuous. If it can alter the body chemistry in some desired fashion it must also, either incidentally or because of misuse, be capable of producing undesirable, or dangerous, or fatal effects.

Jane Whitman (not her real name), a former operating nurse at a private hospital in San Francisco, quit her job in disillusionment. She told us, "Working in the operating room was like having a continual nightmare. The patients are completely snowed. They have so much premedication that they don't even know they're in the operating room. General anesthesia is given for almost every case — the patient can be having a procedure on his big toe and still get a general anesthetic. I think they overload the patients incredibly with drugs. They think nothing of overdosing with anesthesia because they have the drugs that will reverse its effect. They give both drugs with abandon and have no thought of what this does to the body on the cellular level for months. Nobody understands what all these drugs do to all the incredibly fine things in the body. The operating room is a product of a salesman's mind."

When the color of the pills you've been getting regularly

changes, tell the nurse. Most hospitals buy drugs generically instead of by brand name (for example, aspirin is a generic name and Bayer is a brand name) because it's cheaper. So it could be that the hospital is dispensing a new batch of a differently colored brand of the same drug. And again, it could be a mistake.

Although an elaborate system of checks and balances exists to get the right drug to the right patient, mistakes happen. The drug company can make a mistake in manufacture, storage or delivery. The hospital pharmacy can contaminate a batch of a sterile drug when it measures out a supply for each floor. The nurse can give the patient in bed A the pills for the patient in bed B and vice versa. Of course, you can't control all of these mistakes, but you can help prevent some of them by saying that you've been getting capsules when the nurse brandishes a syringe, or that you've only been taking 1 green pill when she gives you 3 blue ones.

A study published by the Pittsburgh Institute of Legal Medicine in March, 1974, said research shows the error rate of medications in U.S. hospitals is 1 in every 8 administered.

Many hospital patients complain bitterly that they are awakened to take sleeping pills. What's happened here is that the doctor has ordered the medication for you and the nurse follows his orders. If you refuse to take it, she must make a note of it on your chart and destroy the medicine in front of a witness. You can eliminate this problem by asking your doctor if he will order you pain pills, sleeping pills and so forth "p.r.n.," or as necessary. Then the nurse will only give them to you if you ask her or say yes when she asks if you want them.

When you leave the hospital, ask how long you need to continue taking drugs. Keep taking them as long as the doctor says, because discontinuing them too soon could harm you. If you stop taking antibiotics for an infection as soon as your symptoms disappear, but before all traces of infection are gone, you could get a recurrent infection.

Because the doctor is busy or doesn't want to alarm you, he might not tell you about the drug's possible side effects. They can be important. Demerol, a brand name for meperidine, a first cousin to morphine, is often prescribed as a pain-killer for postsurgical patients. But you might be too fuzzy to drive or operate machinery after you take it. That's why you should always ask the doctor or the pharmacist to give you the package insert, which contains detailed information about the drug. The FDA requires drug companies to provide inserts with drugs. The insert may be technically written, but you can probably understand the essentials with the help of your surgeon or a medical dictionary.

Whenever symbols on the doctor's prescription pad bewilder you, ask him to translate. Chances are it's an abbreviation of a Latin term. For example, "c" is short for "cum," which means "with" and "g" for "gutta," which means "drop." Make sure you understand when and how you are supposed to take the pills when you go home from the hospital. If a pill is to be taken before a meal, don't take it with the meal or after. If you do, it might be absorbed more slowly because it stays in the stomach longer, or its effects might be destroyed by gastric acids. If it's to be taken with a meal and you take it alone because you're skipping lunch, it could irritate your stomach. Some pills are coated so that they dissolve in the intestine, not the stomach, and vice versa.

Save yourself money by asking the doctor to prescribe the drugs you need after hospitalization by generic name, and buy them at a drugstore instead of the hospital pharmacy, which is perhaps more convenient but also more expensive.

Pills and shots aren't the only ways to get medication in the hospital — some medicines come in the form of nose, eye and ear drops, salves and creams, rectal, vaginal and urethral suppositories, and inhalant mists and gases. The advantage of medication taken orally is that it's reversible if you have disastrous side effects — you can have your stomach pumped. Available in the forms of liquids, tablets, capsules and powders, oral medication can be swallowed or dissolved in the mouth, under the tongue or between the gum and cheek.

Medication given by injection cannot be recalled. Methods of medicating by injection include: *intramuscular* injections, which go into the layers of muscle, are fast acting and are not painful because muscle has few nerve endings; *subcutaneous* injections, which go into the connective tissue just under the skin and are used for small amounts of highly potent and soluble medicines; *intravenous* injections, which go through the skin and directly into the vein, sending drugs into the bloodstream for rapid absorption; *intradermal* or intracutaneous injections, which go into the skin for local effect; *intrathecal* or intraspinal injections, which go into the spinal fluid and are used for local anesthetic or to fight infection in meningitis; and *intrasynovial* and intra-articular injections, which go into the joint to reduce inflammation and usually cause local discomfort.

If you are getting shots repeatedly in the same hip, arm, thigh or buttock, you may get sore. Tell the nurse which side you had your last shot in when she comes in to give you another one. You may tense up in expectation of a shot, which makes it feel worse. Try to think about anything but the injection. A good nurse can flip the needle in before you can blink.

Can you see your chart? Until recently, most Americans have had no legal right to view their own hospital records unless they are going to sue the hospital. Then they can subpoena the records for court evidence. A small but growing number of states are now beginning to grant patients the right of access to information in their hospital records. If you want to see yours, ask the surgeon beforehand if you may or if he will at least send a copy to your family doctor after your hospital stay. After you have been out of the hospital a couple of weeks, the necessary notations from various departments should have been made and your chart will be complete.

Reasons surgeons and other hospital personnel give for not allowing patients to view charts are that:

- patients of modest or limited intelligence might not understand them.
- patients can't handle portions of them without a doctor there to explain.
- the doctor would lose control of the situation.
- patients might use material from the charts to bolster a malpractice suit.

But when 2 Australian researchers tested a group of 25 patients who had seen their charts and a group of 25 who had not, there seemed to be little difference between the 2 groups. In some cases, though, those who had seen their charts were reassured. Two patients who suspected the doctors were keeping the diagnosis of cancer a secret from them found that they did not have the disease. And in one case, a pregnant woman alerted the staff to a potentially dangerous mistake — she had an Rh incompatability and her blood type was incorrectly listed (*Annals of Internal Medicine,* April, 1977).

Even in uncomplicated cases, surgery requires a deluge of paperwork for every patient. Your chart will include everything from requisitions for your x-rays to tallies of the amount you urinated for several days after surgery. You might want to ask the surgeon if you can see photocopies of portions that interest you — perhaps the overall summary of your diagnosis and treatment, your prognosis (forecast of the probable outcome of the disease), the operative record (a form that the doctor fills out after surgery telling what he found and what he did about it) and the pathologist's record. Then with a few minutes of his time and a good medical dictionary, you can arrive at a good understanding of what ailed you.

Going Home

As anxious as you may be to leave the hospital, you may also be a little apprehensive about going home, especially if you live alone. If you anticipate any problems with home recovery — a need for child care, housekeeping or nursing services — find out if the hospital has a home care program. Under such programs, if you are well enough to leave but not totally able to take care of yourself, you can go home. Lab technicians are sent to your home to draw blood for follow-up tests and nurses are sent out to change dressings. Even if the hospital has no such program, another nearby hospital's home care program might accept referrals from the one you are staying in.

Other places you might go for help are the local chapter of

the national Visiting Nurses Association, local government health department or the social service department of the hospital. If you do not feel able to do housekeeping, try the United Fund Homemakers, classified ads of the newspaper or local employment agencies, which sometimes keep lists of cleaning women and men.

Sometimes, the surgeon pops into your hospital room, consults your chart, decides you're looking and feeling well and decides on the spur of the moment you can go home. You might not have had time to make preparations. That's why it's a good idea to ask approximately when you'll go home from the outset and keep asking every few days. If you are going home soon, remind the surgeon if you still need to be taught a diet, exercises, or how to give yourself an injection or change a dressing. If you still have any questions about the lab report of the material removed for you or your postoperative instructions, now's the time to ask them.

Unless an emergency arises and you are unable to reach him, return to the same surgeon for your postoperative care. If the surgeon is in group practice, for example, you might be ushered in to see one of his associates instead of him during your postoperative visits. That's why you should specify to the receptionist which doctor you want to see. Then report all your symptoms — bleeding, pain, swelling, possible side effects from drugs and so on. Don't be afraid to call before your appointment if anything goes wrong.

When you do get home, don't be so afraid of hurting yourself that you are waited on hand and foot. You'll feel better sooner if you gradually work up to your former levels of activity. If you're unpleasantly tired at the end of the day, you probably overdid it.

Our patient, Carl, has a fairly smooth home recovery. His gas pains gone, he is reading in a chair by his hospital bed when Dr. Morris arrives.

"You're looking chipper today, Carl."

"I feel chipper, too. Whatever you did helped me out."

"Would you like to go home?"

"Would I!" Carl exclaims.

"Fine. I'll sign your discharge papers and you can leave this morning. Call my nurse for an appointment in about 10 days — let's see, that would be the 22nd. Any questions?"

"How soon can I go to work?"

"We'll talk about that at your next appointment."

Luckily, Alice is home when Carl calls and she comes to pick him up. Despite his soaring spirits, he feels exhausted by the time he signs out of the hospital. He waits for Alice in the car while she goes in the drugstore to fill his prescriptions. When he gets home to his own bed, he is even too tired to finish reading his spy novel, the climax of which he had just reached when Dr. Morris appeared unexpectedly in his room. His only real problem occurs a couple of days later, though, when Alice serves French onion soup with dinner.

Although onions had given him indigestion in the past, Carl thinks removal of his gallbladder will have given him immunity from such problems in the future. It tastes so good to him he has 2 bowls. Dr. Morris has neglected to mention that although some patients can eat foods that previously triggered problems before gallbladder surgery, other can't, at least not for a while. Some patients can eat some, but not all, of the foods that bothered them before surgery and others can eat those foods in moderation. The only way to find out is to try a few bites of the foods and see what happens. After eating the soup, Carl has gas pains almost as severe as those he had in the hospital. Alice urges him to call the doctor, but he decides instead to forego onions in the future.

"I'll wait until my appointment," he tells her.

By the time Carl's appointment rolls around, he's already taking the dog on long walks and itching to get back on the golf course. The doctor looks him over quickly, says he seems to be doing well, tells him he can go back to work in another 10 days and sends him home. Carl completely forgets to ask about the onions, a vegetable he will view with suspicion for the rest of his long and healthy life.

9
Nutrition for Surgery Patients

We've all heard a story about someone who goes through surgery without a hitch, only to run into big trouble during recuperation. The anesthesia may take an unusually long time to wear off, and leave him weak and confused. His cheeks become hollow and frighteningly pale. As days pass, sometimes weeks, he doesn't seem to be healing up on schedule. The incision remains red and raw as if the surgery had only been performed that same day. He picks up an infection that his body seems unable to deal with, and as more and more drugs are administered, he seems to become progressively weaker. He may develop bedsores. Pneumonia may even set in. He is encouraged to eat, but his appetite is poor and the hospital food seems unappetizing at best. When he is finally discharged, it takes many long weeks until he feels even close to being back to normal.

Ever heard such a story? Probably, you've *seen* such things happen to a friend or relative. And perhaps you're unfortunate enough to have *lived* through these circumstances.

There are, of course, many factors which determine how quickly and how well a person recuperates from surgery. But in recent years, doctors have learned that nutrition plays a bigger role in the recovery story than most had imagined. It seems that surgeons seldom *saw* nutritional deficiencies complicating recoveries because they seldom *looked* for such causes, too often ascribing poor recovery to lack of "strength" or simply the result of "age." But now that doctors, at least some of them, have begun actively looking for signs of malnutrition — both the kind that you can see in a hollow face and the kind that only shows up on blood tests — they have sounded the following alarm: *even in the biggest and best hospitals, malnutrition is shockingly common, sometimes even extreme malnutrition, with the result that many patients are forced to endure a period of convalescence far longer and more stressful than would be otherwise necessary.*

While the recognition of nutrition's importance steadily increases, the situation still leaves much to be desired. One unfortunate development is a much greater interest in intravenous feeding than plain old eating, perhaps because surgeons can control the former while only the patient can control the latter. On the other hand, this is a clear mandate to the patient to look after his own nutrition as best he can, both before and after surgery, to insure that he is giving his body everything it needs to return to full health. One study we'll mention later suggests that well-nourished patients may spend fully one-third less time than poorly nourished patients recuperating in the hospital.

Perhaps you're wondering why it is that surgery puts nutritional health to such a severe test. What is so difficult, after all, about lying in bed? But the seemingly peaceful inactivity of bed rest is deceiving. While you may hardly be moving, your body is frantically mobilizing all resources available in response to what it perceives as a brutal, life-threatening injury rather than medical treatment. Temperature, pulse rate and blood pressure all rise; hormone and fluid levels fluctuate; and the metabolism in general shifts into high gear to cope with the work of repairing injured tissues and defending against infection. Vitamins, minerals and protein, all required just to carry on normal day-to-day body maintenance, are suddenly called on to participate in emergency repairs and defense as well. What's more, all these nutrients can only work as a team, which means that the recuperation process may only be as effective as the weakest link in that team. Good protein reserves, for instance, will help your incision heal more quickly, but if vitamins that feed the body's immune system are in short supply, an infection may result that will prevent the skin from healing. The closed wound itself is an ideal breeding site for bacteria which thrive in a warm, moist, oxygen-free environment, so you can see that your natural healing potential is being challenged to the utmost.

From all this, it's easy to see how low nutrient levels, created by poor diet at home, and compounded by missed meals, poor appetite and heavy medication in the hospital, can swiftly result in malnutrition that retards healing, drains your strength and prolongs recovery.

Protein – Calorie Needs

It may be difficult to believe that you are burning up more calories while lying in a hospital bed than you would be going about your normal activities, but it's true — sometimes dangerously true. Your metabolism is running at full throttle and if the calorie and protein supplies don't meet the demand, the system begins to sputter and break down and you are in trouble. You feel weak, wounds don't heal, swelling increases, and so does your hospital bill.

All that energy can only come from 2 sources: the food you eat, and the carbohydrates, fats and proteins stored in your body.

The body first uses up the available carbohydrates for energy. Within 8 to 16 hours after eating your last meal (6:00 P.M. of the evening before surgery), total carbohydrate stores will be completely exhausted. Under normal circumstances, the body would then resort to breakdown of fat into usable carbohydrates. (The average person has enough stored fat to sustain his calorie needs in this way for about 2 months.) However, protein itself is vitally needed not only for day-to-day survival but for emergency tissue repair, and cannot be manufactured either from stored carbohydrates or fats. If dietary intake is inadequate to meet increased repair needs of surgery, the body steals protein from its muscles.

Most healthy men need about 55 grams of protein (the amount in about 6 ounces of lean chicken) daily for normal body function; most women, about 45 grams. Postsurgical patients need much more for urgent tissue repair: at least 100 grams a day or more, depending on the extent of the operation.

For each gram of protein to be properly utilized by the body, it must be accompanied by 25 calories from fats and/or carbohydrates. That's a minimum of about 3,000 total calories a day. (Those protein–calorie needs are doubled in the patient who has had very serious surgery, uncontrolled infection or fever.)

So why not just eat more during your hospital stay and recuperation? That sounds like the simple and obvious solution. But in fact, a great number of surgical patients are actually starving — even if they are overweight, due to a combination of factors: the fruit-juice-gelatin-missed-meals syndrome; poor appetite due to disease itself, presurgery jitters, hospital food that doesn't particularly suit them; prescribed drugs; being deliberately kept off foods ("n.p.o.") for lab tests, or meals missed because of lab tests scheduled at mealtime.

With low intake of protein and calories (and often vitamins and minerals), the body can't do its repair job, much less thrive. Such malnutrition significantly lowers chances for speedy and successful recovery. (Don't eat for 12 hours when you're *well* and see how you feel!)

The specific problem of protein deficit is compounded by a phenomenon called "negative nitrogen balance" that is almost inevitable in all surgery patients. For about 2 to 5 days after surgery, the body begins breaking down body protein.

Eventually, the body will adjust to a prolonged period of total starvation, stop using its own protein, and automatically revert to breakdown of fat for energy. But until that happens, the body literally begins to consume itself; the patient is weak, healing is slowed down, and chances of widespread infection go way up.

Surgeons discovered about 12 years ago that what nature can do by itself after prolonged starvation can be stimulated by continuous doses of concentrated carbohydrate (such as sugar), fed by way of a vein in an arm. Fuel provided that way bypasses the gastrointestinal tract and directly floods tissues with carbohydrate-derived energy, which the body agrees to accept rather than to continue to break down stored muscle protein for energy.

Intravenous carbohydrate will significantly cut nitrogen losses in the patient who doesn't eat properly — or at all — for several days, sparing him great losses of body protein. And it provides an extra 600 calories or so, boosting his energy supply. Recently, amino acid (protein) solutions have been introduced as an option, but for now intravenous sugar is the common "convenience food" of the surgical ward. One doctor commented, "We'd like to give chicken soup through the IV, if we could only figure out how to get the matzoh balls through the tube."

Alcohol used to be given as a fuel in IVs, but serious deficiencies of the B vitamin folate developed. (That will come as no surprise to anyone familiar with the fact that B vitamin deficiencies are common in alcoholics.) A study conducted by Dr. C. A. J. Wardrop and colleagues at the University Hospital of Wales blamed severe folate deficiencies in surgical patients there on the fact that they were getting the equivalent of 3 martinis a day on 10 days of IV solutions (*Lancet*, October 4, 1974).

Total IV feeding is only justifiable in about 10 percent of surgical patients. Some patients reach nutritional depletion a lot faster than others, depending on the age of the patient and the severity of the operation. After routine elective surgery, the phase of IV feeding is short; the body automatically reverts to positive nitrogen balance and you should be taken off IV nutrition and steered back to a regular oral diet as soon as possible. Feeding by a vein in the arm can only support the addition of an extra 600 calories, and a patient can eventually starve for lack of protein. Most undernourished patients can be fed either real food by mouth or the chemical equivalent of real food by nasogastric (nose-to-stomach) tube. (As one doctor puts it, "Man was not made to be fed by vein alone. If the G.I. tract works, use it!")

In a British study of 47 patients undergoing cardiac surgery, those patients who ate earliest in the postoperative period lost the least body protein and potassium, common indicators of postop nutritional status (Walesby et al., *Journal of Thoracic and Cardiovascular Surgery*, April, 1979).

Following major surgery, or in the presence of severe concomitant infection or disease, it may be impossible for the patient to be fed orally, by arm vein, or by tube. In those critical cases, weeks of nutritional support can only be provided by means of large formulas of amino acids, calories and fluids — total parenteral nutrition (TPN) — pumped through a catheter into a major vein under the collarbone.

Other uses for the ubiquitous arm-vein IV are to replace body fluids, supply emergency blood transfusions, or administer drugs that cannot be absorbed by the gastrointestinal tract. However, the commonly touted role of the IV to provide readily available access to the bloodstream in the event of an unexpected complication is unjustifiable because quick insertion of a special needle into the scalp, if needed, will do the job in these rare cases.

In fact, there is evidence that IVs are overused in many, many cases. Very few patients escape the IV no matter what the reason for their hospitalization, observes John F. Viljoen, M.D., of the UCLA School of Medicine. In an outspoken letter-to-the-editor in the *Journal of the American Medical Association,* Dr. Viljoen writes, "It appears that the normal route for the assimilation of fluids is abruptly terminated at the hospital admitting office. Those of us involved in the care of the surgical patient are particularly guilty of this. While the infusion of fluids into a vein has undoubtedly saved countless lives, it is high time to reexamine our compulsion to start IV infusions in every patient." Dr. Viljoen goes on to point out that aside from the discomfort of IV feeding, there are very real potential hazards, including introduction of foreign particles and bacteria into the puncture, hemorrhage after the tube is removed, blood clots and accidental use of wrong drugs. Dr. Viljoen cautions, "Intravenous infusions should be initiated only when clear-cut indications exist" (May 21, 1977).

In spite of the use of IVs and TPN, protein-calorie malnutrition (PCM) is common among hospital patients. Until recently, PCM has been largely identified as a severe medical problem common to nutritionally deprived children and widespread in underdeveloped areas of Asia, Africa and Central America. Studies now reveal alarmingly high rates of PCM among adult medical and surgical patients in large city hospitals in the United States and England. One study conducted by Bruce R. Bistrian, M.D., M.P.H., and George L. Blackburn, M.D., Ph.D., found that half the patients in a municipal hospital had moderate to severe protein-calorie malnutrition (*Journal of the American Medical Association,* November 11, 1974). Follow-up studies in other cities showed similar rates, and others suggested that vitamin deficiencies are also common.

If we are supposed to have the best medical care available in the world, why do we share this dread condition with starving children in Biafra and Bangladesh? An editorial accompanying the published report by Drs. Bistrian and Blackburn calls such high rates of malnutrition "shocking" and places the burden of responsibility for the nutritional status of hospitalized patients on the shoulders of the physician.

"In other words, if protein-calorie malnutrition isn't present when a patient comes in, we do everything we can to induce it," said Joel Freeman, M.D., at the Third Annual Nutrition Symposium at University of Pennsylvania School of Medicine in April, 1979. Dr. Freeman expanded on that wry comment in a telephone interview: "When the patient is in the hospital for the preop period of lab tests, not eating or on IV, malnutrition is provoked. Every single patient, elective or otherwise, is subject to this, although it is not as significant in elective patients as in the critically ill. Regardless of his nutritional state when he comes in, any malnutrition is compounded by the hospital stay."

How Vitamins and Minerals Help the Body Heal

Soaring needs for protein and calories due to surgery are accompanied by needs for the vitamins and minerals necessary for extensive tissue repair. Normally, all tissues require vitamins and minerals to varying degrees, and requirements are higher when there is repair work to be done.

Most of these small, active compounds cannot be synthesized from scratch inside the body, but occur naturally in the plants we eat or foods from animals, which eat those plants. Tables 1 through 8 show vitamin and mineral requirements for some of the key healing vitamins and minerals during optimum health, requirements raised by injury such as surgery, and serving-size portions of some foods high in particular nutrients. In many cases, diet alone cannot possibly meet the therapeutic requirements, and supplements may be necessary to augment dietary supplies.

Nutritional data used in charts throughout this chapter are adapted from the following sources. Tables 1 through 8 deal with requirements of several crucial vitamins and minerals and their common dietary sources. Tables 9 and 10 deal with protein and fat in foods.

Burton, Benjamin, Ph.D., *Human Nutrition,* Third Edition, McGraw Hill Book Company, 1976.

Dunphy, J. Englebert, M.D., and Lawrence W. Way, M.D., et al., *Current Surgical Diagnosis and Treatment,* Lange Medical Publications, 1977.

Food and Nutrition Board-National Research Council, *Recommended Dietary Allowances,* National Academy of Sciences, 1979.

Freeland, Jeanne H., Ph.D., and Robert J. Cousins, Ph.D., "Zinc Content of Selected Foods," *Journal of the American Dietetic Association,* vol. 68, June, 1976.

Murphy, Elizabeth W., et al., "Provisional Tables on the Zinc Content of Foods," *Journal of the American Dietetic Association,* vol. 66, April, 1975.

Perloff, Betty P. and R. R. Butrum, "Folacin in Selected Foods," *Journal of the American Dietetic Association,* vol. 70, February, 1977.

USDA Handbook No. 8, *Composition of Foods,* October, 1975.

USDA Handbook No. 456, *Nutritive Value of American Foods in Common Units,* November, 1975.

USDA *Home and Garden Bulletin* No. 72, April, 1977.

Vir, Sheila C., M.Sc., Ph.D., and A. H. G. Love, M.D., "Vitamin B_6 Status of the Hospitalized Aged," *The American Journal of Clinical Nutrition,* vol. 31, August, 1978.

Vitamin C (ascorbic acid) is the chief healing vitamin because it is essential for the manufacture of collagen, a tough, fibrous substance which gives strength to new tissue by cementing cells together, making healing possible and preventing the layers of the wound from splitting apart. Vitamin C also heals wounds indirectly by encouraging capillaries to renew themselves in the wound area, bringing with them red blood cells, nutrients and antibodies that fight infectious bacteria.

Large amounts of vitamin C are normally stored in the adrenal cortex, and promote overall recovery by helping that gland to

Table 1. Selected Food Sources of Vitamin C (Ascorbic Acid)

Recommended Dietary Allowance *(milligrams)*	Therapeutic Requirement *(milligrams)*
60	500–3,000 or more

Selected Food Sources	Quantity	Vitamin C content *(milligrams)*
Broccoli	1 small stalk	128
Orange juice	6 ounces	93
Cantaloupe	½ melon	90
Strawberries	½ cup	88
Brussels sprouts	4 sprouts	73
Green peppers	½ cup	64
Cauliflower	½ cup	33
Tomato juice	6 ounces	29
Tomato	1 medium	21
Potato	1 large	31
Mung bean sprouts	½ cup	10

produce certain hormones which protect the entire body against all types of stress, including surgery. However, those stores are rapidly depleted not only by the increased stress of surgery but also by any disease, fever or infection which may accompany it. In fact, the more severe the stress, the faster the rate of vitamin C depletion. If your stores are inadequate, your recovery could be prolonged a week or more.

The minimum required dose of vitamin C for wound healing is 500 milligrams a day, compared to the Recommended Dietary Allowance of 60 milligrams daily for the healthy individual. Needs may go up to 3 grams (3,000 milligrams) a day or higher, as the anesthesia wears off and during the initial stages of healing. Because vitamin C is water-soluble and the excess beyond tissue saturation is passed out in the urine, doses should be given at several intervals throughout the day rather than in one lump quantity.

Just as vitamin C sparks collagen formation, vitamin A influences the rate at which the collagen is laid down between cells, and so it, too, encourages the growth and repair of tissues. Vitamin A's larger role is the maintenance of the epithelium, tissues that line organs and cover the body. When those tissues are wounded, epithelial cells at the edge of the wound begin to migrate over the wound in leap-frog fashion.

The body manufactures vitamin A from carotene in green leafy and deep yellow vegetables, carrots, squash, and sweet potatoes, or obtains it directly from animal products such as beef liver, cheese, eggs and milk. The addition of supplemental amounts of vitamin A to the diet have been shown to enhance the process of wound healing. Doses of 10,000 International Units a day meet the approximate needs of surgical patients. (See Table 2, p. 144.)

Because the B vitamins are important to efficient metabolism, the speedup in metabolism prompted by surgery increases the need for most of the B complex, which includes folate, thiamine (B_1), riboflavin (B_2), pantothenate, pyridoxine (B_6) and vitamin B_{12}. Needs for all the B vitamins go hand in hand, which is not surprising in light of the fact that they occur together naturally in foods. But specific B vitamins serve specialized functions in surgical healing.

Table 2. Selected Food Sources of Vitamin A

Recommended Dietary Allowance (*International Units*)	Therapeutic Requirement (*International Units*)
5,000 (men) 4,000 (women)	10,000 (all adults)

Selected Food Sources	Quantity	Vitamin A content (*International Units*)
Beef liver*	3 ounces	45,390
Sweet potato	½ cup	10,075
Cantaloupe	½ melon	9,240
Dandelion greens	½ cup	6,145
Swiss chard	½ cup	4,725
Winter squash	½ cup	4,305
Beet greens	½ cup	3,700
Broccoli	1 small stalk	2,835
Peach	1 medium	2,030
Endive	1 cup	1,650
Tomato juice	6 ounces	1,460
Onion tops	¼ cup	1,000

**Liver should be limited to 1 serving per week.*

Both folate and vitamin B_{12} help maintain the red blood cells which deliver vital nutrients to all cells, including those involved in wound healing. Either because of increased demands or decreased dietary intake, deficiencies of those 2 B vitamins are most likely to crop up in hospital populations, particularly among the aged. A Danish study by Drs. Ib Hessov and Lars Elsborg showed that out of 46 elderly long-term surgical patients in one hospital ward, most had borderline intakes of vitamin B_{12} and definite folate deficiency. Evidently, the patients' preference for snacks and tidbits over regularly served meals compounded preexisting vitamin deficiencies (*International Journal of Vitamin and Nutrition Research,* October 26, 1976).

More recently, a survey of the nutritional status of medical patients in one American hospital showed that 69 percent of those patients admitted *entered* the hospital with low blood folate levels. Furthermore, after 2 weeks of hospitalization, serum folate fell by an average of 48 percent in those who had had normal levels at time of admission. Roland L. Weinsier, M.D., D.P.H., and Charles E. Butterworth Jr., M.D., and other researchers in the study, mention that even when multivitamin supplements are occasionally given to patients, folate is usually missing from the formula (*American Journal of Clinical Nutrition,* February, 1979).

Thiamine, along with folate, liberates energy from stored or dietary carbohydrates. The more carbohydrates in your diet, the more thiamine you need. Studies have shown that people on IV fluids, which are ultrarefined carbohydrates, can develop a thiamine deficiency in as short a time as 4 or 5 days. And long before a really severe deficiency develops, symptoms show up such as loss of appetite, irritability, pain and lack of interest in important matters — just the kinds of things that can make a convalescence miserable.

Both pyridoxine (vitamin B_6) and pantothenate seem to play an important role in the formation of antibodies — special substances the body must manufacture to fight off harmful foreign invaders such as bacteria and poisonous toxins. By encouraging production of antibodies, therefore, those B vitamins help to brace the body against anesthesia, drugs and possible infection. Needs for vitamin B_6, in particular, increase for a person on a high-protein diet.

Riboflavin (vitamin B_2), too, is necessary for the utilization of protein. Niacin (or its alternative form, niacinamide) is necessary for the utilization of both protein and carbohydrates.

B vitamins are water-soluble, which means they are not stored well in the body and must be supplied daily in the diet.

Tables 3 and 4 list dietary needs and sources. Note that some values are expressed in milligrams, others in micrograms. Keep in mind that 1 milligram is equal to 1,000 micrograms when you choose a B complex supplement to meet your surgical needs.

Table 3. Selected Food Sources of Major B Vitamins (Boldface numbers indicate especially high values)

		Thiamine (B_1) (*milligrams*)	Riboflavin (B_2) (*milligrams*)	Niacin (B_3) (*milligrams*)
	Recommended Dietary Allowance	1.4 (men) 1.0 (women)	1.6 (men) 1.2 (women)	18 (men) 13 (women)
	Therapeutic Requirement	5–10 (adults)	5–10 (adults)	100 (adults)
Selected Food Sources*	**Quantity**	**B_1 content** (*milligrams*)	**B_2 content** (*milligrams*)	**B_3 content** (*milligrams*)
Beef liver	3 ounces	0.22	**3.56**	**14**
Brewer's yeast	1 tablespoon	**1.25**	**0.34**	**3**
Chicken, dark meat	3 ounces	0.10	0.16	**4.5**
Chicken, light meat	3 ounces	0.07	0.08	10
Buttermilk	6 ounces	0.075	**0.33**	0.15
Wheat germ	¼ cup	0.44	0.20	1.2
Haddock	6 ounces	0.06	0.12	**5.4**
Yogurt	½ cup	0.5	**0.22**	0.1
Turkey, light meat	3 ounces	0.04	0.12	**9.4**
Peanut butter	1 tablespoon	0.02	0.02	**2.4**

**Foods listed are cooked, when applicable.*

Table 4. Selected Food Sources of Other B Vitamins

Pyridoxine (B_6)

Recommended Dietary Allowance	Therapeutic Requirement
2 milligrams	2–25 milligrams

Selected Food Sources	Quantity	B_6 content (*micrograms*)
Banana	1 medium	560
Beef liver	3 ounces	560
Brewer's yeast	1 tablespoon	390
Cod	3½ ounces	340
Carrot	1 medium	140
Halibut	3½ ounces	110
Flounder	3½ ounces	100
Wheat germ	1 tablespoon	74

Pantothenate (Pantothenic acid)

Recommended Dietary Allowance	Therapeutic Requirement
4–7 milligrams	20 milligrams

Selected Food Sources	Quantity	Pantothenate content (*micrograms*)
Sweet potatoes	½ cup	1,099
Broccoli	½ cup	1,080
Chicken, all sections	3½ ounces	715
Mushrooms	½ cup	595
Peas	½ cup	576
Cauliflower	½ cup	529
Banana	1 medium	525
Oats, before cooking	⅓ cup per serving	351
Peach	1 medium	245
Whole wheat bread	1-ounce slice	160
Wheat germ	1 tablespoon	120

Table 4—*Continued*

Folate (Folacin, Folic acid)

Recommended Dietary Allowance	Therapeutic Requirement
400 micrograms	1 milligram (1,000 micrograms)

Selected Food Sources	Quantity	Folate content (*micrograms*)
Brewer's yeast	1 tablespoon	313
Black-eyed peas	6 ounces	230
Beef liver	3 ounces	123
Orange juice	6 ounces	102
Romaine lettuce	1 cup	98
Cantaloupe	½ melon	82
Beets	½ cup	67
Brussels sprouts	8 sprouts	56
Broccoli	½ cup	50

Vitamin B_{12}

Recommended Dietary Allowance	Therapeutic Requirement
3 micrograms	4 micrograms

Selected Food Sources	Quantity	B_{12} content (*micrograms*)
Brewer's yeast	Content varies with product	
Beef liver	3 ounces	64
Tuna, drained	½ cup	2.4
Sole	6 ounces	2
Haddock	6 ounces	1
Whole milk	6 ounces	0.9

Vitamin K is especially vital to proper blood clotting. That is, it prevents you from bleeding to death. Because it is so crucial to survival, vitamin K is one of the few vitamins synthesized in the body; it is produced by tiny organisms in the intestine. It is then used by the liver to produce prothrombin, a substance which is necessary for blood coagulation. If blood flowing freely in the area of the surgical wound doesn't clot when vessels are cut, the blood will flood the wound uncontrollably, delaying healing.

Only prolonged use of antibiotics without supplementation, absorption problems or liver disease will create a life-threatening deficiency of vitamin K. Eating a diet that includes a wide variety of green leafy vegetables will help insure against clotting malfunction from vitamin K deficiency; supplements probably won't be necessary.

Table 5. Selected Food Sources of Vitamin K

Recommended Dietary Allowance	Therapeutic Requirement
50–140 micrograms	1 microgram per kilogram of body weight, daily
	57 micrograms for a 125-pound adult
	68 micrograms for a 150-pound adult
	82 micrograms for a 180-pound adult

Selected Food Sources	Quantity	Vitamin K content (*micrograms*)
Widely distributed in green leafy vegetables		
Cauliflower	½ cup	157
Soybeans, before cooking	¼ cup	100
Cabbage, shredded	½ cup	88
Potato	1 large	50
Oats, before cooking	⅓ cup	20

One other member of the wound-healing team well worth mentioning is vitamin E, which relieves wound inflammation and consequently pain and itching. When applied topically as an ointment, vitamin E oil or wheat germ oil (a commonly used medium for vitamin E) may reduce the pain and redness of surgical scars. One person described her success with wheat germ oil for scar healing this way:

> I had open-heart surgery. The scar was painful and sore. I finally tried vitamin E oil which eased the soreness temporarily. But I had to reapply it often. The middle section was red, thick, sensitive and slow to heal. I reached a point of desperation. I tried an ointment of wheat germ oil plus vitamin E, and the improvement was miraculous! The scar is no longer painful nor red.

Minerals, too, are basic to the healing process. Trace amounts of 13 inorganic compounds are necessary for normal metabolism. They are absorbed via the gastrointestinal tract from the foods we eat; surgery enhances the need for certain major ones.

Zinc holds a pivotal role in wound healing, probably because it sparks the release of vitamin A from the liver and enhances that vitamin's role in healing. Zinc is also fundamental to reproduction of new cells and metabolism of protein for tissue repair. One study found that surgical patients given a zinc supplemented diet had pinker, cleaner, healthier-looking new tissue in their rapidly healing wounds. Zinc is also important to infection control.

Deficits of zinc can impair healing. The Recommended Dietary Allowance is 15 milligrams — double that amount may be necessary to insure optimum wound healing. Guidelines to zinc requirements appear in Table 6.

When zinc deficiency does occur, it is quite likely to go hand in hand with a deficit of copper, which is essential to health because it is needed to forge myelin, the protective sheath which surrounds nerve fibers. Copper also stimulates iron absorption.

Table 6. Selected Food Sources of Zinc

Recommended Dietary Allowance (*milligrams*)	Therapeutic Requirement (*milligrams*)
15	30

Selected Food Sources	Quantity	Zinc content (*milligrams*)
Beef liver	3 ounces	4
Turkey, dark meat, without skin	3 ounces	4
Brazil nuts, shelled	½ cup	2.4
Turkey, light meat, without skin	3 ounces	2
Fish, cooked (white varieties)	6 ounces	2
Wheat germ	1 tablespoon	1
Chick-peas (garbanzos)	½ cup	1
Black-eyed peas	½ cup	1

Textbooks have traditionally stated that the average diet provides more than enough copper to meet the 2 milligrams needed to replace daily losses through excretion. But many hospital patients, including those on some therapeutic diets, are getting seriously low amounts of both zinc and copper in their diets. A study by Leslie M. Klevay, M.D., and other researchers, conducted for the U.S. Department of Agriculture and the University of North Dakota, looked at 20 hospital diets as well as diets consumed by the general public. The startling results showed that hospital diets averaged 0.76 milligrams of copper per day (60 percent below the 2-milligram requirement) and zinc levels averaged 9.4 milligrams per day (35 percent below the 15-milligram requirement). Not only are the researchers convinced that the average diet consumed by most people both in and out of hospitals is quite probably low in both zinc and copper, but Dr. Klevay feels that the discovery of significant deficits of those 2 minerals strongly suggests that other trace minerals should also be investigated (*Journal of the American Medical Association,* May 4, 1979).

Dr. Klevay told us that a person facing hospitalization for surgery (or any other procedure) can best avoid a dual deficiency of zinc and copper by eating those foods high in both minerals (see Tables 6 and 7). He emphasized, "Beef liver is the number 1 source of both zinc and copper, in an excellent ratio." (We'll explain further about how to incorporate such nutrient-rich foods into your diet later in this chapter.)

Copper stimulates the absorption of still another mineral, iron. Iron delivers vital oxygen to the cells by way of red blood cells. People who suffer from bleeding hemorrhoids or peptic ulcers, or women who have excessively heavy menstrual periods, are candidates for iron depletion due to blood loss. Poor diet,

Table 7. Selected Food Sources of Copper

Recommended Dietary Allowance	Therapeutic Requirement
2-3 milligrams (2,000-3,000 micrograms)	Not established

Selected Food Sources	Quantity	Copper content (*micrograms*)
Beef liver	3 ounces	2,384
Halibut	6 ounces	392
Beans, dry	¼ cup	389
Mushrooms	½ cup	350
Whole wheat flour	½ cup	300
Banana	1 medium	298
Chicken, dark meat, without skin	3 ounces	188
Chicken, light meat, without skin	3 ounces	119

combined with surgery for a condition involving bleeding, puts an additional strain on iron reserves, which play a big part in the body's total immune system. (Incidentally, vitamin C, also known for its defense abilities, improves the absorption of iron.)

Good food sources of iron are lean meats, beans and legumes, nuts, green leafy vegetables, and whole grain cereals (see Table 8).

Potassium is a determining factor in the complicated process of regulating fluid intake and output and acid–base balance in the body. Either too much or too little potassium can be a problem, because abnormal levels interfere with normal action of mus-

Table 8. Selected Food Sources of Iron

Recommended Dietary Allowance (*milligrams*)	Therapeutic Requirement (*milligrams*)
10 (men) 18 (women)	10 (men) 18 (women)

Selected Food Sources	Quantity	Iron content (*milligrams*)
Beef liver	3 ounces	7.5
Soybeans	½ cup	2.5
Raisins	½ cup	2.5
Lima beans	½ cup	2
Turkey, dark meat, without skin	3 ounces	2
Haddock	6 ounces	1.8
Cod	6 ounces	1.8
Brewer's yeast	1 tablespoon	1.4
Turkey, light meat, without skin	3 ounces	1
Endive or escarole, shredded	1 cup	1
Whole wheat bread	1-ounce slice	0.8

cles, including the heart. It is found in many foods. Potassium in food enters the body, mingles with other minerals in the blood and cell fluids for a few days, and is eventually excreted by the kidneys. Normally, the turnover rate is stable, and input about equals output.

Following the stress of surgery, the nitrogen losses through urination are accompanied by increased potassium losses. Potassium can also be flushed out of the body by long-term use of drugs such as diuretics and steroids, or chronic diarrhea, vomiting and fever, because fluid leaving the body carries potassium along with it. (More rarely, the potassium can be left behind, overloading the body. Either of those abnormalities is a threat to health.)

Potassium can easily be added to an IV formula if absolutely necessary, but the preferred route is by mouth, since many foods contain adequate potassium to bring the body's potassium levels back into balance. Supplements are not usually necessary except for patients taking diuretics. Good food sources are lean meats, fish, poultry, bananas, raisins, dates, tomato, orange and pineapple juices, yams, squash, potatoes, Brussels sprouts, cauliflower, lentils and broccoli.

Slightly less crucial but still important minerals are magnesium and calcium. Magnesium levels, which are essential to muscle tone (including heart muscle tone) and enzyme reactions, are disturbed by surgery. Supplementing the diet with magnesium is the best way to counteract the effects of surgery. Donald E. Reiner, M.D., a general surgeon in Santa Maria, California, customarily prescribes 75 milligrams of magnesium, in combination with 150 milligrams of calcium, 3 times a day for his surgery patients, beginning 1 or 2 weeks before surgery, to insure against inadequate intake. Calcium is essential for fracture repair and to help prevent fractures in bedridden patients who may have falls when they do get up. However, inactivity significantly prompts calcium losses from bone regardless of intake; so the best way to avoid brittle, and therefore easily broken bones is to walk around as much as possible after surgery.

Building up your diet with fresh foods and supplements is your best defense against surgical stress. When you're wheeled into the OR, knocked out, and the surgeon asks, "Is the patient ready?" — you'll be ready. When he reaches for his scalpel, the B vitamins bolster you. When the nurse hands him a sponge, vitamin K will be there to do its job. When he sutures you up, zinc and vitamin A take charge. When your stunned body begins to realize what's hit it, vitamin C bolts to the wound site.

The Problem of Overweight

The shape your body is in when you face the surgeon's knife significantly influences your chances for a speedy and uncomplicated recovery.

When asked what advice they would give to their patients facing any kind of elective procedure, the surgeons we spoke to unanimously said, "Lose weight!" (Even people facing intestinal bypass operations for extreme obesity are put on a 6-week weight loss program to prepare them for the operation!)

Surgeons hesitate — even refuse — to operate on fat people for some very good reasons. They are more prone to heart and circulatory disease and digestive tract problems. Furthermore, excess fat prolongs the operation by getting in the way of the surgeon's scalpel and putting more pressure on the incision area. Anesthesia is more difficult to administer to an obese patient, and the longer the operation, the greater the amount of anesthesia that must be given to the patient.

Postoperative wounds don't heal quickly in an overweight person. Stitches don't hold up as well and are easily pulled apart by sagging flesh. Wound infection is more likely. There is greater possibility of a blood clot developing and lodging in the main artery leading to the lung — an event called formation of a pulmonary embolism, which carries the risk of death.

Getting up and around after surgery is delayed in a hefty person; prolonged inactivity increases the risk of pneumonia and ileus (abdominal pain, distention from gas bubbles and constipation). The chances of respiratory complications setting in are greater in obese people.

Most surgeons prefer to delay elective surgery until the patient loses weight. Keep it in mind — if you are overweight and ever need emergency surgery, your risk of all those postoperative complications is much greater than that faced by a normal-weight person.

Drugs and Surgical Nutrition

Aside from surgery itself, certain drugs which may be part of your treatment affect your nutritional state by suppressing appetite or interfering with normal absorption, utilization or excretion of vitamins and minerals. Those drugs include antibiotics, sedatives, cholesterol-lowering agents, anticoagulants, thiazide diuretics, laxatives, antacids and chemotherapy drugs, among others.

Chronic aspirin use, for example, can cause iron deficiency as a result of bleeding in the gastrointestinal tract. Both aspirin and barbiturates increase vitamin C requirements. Antibiotics block formation of vitamin K, essential to adequate blood clotting. Any one of a number of drugs can induce multiple deficiencies of B vitamins, such as folate and vitamin B_{12}, or iron deficiency secondary to folate, B_{12} or B_6 deficiency.

Cortisone, taken to suppress inflammation, also inhibits the normal process of wound healing. Vitamin A, taken internally or applied directly to the wound as an ointment, can counteract that effect and restore the body's normal healing ability.

Some anesthetics cause the body to draw on its vitamin C stores for detoxification and excretion. In fact, coming out of anesthesia can be eased considerably by the intravenous infusion of massive doses of vitamin C because of its ability to sweep away the toxic effects of anesthetic drugs. Dr. Donald Reiner adds 10 to 12 grams of vitamin C to the intravenous formula administered to patients immediately after surgery. As a result, he reports his patients suffer less grogginess and are more alert and comfortable when they awake. Lesser doses of vitamin C are continued for a couple of days to ease the stress of wound repair.

If you have regularly been taking medication before admission for surgery, the odds of your having lowered levels of certain nutrients go up. If you are taking more than one drug, your nutrition gauge may be vulnerably low.

Nausea and vomiting which sometime accompany heavy medication further deplete your nutritional status. If your vitamin and protein intake is low because of postoperative starvation, the toxic effect of drugs is enhanced because of the body's reduced ability to detoxify and eliminate the chemicals.

Don't forget that household items like alcohol and caffeine are also drugs. Used on a daily basis, they may block absorption of B vitamins that your body urgently needs for surgical healing. Adding several cups of coffee and tea to powerful drugs racing through your body puts hazardous strain on the nervous system.

Drug-induced deficiencies, compounded by the stress of surgery or long-standing illness, can certainly leave you at your worst to begin recuperation.

Getting Yourself Ready for Surgery

Isn't it logical to assume that knowledge of the effects of surgery and medication on nutritional reserves would make the hospital staff alert to the need for an extensive nutritional evaluation of every patient admitted to the hospital? Don't be too sure.

The responsibility for your nutritional welfare is fragmented among the physician, nurses and dietitians. The physician usually quickly glances at the patient from bedside, jots down a quick judgment of "well-nourished," and that's that. Height and weight measurements are often omitted from patient charts. Lab tests are often not even available, or not utilized when they are.

In the absence of any obvious signs of gross, single-deficiency diseases such as scurvy or beriberi, vitamin and mineral levels are presumed to be normal when, in fact, that may be far from the truth. In a study of 67 patients in 2 teaching hospitals, 46 patients had vitamin or mineral deficiencies but only 18 were given supplements. In fact, 91 percent of the patients showed either actual or potential malnutrition, according to researchers Alice L. Tobias, Ed.D., R.D., and Theodore Van Itallie, M.D., of the Institute of Human Nutrition, Columbia University, New York (*Journal of the American Dietetic Association,* September, 1977).

Erroneous assumptions as to the vitamin and mineral status of patients, along with protein-calorie malnutrition, contribute to the epidemic proportions of iatrogenic (physician-induced) malnutrition in hospital patients. Basing his conclusions on broad hospital experience, Charles E. Butterworth Jr., M.D., director of the nutrition program at the University of Alabama and former chairman of the Council on Foods and Nutrition of the American Medical Association says, "I suspect, as a matter of fact, that one of the largest pockets of unrecognized malnutrition in America . . . exists not in rural slums or urban ghettos, but in the private rooms and wards of big city hospitals." Dr. Butterworth adds, "I am convinced that iatrogenic malnutrition has become a significant factor in determining the outcome of illness for many patients" (*Nutrition Today,* March/April, 1974).

How extensive is the research on the effects of presurgical levels of such vitamins as A and C, or zinc, and actual recovery rates? Unfortunately, definitive studies have yet to be done. But when asked about the logic behind a patient building himself up on vitamins and minerals before surgery to increase his chances of speedy and successful recovery, James L. Mullen, M.D., head of Nutrition Support Services, Hospital of the University of Pennsylvania, said, "It makes perfect sense."

A few research projects are now beginning to delve into that relationship. In one study of 47 randomly selected cardiac surgery patients, conducted by R. K. Walesby and associates in London, the length of postop hospitalization of well-nourished patients was compared to that of nutritionally depleted patients. "The mean [average] stay of the 21 nutritionally normal patients was 17 days . . . while that of the nutritionally depleted patients was 27 [days]. The difference is significant," the doctors said (*Journal of Thoracic and Cardiovascular Surgery,* April, 1979). Actually, the difference amounts to more than a third, with well-nourished patients spending 37 percent less time in the hospital.

But you can't afford to wait for reams of formal test results before taking personal responsibility for the shape you're in when the orderly wheels you into the OR. Just as you wouldn't think of undergoing surgery without financial insurance, there are easy, specific steps you should take to add nutritional insurance to your medical coverage.

Take stock of your diet as far ahead of time as possible to make necessary adjustments in good time. Two weeks to a month is best; you may have even more time for preparation if your surgery is tentatively scheduled far in the future. In fact, you may want to postpone surgery until you feel that you are well enough prepared.

An easy-to-use food guide: the picture of health. You shouldn't think solely in terms of assigning single, specialized tasks to each vitamin and mineral and eating one food per vitamin per task. Protein and other nutritional elements don't work alone, independent of each other. All are important as team members; their tasks overlap and are coordinated to keep the body in working order and to make necessary repairs. You should think in terms of the total effect of your diet.

Because endless lists of foods and nutrients can be unwieldy sources of information, it's simpler to form one commonsense mental picture of the best foods for health as a guide to choosing a diet that provides the wide range of nutrition your body needs to brace itself for the operating room.

The Food Target Guide in Figure 1 takes into consideration the balance of protein, carbohydrates, fats, calories, vitamins, minerals and fiber, and makes meal-planning before and after surgery much easier.

Aim for the center circle of food choices, and you'll get exactly what you need. Foods in the second ring are basically healthful but many tend to be high in fat and should be eaten less often than those in the center. Following surgery, foods in the second ring should occasionally be added to the diet to help meet increased protein and calorie needs of wound healing. Choosing from among those foods in the 2 center circles will reduce your chances of developing nutritional deficiencies that blockade healing and prolong the recovery process.

Foods in the outer ring should be selected rarely and those outside the target, never.

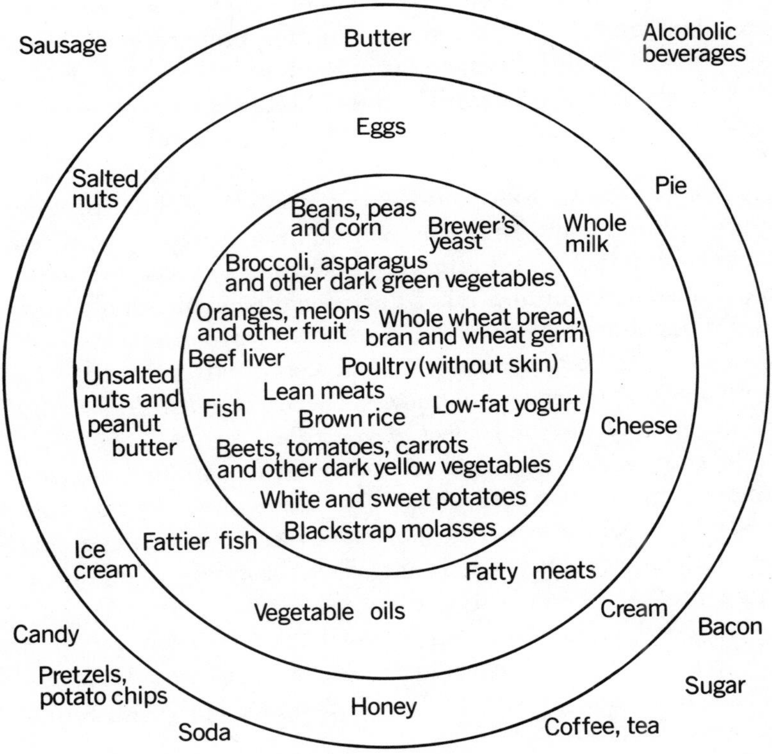

Figure 1. ***Food Target Guide for Before and After Surgery***
Eat foods from the center circle for the best in surgical nutrition. Foods in the second ring should be added to the diet occasionally; those in the outer ring, rarely, and those outside the target, never.

Protein and fat plague. Protein, fats and carbohydrates do not naturally occur in isolation; rather, each exists combined in varying proportions with one or both of the others, plus a good deal of water. Just how much and what proportion of these 3 nutrients we get in our diets is crucial to general health and well-being, but especially critical to the surgery patient.

August Daro, M.D., practicing in Chicago, is one of the physicians to whom we spoke who pays close attention to the nutrition of his presurgery patients. "Foremost," emphasized Dr. Daro, "is the importance of a sound diet. Eating the wrong foods will give you far too many calories and not enough protein, which heads you straight for protein malnutrition that is so common in hospital patients. Be sure to eat enough protein."

Eating enough protein itself presents no great problem. Some forms are cheaper than others, but protein is easily available from both animal sources (beef, pork, poultry, fish, cheese, eggs, milk) and plant sources (beans, nuts, grains, legumes). The problem is that the forms of protein we eat most of — animal sources — arrive on our dinner plates with unwanted amounts of extra fat. So we can't talk about protein without talking about fat.

"The American diet is probably the fattiest diet that has ever been in existence in an urban society since the beginning of time," said David Capuzzi, M.D., Ph.D., at the Nutrition Symposium at the Hospital of the University of Pennsylvania in April, 1979. Dr. Capuzzi, associate chief of staff research at the Philadelphia VA Medical Center, added, "The only other diet which approaches this high fat intake is that of the Finns, who along with Americans lead the world in deaths from coronary artery disease."

Those glaring facts strongly suggest that our diet is not exactly "the best diet in the world," as some people boast. While it's true that the average American has *available* the best diet in the world, whether he *eats* the best of what's available to him is quite another story. Dr. Leslie M. Klevay, who uncovered the surprising zinc and copper deficits in diets in and out of hospitals, feels the medical world is just beginning to face that reality and our food choices should be reexamined.

A statement from a surgical text describes the optimal diet this way: "For Western societies to meet these criteria for an optimal diet, consumption of fat would have to decrease . . . and carbohydrates (principally complex carbohydrates such as potatoes and breads) would have to increase. As a source of protein, meat is presently overemphasized at the expense of grains, legumes and nuts." In addition, no more than 10 percent of the fat should be of the saturated type that is found in animal products (*Current Surgical Diagnosis and Treatment,* Lange Medical Publications, 1977).

You need "the best diet in the world" more before and after surgery than at perhaps any other time. Get the required 45 to 55 grams of protein from the best sources — it is very wise to choose from various plant and animal sources that carry the least fat baggage. When you think protein, don't automatically think steak. Choose the forms that add fewer fat-derived calories and more protein-carbohydrate-derived calories. Both the Food Target Guide in Figure 1 and sources of dietary protein in Table 9 should be helpful.

You may also wish to keep in mind that the lighter the meat, the better the protein-fat ratio. Fish and poultry derive only half as much of their total calories from fat as do certain cuts of beef and pork. Nearly half of a sausage, for instance, is fat, and that fat yields 82 percent — far more than its share — of calories in that piece of meat. Even though muscle meats contain fair amounts of unremovable fat, certain cuts of beef, if very carefully trimmed of every visible shred of fat, can approach the lower fat-calorie levels of poultry and fish, which fill the protein bill quite nicely.

Dr. Donald Reiner, the surgeon in Santa Maria, California, emphasizes fish and poultry in the high-protein regime he prescribes for his patients. Low-fat varieties of fish like cod, flounder, haddock, perch, pollack and sole take just 10 minutes or so to broil and are practically pure protein, with plenty of vitamins and minerals. Look for a supermarket that is known for its fresh fish or seek out a fish store in your neighborhood, and shop there

(*Continued on page 165*)

Table 9. Selected Food Sources of Protein

Food (*cooked, where applicable*)	Quantity	Protein (*grams*)	Calories	Fat (*grams*)	% of total calories from fat
Lentils	½ cup	8	106	trace	less than 1
Buttermilk	6 ounces	7	66	0.2	2
Milk, skim	6 ounces	7	66	0.2	2
Split peas	½ cup	8	115	0.3	2
Cottage cheese, dry curd	½ cup	12	63	0.2	2
Brewer's yeast	1 tablespoon	3	23	0.1	4
Lima beans	½ cup	6.5	95	0.5	4
Navy (pea) beans	½ cup	7.5	112	0.5	4
Kidney beans	½ cup	7	109	0.5	4
Shrimp	10 large	14	67	0.6	8
Scallops	6 ounces	35	169	2	11
Turkey, light meat, without skin	3 ounces	28	150	3	18
Chicken, light meat, without skin	3 ounces	49	275	7	23
Cod	6 ounces	49	288	9	28
Yogurt from skim milk	1 cup	8	123	4	29
Chicken, dark meat, without skin	3 ounces	27	167	5.9	32
Sirloin steak, trimmed of fat	6 ounces	55	352	13	33
Haddock	6 ounces	34	282	11	35

Table 9—*Continued*

Food (*cooked, where applicable*)	**Quantity**	**Protein** (*grams*)	**Calories**	**Fat** (*grams*)	**% of total calories from fat**
Flounder	6 ounces	51	342	14	36
Turkey, dark meat, without skin	3 ounces	26	173	7	36
Tuna in oil, drained solids	½ cup	23	158	6.5	37
Halibut	6 ounces	43	288	12	38
Soybeans	½ cup	10	117	5	38
Ham, lean, trimmed of fat	3 ounces	25	184	8.5	41
Beef liver	3 ounces	22	195	9	42
Ground beef, lean	3 ounces	23	186	10	45
Yogurt from whole milk	1 cup	7	152	8	47
Milk, whole	6 ounces	6	119	6	48
Salmon (sockeye)	3 ounces	23	188	10	48
Sardines	4 fish	12	96	5	49
Prime rib of beef, trimmed of fat	6 ounces	48	410	23	50
Pork chops	5.9 ounces	51	454	26	52
Tofu (soybean curd)	1 piece, 2½ × 2¾ × 1″	9.5	86	5	52
Mackerel	6 ounces	37	402	27	60
Ground beef, regular	2.9 ounces	20	235	17	65

Table 9—*Continued*

Food (*cooked, where applicable*)	**Quantity**	**Protein** (*grams*)	**Calories**	**Fat** (*grams*)	**% of total calories from fat**
Egg, hard-cooked	1 large	6.5	82	6	66
Cheddar cheese	1 ounce	7	113	9	72
Sirloin steak, not trimmed of fat	6 ounces	39	658	54	74
Corned beef	3 ounces	21	337	28	75
Salami	3 1-ounce slices	15	264	22	75
Bologna	3 1-ounce slices	10	258	23	80
Prime rib of beef, not trimmed of fat	6 ounces	34	748	67	81
Sausage	3 links	7	186	17	82
Frankfurters	2 franks	14	352	32	82

often. (Shellfish are low in fat but because of environmental contamination are not a highly recommended source of protein.)

Chicken and turkey, minus their skin and giblets, not only provide excellent protein without copious amounts of fat, but the darker portions are especially rich sources of B vitamins.

If there is one red meat that should be included in your surgery bill of fare, that meat is liver. Liver is such an excellent source of vitamin A, B vitamins, iron, zinc, copper and potassium that it is truly an antistress, healing and strengthening food.

Liver doesn't have to be the tough stringy piece of dinner meat you battled with as a child. First, be sure your raw liver is tender. Ask the butcher to slice it really thin. Before you actually cook it, soak it for about an hour in its own juice and a little water, perhaps adding a minced clove of garlic and a few onion slices to the marinade.

To cook liver, preheat the frying pan so it's good and hot. Sprinkle a few drops of oil on the bottom, and cook the slices for 30 seconds or so on each side.

If liver prepared that way still doesn't appeal to you, try desiccated liver. That's a concentrated form of liver made by removing the fat and then drying the liver in a vacuum. Desiccated liver is available in tablets and capsules. Buy only desiccated liver which clearly lists Argentinian beef as its source. Cattle raised in that South American country are not fed growth hormones because there they are prohibited by law.

Dairy products can be friend or foe in the nutrition game. While milk, cheese and eggs are rich sources of protein, calcium, vitamins A and B_{12} by themselves and augment the quality of plant protein, they are too high in saturated fat to be given starring roles in your program. Low-fat yogurt and uncreamed, dry curd cottage cheese are your best bets in the dairy department, with eggs allowed occasionally if you use yolks sparingly.

Low-fat dairy products as well as grains, can be added to beans and other legumes (peas, chick-peas, soybeans, limas) to augment the protein value of those plant proteins, which have no more than mere traces of unsaturated fat. You don't have to prepare complicated entrees in order to work bean dishes into your menus. Reserving one day a week for split pea or lentil soup with whole wheat bread, adding chick-peas to your salads, or quickly making up a batch of 3-bean salad on the weekend, are some effortless ways to add plant proteins to your diet. (If flatulence is sometimes a problem for you, it might be a good idea to avoid beans for the few days immediately before surgery.)

Do you know where your fat is coming from? Table 10 lists food "extras" which win no prizes for vitamins or minerals and derive their calories largely from fat. Cutting way down on those items will lop plenty of "fat calories" from your daily total calories; protein or complex carbohydrate calories should be substituted for these "fat calories."

You will notice that french fries and gravy do not appear as recommended dietary sources of zinc and vitamin A — or of anything else. They *are* excellent sources of extra grease, though — the one item the surgery patient needs the very least of.

The problem with butter and margarine is not only that they are total fat, but also that they show up on so many otherwise honestly good, wholesome foods: broiled fish, baked potatoes, broccoli, whole wheat toast and muffins, peas and carrots, corn on

Table 10. Fat Content of Selected Foods

Food	Quantity	Calories	Fat (*grams*)	% of calories from fat
Butter or margarine	1 pat	36	4	100
Lard	1 tablespoon	117	13	100
Vegetable oils	1 tablespoon	120	14	100
Mayonnaise	1 tablespoon	101	11	98
Tartar sauce	1 tablespoon	74	8	97
Cream, heavy whipping	1 tablespoon	53	6	95
Cream cheese	1 tablespoon	52	5	92
Sour cream	1 tablespoon	31	3	87
French dressing	1 tablespoon	66	6	85
Cream, light	1 tablespoon	32	3	84
Cream, half-and-half	1 tablespoon	20	2	81
Egg yolk	from large egg	59	5	79
Egg, whole	1 large	82	6	64
Ice cream	½ cup	135	7	47

the cob, and sometimes even rice! If you can recall looking down at your last dinner plate and seeing everything except your salad swimming in butter, you're in trouble. Learn to love those steaming spuds with just a dab of low-fat yogurt and chopped parsley. Sprinkle apple cider vinegar on beans and broccoli, if you must add something. But never, never, say "Please pass the butter," without stopping to ask yourself, "Do I really need that?" (If you're absolutely convinced you do, try to use as little as possible.)

"Carbohydrates" has traditionally been a dirty word in the diet lexicon. Simple, refined carbohydrates (sugar alone, or products such as candy, soda and cake) *are* villains. But unrefined, complex carbohydrates are much closer to the state in which nature manufactured them; they should be the principal suppliers of the fuel used by your body. Fresh fruits and vegetables, whole grain cereals and breads, potatoes, peas, beans, nuts and seeds are all complex carbohydrates.

Learn to shop with an eye for dark green and yellow vegetables, ripe fruits, and potatoes that come in skins, not boxes. Once you've got them in your kitchen, don't overprocess them on the range or in the oven. Overcooking destroys much of the superhealing vitamin C in vegetables, and cooking draws out both C and important B vitamins, especially folate. When you must cook vegetables, steam them in a vegetable steamer or cook them very quickly in as little water as possible.

Eating several servings of raw vegetables a day is the best way to get as much out of your vegetables and into your presurgical body as possible. The easiest way to incorporate raw vegetables into your daily menu is to make yourself a large salad every day. That doesn't mean a few sorry leaves of pale lettuce, a soggy wedge or two of truck-ripened tomato and a slice of mushy cucumber, topped with bacon dressing. That's the salad equivalent of junk food: lots of fat and practically no vitamins.

Make yourself a real salad. Include dark leafy greens such as romaine lettuce, chicory, endive or escarole (vitamins A and K, and iron) as your salad base. Load it up with fresh, tender carrot shreds or zucchini chips (more vitamin A), green peppers (precious vitamin C), raw mushrooms (copper), cauliflowerets (the B vitamin pantothenate) and sprouts (protein plus magnified quantities of healing vitamins). Top it with a tablespoon of wheat germ (vitamins B and E, and zinc) and sprinkle it with lemon juice (more C). That's a salad your body can use, down to the last crisp morsel.

Don't let eating out deprive you of your salads. Choose restaurants that are known for their bountiful self-service salads, then march right up to the salad bar, grab a bowl, and heap your greens with beets, garbanzos, cottage cheese, onions, mushrooms and green beans. Sidestep the oily or creamy dressings and sprinkle your harvest with tangy vinegar.

A chilled glass of smooth Super Vitamin Cocktail will add extra vitamins and minerals to your daily intake of vitamin C and iron. Most of the ingredients are available in supermarkets year-round. Keep a pitcherful in the refrigerator and drink it often, especially if pickings are slim in the produce market in the weeks before your surgery.

Super Vitamin Cocktail

- 4 cups tomato juice
- 2 tablespoons lemon juice (juice of 1 lemon)
- 2 stalks celery, with leaves, chopped
- 1 teaspoon parsley, minced
- 1 tablespoon onion, minced
- 2 tablespoons green pepper, diced
- ¼ teaspoon celery seed

Combine 1 cup of tomato juice and remaining ingredients in blender. Blend at high speed until smooth. Add remaining juice, continuing to blend until thoroughly mixed. Chill well before serving. Yield: almost 5 cups

Vitamin and mineral supplements. A quick review of Tables 1 through 8 which appear earlier in this chapter suggests that even the food sources richest in nutrients may not be able to meet therapeutic requirements raised far above the Recommended Dietary Allowances (RDA) by the demands of surgery.

The key to a hastened recovery, then, is wise choice of the foods you *are* able to eat, supplemented by at least the RDA of vitamins and minerals, starting at least 2 to 4 weeks ahead of surgery, if possible. (Therapeutic dosages should be begun immediately after surgery, at the latest.)

A review of several studies which looked at the relationship between vitamin C levels in the blood of patients before and after various types of surgery supports the use of vitamin C supplements: "Surgical operations were inevitably followed by an authentic increase in ascorbic acid requirements, since . . . [blood levels] fell by 42 percent on the third day [after surgery]." That same article cites the daily use of 1 gram (1,000 milligrams) of oral vitamin C for 3 days in the successful treatment of bedsores in hospital patients who did not necessarily show deficiencies of the vitamin, demonstrating vitamin C's helpful role in nonsurgical wound healing as well (*British Medical Journal,* February 17, 1979).

"Supplements are very important," says Dr. August Daro, of Chicago. "I tell my surgery patients to take up to 1,500 to 2,000 milligrams of vitamin C a day, divided into 3 doses, before surgery. (That amount can be reduced if not well tolerated.) Added to that are 3 10-milligram tablets of zinc daily, preferably in chelated form for better absorption, and 10,000 International Units of vitamin A."

In addition to the vitamin C and A and zinc, which are well recognized as crucial to successful healing, Dr. Donald Reiner, of California, prescribes 25 milligrams of iron, 1 to 3 times a day, before and after surgery. Dr. Reiner has also found that vitamin E significantly cuts down on the pain of surgical healing and suggests his patients take 400 International Units, twice a day, before and after surgery.

You'll probably want to boost your B vitamins, especially folate, B_6 and B_{12}, because of the high likelihood of deficiencies of those particular vitamins among hospital patients and the vital roles they play in healing. Be sure to check the units of measure: it takes 1,000 micrograms to equal 1 milligram (see Table 3).

Brewer's yeast and wheat germ are special foods that are so packed with nutrition that they are virtually nutritional supplements in themselves. Brewer's yeast taken as a nutritional supplement is an excellent source of protein, chock-full of B vitamins (including B_{12}, otherwise found only in animal products), and rich in minerals, including iron, calcium and potassium. Powdered brewer's yeast is easy to add to recipes for bread, pancakes, muffins, stews, and vegetable and fruit juices.

Wheat germ is one portion of the wheat grain which has been removed to make the white flour in most people's kitchen canister. It's also absent from the white flour that customarily goes into noodles, macaroni products, cakes, cookies, sugar buns, doughnuts, pastries and ready-to-eat cereals. Returned to your menu as a food supplement, wheat germ replaces the thiamine, pantothenate, vitamin B_6, riboflavin, niacin, vitamin E, iron, magnesium, zinc and potassium lost in processing those products.

Raw wheat germ is higher in nutrition than the toasted kind because it has not been subject to heat. But toasted wheat germ keeps longer, tastes more palatable, and is still a nutritional gold mine. To give raw wheat germ a toasty flavor, put about ½ cup in a 250° oven for about 15 minutes or until it is light brown. Add this toasted wheat germ to a jar of raw wheat germ and the whole batch will taste toasted.

Here are some suggestions for adding the nutritional benefits of wheat germ to your diet: For breakfast, serve wheat germ as your cereal, topped with bananas, strawberries and yogurt. Sprinkle some wheat germ on your poached eggs. In pancake and waffle batters, substitute ½ cup wheat germ for an equal amount of flour. In muffins and breads, replace 2 tablespoons of each cup of regular flour with 2 tablespoons of wheat germ. The easiest way to measure is to put the 2 tablespoons in the cup first, then fill it with flour. Add a few tablespoons of wheat germ to hamburgers, meatballs and meat loaf. Add a tablespoon or 2 to brown rice after cooking. Add a tablespoon to a light dessert of cottage cheese and fruit.

Don't be shy about letting your doctor know you intend to continue your nutritional program in the hospital. Your doctor may even nod in approval at your interest in optimal healing, because more and more physicians recognize the call for more research on the link between nutrition and reduced complications is growing louder. Your supplements will be checked in at the admissions desk, just like medication, and returned to you. Or you can make a list of the specific amounts of each nutrient you are taking so your doctor can order a prescription for you from the hospital pharmacy. (That is likely to cost more than your home supply.)

Making the Most of Hospital Diets

In many cases, it's possible to begin eating regular food for your first scheduled meal after return from the recovery room. But if you have trouble swallowing, if surgery has interfered with normal use of the gastrointestinal tract, or if you've been fed solely by IV for several days, a pre-prepared, fiber-free formula that is the chemical equivalent of food may be introduced through a nasogastric tube. Those elemental diets deliver calories, fluids, protein and nutrients directly into the stomach, leaving the G.I. tract with as little digestive work to do as possible, but preventing starvation. The patient is asked to swallow a tube about the size and flexibility of spaghetti. It is slightly uncomfortable, but generally well tolerated by patients who must depend on it for nourishment. Tube feeding is sometimes used in addition to regular meals, to supply extra nourishment — primarily protein and calories.

Returning to normal diet-by-mouth may begin with the full liquid diet. If you've been on IV as sole source of sustenance for a few weeks, suddenly dumping a lot of hard-to-digest food into the intestines will cause problems, the major one being diarrhea. Full liquid diets consist primarily of strained, semisolid foods that are easy to swallow and absorb. Fortified eggnogs and milk shakes are the mainstay of full liquid diets, if milk is tolerated. Other typical foods include strained juices, tomato juice, broth, strained cream soups, raw eggs, cream, melted butter and margarine, baby cereal, custard, gelatin, ice cream, sherbet, strained vegetables, honey, syrup, sugar, and even soda, coffee and tea. Obviously, this diet is nutritionally poor. Fortunately, liquid diets are ordinarily used only for a few days, followed by the soft diet.

The soft diet is an easily digested, low-fiber intermediary between full liquids and a general diet. Omitted are fried foods, raw vegetables and most raw fruits, whole grain cereals and nuts. Strongly flavored vegetables such as onions, cabbage, cauliflower, Brussels sprouts, cucumber, peppers, turnips, radishes, corn, beans and peas are deliberately excluded, even if cooked. What *are* included in the soft diet are chopped tender meat, mild cheeses, soft-cooked or strained fruits such as apples, peaches, apricots, and pears (without skins), and raw bananas, plus lots of custard and bland pudding. A bit better than the full liquid diet, but no gold medal winner.

Ask the dietitian or a dietitian's aide to explain any modified diet your doctor may have ordered for you. Even within therapeutic diets, personal tolerance and preferences can sometimes be considered. The dietitian can note any problems or suggestions clearly on your chart; in some hospitals, the staff is encouraged to speak directly to the attending physician about a patient's nutritional problems.

The haste with which you are steered back to a normal diet depends on your physician and your condition, but getting back to regular eating as soon as possible is the important goal, because transitional diets obviously fail to satisfy the full range of requirements for protein, calories, vitamins and minerals. As part of the heightened protein and calorie needs after surgery, an extra 40 grams of protein and about 1,000 or so calories will be added to your diet, either as between-meal snacks or larger portions at mealtime.

The logical choices for extra sources of protein are lean meats, fish and cottage cheese, or even milk, if tolerated. The hospital's supply of junk food may be tapped to add needed extra calories. Items which consistently — and astonishingly — appear as "foods allowed" rather than "foods to avoid" on both normal and what are carefully designed to be *therapeutic* diets include: cookies, gelatin, sherbet, jelly, jam, syrup, candy, soda, chocolate milk, ice cream, pudding, cream cheese, angel food cake and vanilla wafers. Many people wouldn't allow those foods in a schoolchild's lunch box, yet the items are common on hospital diets.

Between-meal snacks during the days following surgery aren't served just to break up monotonous hours in the afternoon. Snacks are a bona fide means of providing the extra calories and nutrition needed for surgical repair. Be wary of junk foods. Ask for fruit and whole grain muffins instead of angel food cake, cottage cheese and fruit instead of milk shakes. Other wholesome sources of needed extra calories are dried dates and fruits, whole grain cereal with fruit and yogurt, and pineapple or apple juice. (If your requests aren't readily honored, ask friends and relatives to bring food in to you during visiting hours.) Asking for seconds on potatoes or rice at mealtime, if your appetite is large enough, is another means of avoiding starvation.

Other "foods allowed" that show up 3 times a day are coffee, tea and cola. "Caffeine is probably the most widely consumed drug in the hospital," says dietitian Patricia Stephenson. It is possible for the patient to receive sufficient caffeine to interfere with or act as a potentiator to his other medications — enough to retard recovery, according to Ms. Stephenson (*Journal of the American Dietetic Association,* September, 1977).

You were better off without those caffeinated beverages before surgery, and you certainly can do without them now. Take a variety of favorite herb teas from home into the hospital with you and say, "Hot water, please."

You may have more control than you think over food selection in the hospital. Try to practice the same food selection habits adopted for your home diet prior to surgery. Dietitians we spoke to said patients are welcome to speak up about personal preferences and will be accommodated to the best of the dietary department's abilities, which vary from hospital to hospital. The rationale is that if you don't like it, you won't eat it. And if you don't eat, recovery is next to impossible. (Diet manuals provide for kosher, vegetarian, lactose- and gluten-free diets, as well as for individual likes and dislikes.)

The alert patient can take every opportunity to steer himself away from the trap of greasy chopped hamburger, mashed potatoes swimming in butter, pasty white crescent rolls, artificially flavored gelatin and an ocean of tea. Chicken and fish are nearly always available; if you want sole instead of meat loaf or pork chops, indicate it on your menu. Check off "baked" instead of "fried" or "au gratin" for your potato choice. If you can't get whole wheat bread instead of the usual white dinner rolls, have it trucked in from home. (Ditto if your requests for yogurt are futile.) Insist on fruit instead of gelatin for dessert.

If the hospital breakfast juice tastes suspiciously like artificial juice drink, keep a thermos of chilled juice from home on your nightstand. Physician-sponsored requests for bran will show up in a daily allotment of about ¼ cup on your morning tray. Add bran — and possibly wheat germ from home — to your cooked oatmeal. Order poached or hard-cooked eggs in the shell to be sure you're not getting reconstituted egg powder.

The growing trend toward "restaurant-type" menu selection within each hospital patient's physician-ordered regime is growing, and if your idea of what constitutes the right food is slightly different — and better — than the next person's, the food service should be able to accommodate you.

Also, if you are accustomed to eating your large, hot meal at noon rather than at suppertime, it is possible to continue to do so in the hospital. Your appetite may be able to handle the larger portions earlier in the day but only lighter meals in the evening. If so, indicate your preference on your menu. The end goal is to eat as many of the right foods as you can, whenever you can.

Bran and bowel function after surgery. While some drugs cause diarrhea, others cause constipation. And even if medication doesn't slow down your bowel movements, the change in diet or the inactivity of bed rest is very likely either to result in small, hard, difficult-to-pass stools or to stop bowel action almost completely.

Chemical laxatives are artificial means of relieving constipation by stimulating the wavelike motions necessary to push stools out of the bowel. The safe and natural way to insure that things will keep moving along at the right pace is to be sure that there is enough fiber in the digested food to absorb water in the bowel and form soft stools that are easily eliminated.

Fiber is a component of many whole, unprocessed foods like whole grain breads and cereals, peas, beans, fruits and vegetables. The change to a hospital diet (many processed foods from which the fiber has been removed, irregular meals, reliance on IV feeding) means you will probably be getting very little fiber in your diet. (White bread, for instance, has one-eighth the fiber of whole wheat bread.)

The cheapest, safest and most convenient way to normalize bowel function slowed down by drugs, diet and inactivity is the addition of one heaping tablespoon or more of bran to your diet daily. Drink plenty of water with it.

Besides distress and pain, constipation may also be accompanied by loss of appetite, flatulence, headache, insomnia and irritability, making convalescence miserable. Even more critically, an overloaded colon can block the free flow of blood in the legs and permit formation of blood clots that can travel to the heart or lungs and threaten life. Blood clots in the legs (deep vein thrombosis) is a fairly common postoperative complication because anesthesia induces a type of temporary paralysis in the body, during which blood circulation stagnates.

A high-fiber diet before surgery keeps the blood flowing and prevents that secondary complication. Maurice Frohn, consultant surgeon at Bethnal Green Hospital in London, says, "Over the past 4 years I've operated on over 1,500 patients, and not one of them has suffered any postoperative clotting. This is where bran is particularly significant, because it is in the postoperative state that this situation usually arises — often critically."

Benefits of speedy hospital recovery. What are the implications of shortening the number of days you lie in the hospital waiting for wounds to heal, aside from saving yourself a lot of pain, discomfort and frustration?

The cost of short- and long-term hospital stays in the United States has tripled in the last decade, to a point where in 1977 the total cost nationwide was 65.6 *billion* dollars in a total national health care expenditure of 162.6 billion dollars, according to the Health Care Finances Administration, Department of Health, Education and Welfare. Commenting on the escalating heights of hospital care and health care in general, Charles E. Butterworth Jr., M.D., of the University of Alabama, states, "Obviously, enormous savings could be achieved if hospital stays could be shortened by even a day, or prevented altogether (*Nutrition Today,* March/April, 1974).

The amount you spend on nutritional insurance to avoid nutrition-related complications, reducing the time spent waiting for wounds to heal in the hospital, will be minuscule compared to what the surgery and total hospital stay will cost. But you can't attach a dollar sign to the uncomfortable days spent away from your home, family, garden, hobbies, friends and job.

Nutrition for Continued Recovery at Home

Basically, continuing to eat the high-protein, high-complex-carbohydrate diet adopted before you left for the hospital will maximize your chances for full recovery after discharge. At this time, you may not be able to meet stepped-up protein demands adequately by relying on beans and legumes. Lean meats, low-fat dairy products and occasional eggs are reliable sources. To the 45 to 55 grams of protein you were eating presurgery, add an extra serving of turkey, chicken or fish at mealtimes or a high-protein snack like buttermilk, yogurt or cottage cheese between meals.

Don't let calorie intake slip by sleeping through breakfast or munching on toast and tea at lunchtime. Now more than ever, you should eat regular meals chosen from a wide variety of natural food. Have an attractive bowl of fresh fruit placed next to all those cheery flowers from friends, and reach for an apple or banana from time to time. In other words, eat like an athlete on a training diet, not an invalid.

Continue your program until you notice a gain of a pound or two. At that point, your body metabolism has probably slowed back down to normal, having nearly completed its repair work. The extra calories are no longer necessary.

The same rule of thumb applies to supplements, the most important being B vitamins, vitamins A and E, zinc, iron and especially vitamin C. The immediate and rapid depletion of vitamin C stores during those immediate few days after surgery calls for frequent dosages totalling up to about 2 or 3 grams a day. Therapeutic doses of vitamins and minerals can be cut down as you feel yourself gaining strength and vigor. Gradually, over a matter of weeks, your nutritional needs will again return to presurgery levels.

10
Surgical Costs and Insurance Coverage

There's no question that medical costs are going up. So is everything else. But medical costs are skyrocketing when everything else is merely zooming.

In 1977, medical care expenditures in the U.S. exceeded $160 billion. If that's difficult to fathom, it may help to consider that that's 4 times what health costs were in 1965. Since that year, according to the Consumer Price Index, medical care costs have risen faster than any other prices in the cost of living.

Hospital costs are the single largest item in medical care costs, and have risen to the point where the average cost of a day in the hospital in 1977 was $174, says the American Hospital Association. Ironically, though, hospital costs are the expenditure least likely to be felt by most people. While many patients complain about the out-of-pocket cost of routine office visits and treatments from their doctor, few are directly hit by high-priced hospitalization and surgery, which are usually covered by insurance. More than 90 percent of Americans have health insurance provided by either the government (Medicare), Blue Cross and/or Blue Shield, or commercial insurance companies, and it all seems "free" when a third party picks up the tab. So patients are lax about questioning excessive hospital or surgery bills. Half the time they don't even know what the services they're getting cost.

While that ignorance contributes greatly to the patient's peace of mind, it doesn't do much for the nation's medical budget. Have you ever heard Uncle Joe marvel that his bill for a coronary bypass operation and several weeks of hospitalization was only $15 for the phone in his room? Joe may not have realized that it really cost him much more. What about the money his employer diverts to company-paid insurance premiums that might otherwise be returned as income by profit-sharing, higher salaries or bonuses for employees? What about paycheck deductions to help finance federal Medicare and Medicaid programs? Throughout his working life, Joe has probably paid for his operation in full.

Why Does Medical Care Cost So Much?

A recurrent theme in the literature on health care economy is that the widespread availability of medical insurance has contributed to the inflation of health care costs and that consequently, neither the doctors, hospitals nor insured patients have incentives to hold costs down.

Other explanations for the climb in costs point specifically to payroll and overhead expenses for hospitals, combined with the availability and increased demand for a larger number of expensive procedures for diagnosis and treatment; a demographic shift in growth of the population over 65, who are more likely to require those services; and the specter of malpractice claims by a suit-happy public.

After a close look at just what has happened to the health care industry, we'll tell you how the individual patient, as a consumer, may be able to control his own medical expenses and at the same time help to hold down the aggregate cost to all.

More surgery today. There's a mystique about doctors: they've got training you haven't, and they seem to have answers you haven't got. Because of that perception, and the potential life-and-death implications of refusing medical treatment, there's little tendency to question any treatment suggested, especially surgery.

If reimbursement for the operation is assured, the surgeon is less likely to hesitate to prescribe it than if he thinks you're going to have to come up with the cash yourself. And the patient is less likely to think twice about it. Many patients don't even want to look at their hospital or surgical bills. They just sign an assignment of benefits form and never see the charges. Payment goes directly to the provider. Even if there's a mistake on the bill, they won't know it.

Coupled with those unquestioning attitudes is the high degree of specialization in medicine. A hefty supply of surgeons and superspecialists, eager to apply highly sophisticated techniques, could help to explain why surgery increased 23 percent in the first 8 years of the 1970s while the population itself grew by only 5 percent. There's a tendency for doctors to practice what they've been trained for. When a patient who's a borderline case prefers surgery, which is covered by insurance, over more conservative, lengthy treatment, which is not covered, there may not be any great reason for the surgeon not to operate unless it's a high-risk case.

Fee-for-service system of payment to doctors. Should the nonsurgical approach be taken, medical management often means repeated trips to the doctor's office, with a separate fee paid each time he sees you. That system leads to some very high physician incomes, readily justified by staff, equipment, costly malpractice premiums, long hours and the high level of education the profession requires, according to doctors. In some cases, the cost of long-term medical management can approach that of surgery. And if alternate techniques just delay, but do not replace surgery, the total can of course be higher than either one alone.

Physicians' fees rose by 9.3 percent in 1977, 50 percent more than other consumer prices, reports the Council on Wage and Price Stability. Doctors' incomes rose at a faster rate than those of any occupational group. The median income for doctors in 1977 was $65,430 — more than 5 times the income of the average worker. (They're even higher now, of course.) The Council stated that fees were unjustifiably high by economic standards, and that income levels were higher than needed to attract an adequate supply of physicians.

The fee-for-service system, then, has been blamed for placing a strong incentive on treating many patients, many times. (An alternative health care delivery system, the Health Maintenance Organization (HMO), erases that incentive and will be discussed later in this chapter.)

Malpractice and defensive medicine. Doctors see themselves as victims of a suit-happy public. But that's only part of the problem.

"The crisis of malpractice is a product of many forces, including a disturbing level of negligent and improper care, frequently unrealistic patient expectations and the growing 'philosophy of entitlement' which is rampant among Americans," says Charles P. Hall, Jr., Ph.D., president-elect of the American Risk and Insurance Association, in a published paper on medical malpractice.

"Surgeons are particularly hard hit by malpractice threats," Dr. Hall pointed out in an interview. "Surgeons are most often sued, as opposed to GP's and internists, for instance, because cutting procedures offer more opportunities for things to go wrong. Surgeons tend, as a result, to protect themselves. It is unquestionable that there is a tendency on the part of many surgeons to order more diagnostic tests than are always absolutely necessary. A lot of doctors view any patient who walks through the door as a potential lawsuit and will treat him as such." To the extent that this fear leads to unnecessary tests or procedures, it adds to the already serious problem of rapidly escalating health care costs.

Coupled with the increased use of tests are the astronomically high malpractice premiums paid by doctors to get insurance coverage against possible claims. "Firm costs figures are not readily available on a nationwide basis, but it was estimated that the actual cost of medical malpractice insurance in New York alone amounted to about $244 million in 1975. Those costs were projected to rise to $500 million by 1979," cites Dr. Hall in his article. "The initial impact of these premium costs falls on the provider doctor and/or hospitals but it is estimated that 70 to 90 percent of the total costs is ultimately passed on to the consumer." Dr. Hall points out that in some hospitals, malpractice costs account for $15 or more of individual daily hospital charges (*Annals of the American Academy,* May, 1979).

A good part of the swell of malpractice claims has nothing at all to do with actual negligence or error. Rather, a fair amount of litigation in the malpractice area has more to do with "maloccurrence"; that is, the outcome isn't exactly what the patient expected or wanted.

"Some of these doctors are being sued when, if they hadn't intervened and tried their best, the patient who's suing wouldn't even be alive," adds Dr. Hall. "The cases are often after-the-fact suits that reflect disappointment, frustration, anger. . . and the only persons to direct it toward are the doctor and the hospital. The doctors see themselves as victims of an unreasonable public that expects perfection and of a greedy legal profession that's eager to get a contingency fee from a large judgment in favor of any patient who experiences anything less than prompt, complete recovery from injury or disease. So it's in that environment that doctors practice defensive medicine."

Are doctors and hospitals technology-happy? Aside from overuse of diagnostic tests as a defense mechanism in medicine, there is widespread belief that doctors are fascinated by new equipment and push hospitals to buy the latest in fancy equipment, whether or not that same equipment is available at a nearby facility, thereby making the high cost unjustifiable in terms of need.

No one would argue that devices that keep premature babies alive, allow for open heart surgery and preserve the lives of those with kidney failure are anything short of miraculous. Half the increase in hospital costs over the past decade is due to such new technology. But do doctors, in fact, generally gravitate to more and more technology?

Some do, but they're more likely to be hospital-based physicians, such as those in teaching positions or acute care facilities, rather than the average community office practitioner. Overall, physician-pressured purchases appear to be a myth, according to one study conducted by the Urban Research Center, University of Wisconsin, in Milwaukee. On the whole, physicians interviewed tended to be skeptical of new procedures. Community physicians felt obliged to keep up with developments in their fields but were generally suspicious of claims made about new procedures (*Hospital Medical Staff,* June, 1979).

A controversial bit of gadgetry is the computerized axial tomography (CAT) scanner, used to diagnose brain damage and other internal disorders without operating. At a cost of $600,000 and up, purchase can only be justified on a cost-benefit basis if the unit is used at least 2,500 times a year. Many medical economists believe that more have been sold than are needed. Critics say that where there is insufficient demand for one, doctors will prescribe its use more frequently than would otherwise be the case: patients bear the cost of diagnosis they don't need, or the purchase cost will be passed on to all patients in the form of higher charges for other services. One hospital president maintains that even though there are other CAT scanners in his area, a recent purchase of one by his hospital was necessary because it is a teaching hospital for a nearby medical school.

Most hospitals employ some form of "utilization control," by which use of equipment is reviewed for appropriateness by independent health planning agencies. A common suggestion is that pieces of ultrasophisticated equipment be made available in central locations, and that patients then be brought in from surrounding areas for treatment. This would maintain service and avoid unnecessary purchases by area hospitals.

Unoccupied beds. Until recently, every community — no matter how small the patient supply — wanted a hospital. Some hospital board members and prospective patients in communities still pressure local health planning commissions for prestigious additions and special units, needed or not. In 1977, health planners at the Department of Health, Education and Welfare estimated that there were 100,000 unneeded hospital beds in the U.S. Consequently, they suggested standards that would reduce the number of beds from 4.5 to 4 per 1,000 people.

To stay open under those suggested HEW standards, hospitals would have to run at a recommended 80 to 85 percent occupancy, with the remaining percentage of unoccupied beds allowed for epidemics or seasonal illnesses. Even though those standards are now law, hospitals can no longer get government funds for building, renovating or expanding without a "certificate of need." In meetings with Health Systems Agencies at the local level, hospitals must prove that the community really needs the proposed construction. Only then will the plans be sent for higher government approval.

An occupied bed is an income source; an unoccupied bed is not. By some estimates, an empty bed costs 20 percent as much to maintain as an occupied bed. Expenses such as payroll, which itself accounts for half the cost of running a hospital, remain constant, regardless of daily fluctuations in patient load. Other overhead costs to be met are heat, electricity, maintenance, building financing, fire insurance and so forth. It's been charged that some hospitals admit patients who could be treated as outpatients only in order to generate income, but generally the empty bed count is accepted as an operating cost and is absorbed into charges for caring for inpatients in much the same way a hotel averages all operating costs into its room rates.

Length of stay is another aspect of bed occupancy. The longer you stay, the more profitable it is to take care of you. During the first few days of hospitalization,when a patient is more likely to require intensive care, tests or surgery, more services are required than during the recovery period, when he needs minimal care. To break even, it would be to the hospital's advantage to keep a patient after he's medically ready to go home. That tendency is partly kept in check by review of medical utilization records by PSRO's (Professional Standards Review Organizations) in the area. Also, Medicare and sometimes insurance companies only reimburse up to a certain number of days of hospitalization per procedure.

Some hospitals have maintained cost-effective occupancy by reexamining community needs. In Utah, a hospital has filled excess short-term hospital beds with patients who desperately needed long-term nursing care. In Las Vegas, one hospital is offering lower rates on weekends, when occupancy dips to its lowest point.

How to Get the Most from Health Insurance

Insurance fills a very real need: it lifts a burden from individuals capriciously hit with unexpected medical expenses. It can also provide coverage of some routine medical expenses. For advance payments, called premiums, the insurance carrier will cover whatever medical expenses have been agreed upon in a written contract, your insurance policy. Depending on the arrangement, either the patient, his employer, the doctor or the hospital is reimbursed by the third party carrier when the covered expense is incurred. Coverage is offered either by private carriers (commerical companies or Blue Cross and Blue Shield) or the government (Medicare).

Private insurance carriers. Health insurance is often only one of the services offered by commercial and casualty and life insurance companies. Most don't rely on it for the bulk of their profits; it's only one of several lines of coverage offered, although some commercial companies do offer health insurance exclusively. Aetna, Prudential, John Hancock and Travelers are examples of commercial insurance companies.

Blue Cross and Blue Shield are regarded as the giants of the industry. Established in the 1930s to insure payment of physicians' bills (Blue Shield) and hospital bills (Blue Cross), both have over 70 plans throughout the country, which are affiliated with a single national organization headquartered in Chicago, since the recent merger of the Blue Cross Association and the National Association of Blue Cross Plans. Often marketed as a package, these plans vary from region to region in the premiums they charge and benefits they offer. Occasionally, the 2 compete with each other in the same area for some of the same services.

The Blues often enjoy certain tax benefits because of the special legislation under which they are chartered in many states. Those benefits have, in part, given them the edge in the market. Just under 40 percent of all people with hospital insurance are insured by Blue Cross, which gets discounts on established hospital costs in some places because of its large share of the market.

One reason Blue Cross and Blue Shield are so powerful is that they concentrate solely on health insurance. In addition to several decades of experience, they have traditionally had a chummy relationship with hospitals and doctors. Until 1970, a majority of the board members of Blue Cross plans were physicians and hospital officials. Economists and other critics frequently complain the companies have failed to act to control rising prices and have bowed to hospitals' and physicians' demands for reimbursement.

When employers offer Blue Cross and Blue Shield as part of the employment benefit package, subscribers don't always know what their premiums cost. They are also often shielded from surgery and hospital charges because, unlike most commercial insurers, Blue Cross reimburses the surgeon and hospital directly for services covered when a claim is made.

Medicare and Medicaid. Medicare is a national health insurance program for those over 65 and certain others, such as the disabled.

During your working years, payroll deductions for Medicare are taken from your paycheck as part of the Social Security deduction. Those deductions are matched by your employer and put into a government trust fund, from which you can draw benefits when you reach age 65.

Part A of Medicare automatically provides for hospital expenses, although there is an annual deductible. Part B, which is optional, provides for 80 percent reimbursement of reasonable charges for medical expenses such as lab tests and physician charges. Most people over 65 on Medicare also elect to be covered by Part B, which is paid for by deductions from Social Security checks. For detailed information on Medicare coverage, request the booklet "Your Medicare Handbook" from your local Social Security office or write to the Social Security Administration, Department of Health, Education and Welfare, Baltimore, Maryland 21235.

Medicaid is not insurance, but an assistance program set up to help the aged, blind and disabled. At the option of individual states, through which it is administered, eligibility for Medicaid has been broadened to include those who, because of extraordinary medical expenses at a given time, have become indigent. Some elderly, by virtue of their age and extremely low income, may be eligible for benefits from both Medicare and Medicaid.

Simply because these programs are new and massive, they have suffered growing pains. With their establishment in 1965, a sudden increase in demand for service was created at a time when nothing had been done to increase medical resources in terms of participating physicians and hospitals. There have been problems because the health care system experienced a sudden influx of previously untreated patients which put tremendous pressure on doctors and hospitals. That, in part, caused some of the cost inflation in health care in the late 1960s and early 1970s.

As is true in any national program, there were those who tried to take advantage of the situation and did in fact badly abuse the programs. So-called Medicaid mills, where physicians ran patients through as if on a production line and made a lot of money doing it, got a lot of publicity.

Others managed to give good, legitimate care to large numbers of patients who otherwise had been getting no care at all. Physicians may not have been able to provide the luxury of a 45-minute consultation, but they tried to do what was crucial to meet the patient's basic medical needs. Because Medicare coverage does require some payment on the part of the insured, many elderly also purchase supplementary coverage from the Blues or commercial insurers for uncovered expenses — sometimes called "medigap" insurance.

Understanding Your Insurance Policy

Your policy will discuss exactly what is covered and how much, if anything, you are required to pay before your policy reimburses you or the provider. Because it is a business contract, you should choose a policy wisely to be sure you get the coverage you need, based on what you can afford; then read it carefully to be sure you will not be faced with unexpected out-of-pocket expenses that you cannot possibly pay for. If your company is paying for your policy under a group plan written for all its employees, or if you are eligible for government-provided coverage, it is your responsibility to know where you stand. The following terms and explanations should help.

Basic types of coverage. The 3 basic kinds of medical coverage available are hospital, surgical and medical. Those benefits may be purchased separately or as a package. Roughly, about 90 percent of those who carry hospital carry surgical, and about 80 percent of those with surgical carry medical, which pays for physician services of a nonsurgical nature.

Fee schedules tell you what services are covered and how much the insurer will pay for them. Under Blue Shield, for example, the participating doctor has agreed to accept certain amounts of money as reimbursement for certain covered procedures under certain conditions. If your doctor is a nonparticipating doctor, he has the option of accepting that amount as payment or charging you for the extra. For other commercial insurers, there are no "participating doctors" as such — just a schedule of fees which limits what the insurance company will pay.

Plans that provide for cash payments to the insured (or directly to the provider) for an entire range of services, as long as the charges are "reasonable, usual and customary" for your community, are called "indemnity plans." (Some indemnity plans pay a fixed or "scheduled" amount rather than "reasonable, usual and customary.") Those plans which directly reimburse providers up to specified units of service — x number of days in the hospital, x number of tests — are called "service benefit plans." Blue Cross and Blue Shield, historically, have been primarily oriented toward service benefit plans, but under pressure from commercial competitors, most plans now also offer some indemnity options, at least to group subscribers.

If a surgeon's customary fee for an operation is $450 and the schedule of benefits for that operation covers only $375, a participating doctor will usually consider that lower amount as reasonable and accept it as payment in full; a nonparticipating doctor has the option of charging you the extra $75, but may choose to accept the lower fee as a matter of good will.

One reason for disparities may be fee schedules which fall out of date rapidly. What often happens is that when doctors in a region learn what is considered the "usual and customary fee" for a procedure, the maximum becomes the minimum.

Deductible. The amount you must pay before the insurance company starts picking up the expenses is called the deductible, and usually ranges from $25 to $100. Deductibles can be complicated — separate ones can be applied to different covered expenses. For example, you may have to pay for the first $25 in medical expenses incurred out of the hospital, and again on the first $25 in benefits over a basic hospital-surgical charge. There may be time limits on a deductible, usually 90 to 120 days. That is, within a certain benefit period, that specific amount of expenses, if reached, must be met by you. The insurance then begins to reimburse for any expenses above that amount. At the conclusion of the time period, a new benefit period begins.

Co-insurance is the amount above the deductible that you share with the insurance company up to a maximum, where the company starts paying in full to the limits of the policy. Under a typical co-insurance arrangement, you might have a $25 deductible on any covered expenses incurred. After paying that, you might assume 20 percent of the remaining costs and the insurance company the remaining 80 percent until you hit a maximum of $2,500. The insurance company pays in full for all covered expenses between the $2,500 and the policy's overall dollar limit of, for example, $50,000 in a lifetime.

Major Medical coverage. Besides basic coverage of hospital, surgical and medical expenses, you may carry Major Medical coverage. Characterized by large benefits of up to $250,000 — or no limit — Major Medical may be used as either supplementary coverage to the basic or as a comprehensive coverage, depending on your policy.

Overall maximum dollar limit is the ultimate limit on the amount the insurer will risk. It is calculated on the basis of time, such as the remainder of your lifetime, the length of your illness or a year. Sometimes these factors are combined so that you are allowed a maximum of say, $20,000 per illness and $50,000 in your lifetime. The limit should be reasonably high. Although $50,000 sounds ample to someone who is rarely ill, it can evaporate quickly during the treatment of a serious, chronic disease.

Out-of-pocket expenses could be a surprise unless you know exactly where your coverage stops and what payments could total. Any time an insurance policy calls for co-insurance or a deductible, there is an implication that some out-of-pocket expenses will be faced. Depending on the size of the deductible or the copayment, those costs could potentially be very substantial. The following anecdote, told by a patient being sued by a hospital, illustrates what may happen in the event of serious illness protected by less than unlimited coverage:

> The real problem was the first operation. I had a bypass graft to my main artery for hardening of the arteries. Over a 2-year period, a piece of the plastic from the artificial artery loosened and wrapped its way around my small intestine, eroding it and causing an infection. I worked after the first operation, but it was quite a struggle. I didn't feel a bit good. Then one day I went into shock. I was taken to a hospital for a second operation.
>
> It had taken me 2 years to finish paying off the first operation. My union paid $3,000 and I paid $1,000 to the hospital and $1,000 to the doctor. Then I was feeling so bad

> that I took an early retirement and disability before the second operation.
>
> I had never been sickly before the first operation. I was never told what my fee would be. I was shocked and outraged when the first bill came. And now, I just can't afford to pay this second bill. A man called me from the credit office of the hospital a few months ago and I told him that with the $191 I was getting from Social Security disability payments, I just couldn't pay on it. If I had it, I told him, I'd pay on it. He was real nice and called around to several agencies to see if he could help me. He couldn't, and he said the only thing he could do was to turn it over to the lawyers. It was the first time in my life I wasn't able to pay a bill.
>
> Recently, I received a notice from the sheriff's office that I was being sued by the hospital in court. Now I still can't work — I can't walk because I have such poor circulation in my legs and feet and the hardening of the arteries. Now, I'm getting about $90 a month from the union, too, for disability, and from that money I should be able to start paying about $10 a month on my bill. At that rate, I won't even live long enough to pay it off. I went to Legal Aid and they were good to me, tried to get me to relax, but it's hard to relax with this hanging over me. The lawyers said they wouldn't put me in jail, but they could take my possessions. I don't know what would happen to me then. My things are old — they wouldn't be worth much to anyone — and I don't have much. I live in a small apartment.
>
> I'm not so angry at the hospital as I am at the high prices. You can't afford to get sick anymore. It's cheaper just to die.

In the light of this example, consider your present policy; if the amount that you might have to pay out of pocket is more than you think is safe for you to assume, you might want to change to a policy which calls for lower financial participation on your part and more protection from the insurance company.

Families facing high out-of-pocket medical expenses do have some recourse through tax provisions that permit unreimbursed medical expenses in excess of 3 percent of income to be deducted from income before calculating taxes. That relief only works for those who itemize their tax deductions.

Renewability. A guaranteed renewable policy is not a noncancellable policy. You should be aware of the difference and know what type you carry.

A guaranteed renewable policy does just that — guarantees the renewability, but not the price of the policy. That is, the premiums cannot be adjusted for you alone but they can be adjusted for all policy holders of a given group, or series. As inflation inflicts periodic rate hikes on all policy holders in a series, the healthier members of the group may decide to drop the coverage, thus initiating the possibility of periodic premium increases for the remaining, less healthy, members of the group. The premiums may become prohibitive.

A noncancellable policy guarantees both price and renewability. But it's not as attractive as it sounds. That kind of policy is going to be written with a dollar limit to paying expenses and the guarantee you *don't* get is that the dollar benefit will be enough to pay for treatment, including surgery, at future prices.

Clearly, the guaranteed renewable offers better protection than the noncancellable policy.

Depth and breadth of coverage. Depth of coverage or benefits refers to the dollar amounts that are covered before you have to pay out of your own wallet. Breadth of coverage refers to the range of medical services for which you are insured.

Depth and breadth of coverage vary from one private insurer to the next, including the Blues. People may carry more than one private policy, which overlap or complement each other, or may supplement government coverage through Medicare with "medigap" policies from other insurers.

How Good Is Your Coverage?

It makes sense to evaluate your insurance coverage in light of both your financial situation and health status.

The financial resources of the family, not just the head of the household, help determine what premiums are appropriate to bear. Look at income, assets, savings, pension payments, debts, living expenses and so on. High-income people often deliberately choose a low-premium policy with large co-payments and deductibles because it may be to their advantage to divert money to other investments, and meet a large share of incurred medical expenses on their own, at no great financial hardship. Middle-income families, on the other hand, may prefer to pay a higher premium for coverage of even small or routine medical expenditures, to avoid being hit with unmanageable bills. Low-income people are likely to buy limited coverage simply because they cannot afford the premiums for comprehensive coverage.

The health status of family members and likelihood of any of them running up enormous hospital bills will also influence choice of coverage. Young people with no extraordinary health problems may purposely choose low-premium policies because they are less likely to have large, long-term medical expenses at a time when their income is still limited. Older people are likely to feel that the cost of increasing their coverage is wise in case of a potentially disabling condition in the family.

Group insurance. When Blue Cross or a commercial company insures a group — such as employees of a business — it is able to save administrative and marketing costs and charge lower premiums to group members than to individual subscribers. Benefits provided depend on what the employer has chosen for the group. Since more than 80 percent of people with private coverage are members of group plans, payment of insurance premiums makes the business community the indirect payer of a large part of the national health bill. One medical journal states, "Many observers think that the pressure on health care providers to cut costs and spending may eventually come from business, not from the federal government" (*Postgraduate Medicine,* July, 1979).

Most workers in group health plans are covered for hospital inpatient and outpatient care, surgery, x-rays, post-hospital home health care, medical equipment use, prescription drugs, psychiatric care and family planning. One-third or less are covered for post-hospital skilled nursing care, children's dental care or eyeglasses, and preventive care.

Benefits covered in individual policies, by comparison, fall far below those provided in group policies. Part-time or small-company employees, or those who are retired, self-employed or not covered by a spouse's group policy, find not only that individual coverage is not as broad, but also that the premiums are almost unaffordably high. That's because of the higher costs of selling and administering individual plans, as opposed to group plans where the employer becomes the insurance agent for the company. Insurance companies also worry about what they call "adverse selection" in individual insurance. They say that less healthy people are most strongly motivated to obtain insurance on their own. This problem, they say, doesn't exist with group insurance.

Potential alternatives to individual policies may be possible through membership in fraternal, religious, ethnic, trade or professional associations, such as the American Association of Retired Persons (and its 50–65 division, Action for Independent Maturity), B'nai B'rith, Veterans of Foreign Wars, the National Federation of Business and Professional Women, and some university alumni associations, among many others. Some people join such associations for the sole purpose of the insurance benefits, otherwise unavailable to them. Plans vary from strictly supplemental coverage to more inclusive plans comparable to the comprehensive Major Medical coverage offered by many Blue Cross-Blue shield plans to company employees.

Because more groups are looking into insurance for their members, you may want to investigate such an option before settling on an unnecessarily expensive individual policy. For a complete listing of participating associations and their health insurance benefits, consult your local library for a copy of the booklet, *The Statistics of Fraternal Benefit Societies*, published by the National Fraternal Congress of America, 230 W. Monroe Street, Chicago, Illinois 60606, or write to the NFCA for details on ordering a copy.

If your company is small or cannot afford to offer group insurance on its own, it can often be pooled with others under a Multiple Employer Trust. In this arrangement the participating companies are offered group policies from any one of a number of private insurers as if they were one company. Each of the small companies must have at least 3 employees.

If your present employer or professional or social organization is not presently involved in such an insurance plan, you may want to suggest to your boss, personnel director or an executive officer of your club that he or she contact the following for a list of insurance carriers that administer that type of policy: Professional Independent Mass-Marketing Administrators, 10 S. Riverside Plaza, Suite 644C, Chiago, Illinois 60606. You may even volunteer to investigate such a plan for your group. Rates are competitive with conventional group rates, and considerably lower than individual rates. Benefits, too, may more closely match your needs because of the "likeness" of group members. Teachers, nurses and accountants, for example, may each elect a scope of coverage and co-payment tied to their income brackets, while retired persons may want higher dollar benefits because of their age bracket. The rates for the group are also based on frequency of claims made by its members.

Can Insurance Be Preventive?

Medicine cannot do all that much in the way of prevention. Only people themselves can. And the traditional system of after-the-illness reimbursement of medical expenses does not encourage preventive care.

The preventive steps that have the biggest effect on health — not smoking or abusing alcohol, eating a wise diet and getting enough rest and exercise — are matters which are strictly under the control of the individual. The same people who continue to overindulge, also, as health care consumers, want to magically decrease their days in the hospital, their visits to the doctor and their insurance premiums.

Aside from such obvious things as hygiene and immunization, not much of medicine itself can be termed "preventive." It's more a matter of what you practice than what your doctor can do for you. An EKG is a good example of what people consider to be preventive medicine. It gives certain information about your heart and may lead to helpful recommendations about activity, exercise, weight control and so on. But having an EKG doesn't prevent heart disease. It may help monitor your condition and therefore help *you* to prevent it. By the same token, you may go in for an annual physical, have your blood pressure checked, your lungs x-rayed, and then be told you're in good shape. What does that prevent?

What preventive medicine does, as it is held forth, is to try to contain problems before they reach the crisis stage — at which point they are more costly.

A doctor can tell you to exercise, quit smoking, eat less junk food and relax, but you have the option of following or rejecting that advice. *In terms of insurance, then, why not charge lower premiums for people who indeed practice preventive health care?*

The problem is documentation. A national carrier like Prudential cannot monitor whether or not a customer smokes or exercises or has poor health habits simply by asking and taking his word for it. A small number of "preferred risk" insurance companies are able to offer slightly lower rates to select groups of people in small areas, but for the most part those companies that have tried it have had limited success.

Health Maintenance Organizations (HMOs). HMO plans are the closest thing to preventive medicine. HMOs offer a less traditional form of prepaid health care delivery, which places the incentive on using certain desirable medical services. Regular checkups, for example, are considered preventive medicine and not particularly expensive, but are usually paid for by the consumer rather than by his insurance company. Under customary insurance plans, the services for which the insured is required to pay out-of-pocket because of deductible clauses, are those very services which may help to prevent problems from reaching the crisis stage, thereby requiring more treatment and costing more money.

Under an HMO plan, the subscriber is charged an annual sum, normally paid in monthly installments or weekly payroll deductions, just as conventional insurance premiums are paid. In return, the subscriber (also called a member) is entitled to unlimited amounts of specific physician and hospital services at very little or no charge. That aspect, too, is somewhat similar to the schedule of benefits under traditional insurance. One big difference is that regardless of how often you are sick or how much treatment is needed during the year, the covered service will be provided. Benefit packages are naturally more expensive than Blue Cross, for instance.

Another feature which makes many HMO plans different from the traditional fee-for-service system is that the participating physicians, contracted to treat members of the HMO, are usually paid a fixed salary by the insurer. Essentially, that means the doctor is going to get paid whether he sees you once or 50 times during the year — a marked contrast to fee-for-service, under which you go to any doctor you choose, who charges you each time he sees you.

The financial incentive for the customer is to stick with non-surgical management, even if it means repeated trips to the doctor's office, because the services are prepaid. Evidence shows that HMOs have, in fact, decreased hospitalization of their members, both in terms of fewer admissions and shorter lengths of stay, compared to the fee-for-services practices ("Staff Report on the Health Maintenance Organization and Its Effects on Competition," Federal Trade Commission, July, 1977). In that way, HMOs have real potential for reducing the aggregate cost of health care.

HMOs have met with both praise and skepticism. When the concept was introduced 40 years ago, it was thought the American public would find it overwhelmingly attractive. Acceptance of prepaid health plans, however, has been slow because of both real and anticipated problems.

By definition, an HMO is geographically limited, while the population is very mobile. Because one of the main attractions of the HMO is the reputedly high quality of care by preselected doctors contracted to serve you in your area, that very care to which you are entitled is only available in one location. Originally, HMOs provided coverage only at the home facility, and people were uncomfortable about the question of coverage while on vacation or business trips. Most HMOs today have some provision for out-of-the-area coverage, which is customarily handled on an indemnity basis; that is, your area plan will reimburse you up to a certain amount of money for treatment provided by an outside doctor.

The prospect of being seen by a different doctor at each visit also has turned people off to the HMO. While perhaps true at one time, that practice is disappearing. The modern plan will have you designate one doctor in the practice as your regular doctor, whom you see by appointment. Only if he is on vacation or you have an emergency will you have to be seen by one of his partners. So the criticism of having to see various doctors is no more valid for HMOs than it is for conventional group or solo practices.

The real, underlying problem is that people don't want to break away from the doctor they've been seeing all along. Despite all the criticism of the American health care system, it's still true that people like to see their own, freely chosen doctor. That's the system we were weaned on and seem to prefer. If he joins an HMO, fine. Otherwise, people tend to stick with the doctor they've got.

The most likely candidates for HMO enrollment, in fact, are people who either because they are new to an area or have no real health problems, have no regular family doctor. A classic example would be a couple who has just moved into town and whose children are grown. Perhaps the woman has been going to a gynecologist (GYN) for regular check-ups and her husband has had intermittent minor back problems, but there has been no illness serious enough to require regular medical attention. One day, one of them is rushed to the emergency room for some reason. When asked, "Who is your family doctor?" they go blank. There is no family doctor. Where do they start? That sort of couple is likely to be attracted to the HMO as an appropriate way to meet their medical needs.

One misconception of the HMO practice that has somewhat hindered its growth is fear of long waiting lines in doctors' offices. While in the early days HMOs tended to be run on a production line basis, modern HMOs are no different from the group medical practices you are probably used to. You make an appointment, and the doctor tries to keep to his schedule. Sometimes it works; sometimes you wait. Jammed waiting rooms are no more, no less of a problem in prepaid plans.

Prepaid plans do cost more initially. The premiums are slightly higher than for conventional insurance, because the coverage is more comprehensive, including a larger number of routine procedures such as annual physicals, well-baby care, eye examinations and so on. If your company has been paying the premiums for you under your present plan and the HMO premiums are higher, you must pay the difference if you change. The long-run costs, in light of the broad benefits, may be lower, and the risk of heavy, out-of-pocket costs appears to be smaller than under most conventional plans.

Initially, physicians were vehemently opposed to prepaid plans. Now, reactions are mixed. Many doctors, as a matter of style, cherish the independence offered by the traditional fee-for-service practice. More significantly, some argue that without the financial incentive to see patients for follow-up visits, some doctors will undertreat.

"That potential does exist and warrants concern," says Charles P. Hall, Jr., Ph.D., formerly with the American Medical Association's Department of Economics. "While most of our concern is with overtreatment, especially in terms of costs, the greatest health problems in this country are probably among those who are undertreated rather than overtreated. But there is not, to my knowledge, any clear evidence that HMOs have been guilty of undertreatment."

From the doctor's point of view, the income potential in prepaid group plans is not as high as in fee-for-service practices, although the range is fairly competitive. HMOs compete on appealing nondollar items. Fringe benefits as part of the income offered HMO physicians are likely to include life insurance, a pension, full medical insurance coverage, regular paid vacations, and time off for postgraduate training. Many doctors enjoy the regular hours, opportunities for consultation, and less concern about patient coverage when they themselves are sick or out of town. Much of it is a matter of the personality and work preferences of the individual doctor.

Doctors have voluntarily formed Individual Practice Associations (IPAs) in some areas in direct response to group HMOs. The IPA is an alternate form of HMO which shares characteristics of both prepaid group plans and conventional health insurance arrangements. Subscribers pay the same advance fees in return for the same types of services, but the participating doctors operate independently rather than at a doctor-owned facility, and may serve nonsubscribers as well as HMO subscribers. In that way, the solo fee-for-service practitioner maintains the traditional doctor-patient relationship but agrees to accept the somewhat lower fees set by prepaid plans as payment in full, sacrificing some income for assurance of payment and retaining clients. Like group plans, IPAs seem to lower the rate of unnecessary medical treatment. Less than 4 percent of the insured population of the U.S. is enrolled in HMOs, according to a recent HEW census. They are not as common in rural areas and small towns as in more populated areas. One of the largest and best known is the Kaiser Plan in California, which equals the Blue Cross plans there in enrollment.

Under the Health Maintenance Organization Act of 1973, if there is a federally qualified HMO in your area, and your employer has 25 or more full-time employees, he must offer you the option of HMO membership in addition to whatever other insurance company plan is offered. Medicare and Medicaid recipients can be included in an HMO. With that formal encouragement of federal legislation and consumers' growing awareness of HMO options, it is expected that the number of people joining HMOs is likely to increase substantially in the future.

The mere presence of an HMO in certain areas has reduced medical care costs in entire communities by creating competition, reports the Federal Trade Commission. Competition may take the form of creation of additional HMOs, increased benefit packages in other area plans and stronger efforts to control costs, primarily by cuts in unnecessary hospitalization and shorter lengths of stay. In some areas, Blue Cross plans have reduced hospitalization in response to HMO presence. The trend is for conventional plans, such as Blue Cross, to match many of the popular services offered by prepaid plans by broadening their coverage.

Sponsorship of HMOs varies from hospitals and universities to Blue Cross and commercial carriers. The latter 2 are actively looking into the HMO for several reasons; for them, it may be a matter of survival. Prepaid plans seem to be the direction the industry is taking, and they want to be in on it. In any competitive market such as insurance, it makes good corporate sense to invest dollars and expertise in a style of health care delivery that holds promises of success and profit. As they see the federal government boosting the HMO concept and the political push for national health insurance, carriers are alert to what they see as a major trend.

What You Can Do to Keep Costs in Check

The following are just some of the attitudes, questions, rights and facts that can help you keep a lid on health care costs.

- If you have the attitude that "somebody else" is paying for your care, reconsider. You're paying in the form of higher premiums and prices, if not through outright payments.
- Check your insurance company's rating in the library in the book, *Best's Insurance Reports — Life/Health.*

- Force yourself to read your policy very carefully both when you buy it and when you visit a doctor or hospital.
- Read any insurance forms you are asked to sign.
- Get interim insurance coverage for yourself if you lose your job or are between jobs. Many group plans provide coverage for 30 days or more during lay-off periods.
- Know at what age coverage for your children ends. Some benefits end whenever your son or daughter marries. Others provide coverage up until a certain age as long as they are full-time students.
- Ask your local health department if there is an HMO in your area. Consider joining it if there is.
- If your doctor does not participate in an insurance plan you would like to join, ask him to.
- Ask the doctor or his nurse if he has agreed to accept what your insurance company will pay before you visit him.
- Since insurance companies generally reimburse only for charges that are "reasonable and customary" for the area, find out from the company or a doctor not involved in the case what a reasonable charge would be for the procedure you are about to undergo.
- Ask the physician or his nurse if routine tests (such as a Pap smear in a gynecological examination) will be included in the price of the visit.
- You have the right to refuse treatment you cannot afford and to learn costs, risks and benefits of alternative treatment.
- Find out what outpatient benefits you have before agreeing to be hospitalized for any procedure that could be done in a doctor's office, clinic or outpatient facility.
- If elective surgery is recommended to you, get a second consultation. Find out if your insurance company will cover it and what the charge for the consultation will be.
- If you agree to surgery, ask the surgeon what his fee will be for the operation and what it will include. If he says it is difficult to tell until he starts operating, try to at least get a range.
- Ask the surgeon if preoperative and postoperative visits are included in his fee.

• Ask the surgeon if he will use an assistant at the operation. (If he uses a resident as an assistant, there will probably be no charge. If he uses someone from outside the hospital, there probably will be.)

• If your usual doctor (not the surgeon) will be visiting you in the hospital, ask what he will charge.

• Ask the surgeon if he knows of any aspect of the operation your insurance won't cover. He may tell you, for example, that most local radiologists won't accept what local insurance companies pay for preoperative and postoperative x-rays.

• Ask the doctor when you can go home so you won't remain in the hospital bed an extra day just because someone has neglected to tell you when you can leave.

• Ask what the room rate includes before or when you are admitted. Most likely it includes only room and board — occupancy of a bed and your meals. Laundry could be a separate charge.

• If you are insured, bring your insurance card to the hospital when you are admitted. If you are not, ask the admitting clerk in advance how much cash you should plan to bring or if a check will be accepted.

• Ask if you can keep whatever personal supplies have been charged to you and issued in your name — for instance, rubber rings or sheepskins to prevent bedsores. You can probably reuse them at home.

• If the doctor has ordered medication for you — say, sleeping pills or pain pills — that you don't wish to take, tell the medications nurse that you do not expect to be charged for them. Tell the doctor you don't think you need them the next time he visits.

• If you are given items such as cotton balls or ointments upon discharge, refuse them and ask that your bill be credited for them. You can probably buy the same quality supplies elsewhere in a store for much less money.

• Shop drugstores for lowest prices when you get a prescription after surgery.

- You have a right to privacy about your means of payment, and you have a right to leave a facility without paying your bill.
- Ask to be billed, and tell the billing department you want an itemized bill even if your insurance is picking up the tab. Ask for specifics. For example, if the bill lists $150 in lab charges, ask for a breakdown charge for each test. Try to recall tests you were given (or better yet record them in the hospital) and ask about items you don't remember. Errors do occur.
- Do not go to the emergency room if you do not have an emergency. Chances are your insurance won't pay for it.
- Write the hospital a letter of complaint if you think your bill is unfair, even if your insurance policy has paid it.

Part II

Common Operations – And Your Alternatives

11
Gallbladder Disease

When movie director Tony Richardson set out to find a follow-up for his great success in "Tom Jones," he naturally chose another novel by the nineteenth-century British writer, Henry Fielding. He chose *Joseph Andrews,* and it became one of the best films to do no business in 1978. Why begin a chapter on gallbladder troubles with movies and Henry Fielding? Because soon after shooting began, Richardson was faced with killing off one of his major characters, an old glutton named Lord Booby, and doing it with a disease that was both common and lethal in eighteenth-century England. Because Fielding was a writer who delighted in separating right from wrong, Richardson had to dump Booby with a moral flourish; he had to finish the rich meal of the old boy's life with his just desserts, so to speak. The director chose gout, the disease of high living, broad eating and deep drinking, and he had Booby drown while taking the medicinal waters at Bath for his affliction. Booby slips under the waves when his foot — grown light from rot — and his stomach — grown heavy with food — cause him to bottom-up in a most undignified way.

The reason all this appears in a chapter on gallbladder is that gallstones are the gout of our day. If Richardson wanted to update Fielding's Lord Booby, he'd have to do little more than change his disease (and his clothes). The rich, fatty foods and lazy life-style that gave the Lord pains in his big toe in 1742 would just as surely give him gallstones and pain in his big gut in 1980. The connection between gallstones and gout may have been clear even to eighteenth-century physicians, because one of them, Walter Pope, wrote this gentle sentiment, "May I govern my passion with an absolute sway,/And grow wiser and better, as my strength wears away,/Without gout or stone, by a gentle decay." What's more, a "cure" for gallstones and gout was as available to Dr. Pope as it is to us. Both diseases are among the "advances" of civilization, gout coming at the beginning of the modern age and gallstones bringing up what some would call its rear. The solution to both disasters is a return to "uncivilized" ways in diet and work and the foreswearing of the rich, overrefined foods and sedentary habits we tend to call "progress."

Regular exercise and a diet low in fat and high in fiber could have saved Lord Booby, for, as a Spanish proverb of his time had it, "Gout is cured by walling up the mouth." And the same things would probably cure a modern man's gallbladder disease too. Whether they could have spared his fashionable wife, the chic Lady Booby, is another matter. Modern women are more prone to gallbladder disease than are men, and prevention of the disease among women may not be so simple. The hormones released during pregnancy seem to predispose some women to gallstones. Still, a proper diet would soften the blows of the disease, and the avoidance of any unnecessary additions to natural hormone levels — such as oral contraceptives or estrogen therapy during menopause — can be a great help. Because there is this happy news, this chapter, perhaps more than any other, will concentrate on preventative measures and nonsurgical therapies.

The Detergent Dispenser for Greasy Food

Your normal, healthy gallbladder is 3 to 4 inches long and 1½ inches wide at its broadest point. For some reason, this tiny organ — which hangs just under the liver beneath the arch of the ribs on the right side of the body — is hard to relate to. People compare it to fruits and vegetables when they talk about it. Some liken it to a pear, some to a cucumber and one semipoetic doctor we consulted talked about the "greenish teardrop hanging from the bottom of the liver."[2] One might gather from all this that the gallbladder is always green and wider at one end than at the other. Actually, it looks like a cucumber when empty and like a pear when full. The gallbladder empties and fills, because its job is to receive, store and concentrate bile produced by the liver, its upstairs neighbor, and then release that bile into the duodenum or first section of the intestine when there's food to be digested. Not just any food — fatty foods only. It ignores carbohydrates and most vegetable proteins as it only breaks down fats and oils. At any one time the gallbladder usually holds about 4 tablespoons of liver bile (maybe 2 ounces), whose strength it has increased perhaps 10 times. Over the course of a day, it processes more than a pint of bile. In an emergency — brought on by a pepperoni pizza or an obstruction in the pipes that conduct bile to the intestine — it can swell up to hold nearly 2 quarts.

The gallbladder is connected to the liver, its supplier — and the duodenum, its consumer, by a series of ducts (or tubes) and valves. The hepatic duct carries bile from the liver to the gallbladder, and the cystic duct carries processed bile away from the gallbladder and down to the intestine. It's important to mention these tiny parts of the human plumbing system, because they can both cause trouble and help clear it up. Gallstones — we'll get to them in a bit — can get caught in the ducts and raise the Cain that leads to a surgical removal of the gallbladder. The intricate piping of these ducts also makes gallbladder surgery far more difficult and dangerous than removal of the appendix, another nearby resident of the right side of the abdomen. But, as a compensation, a branch of the hepatic duct bypasses the gallbladder and goes directly to a junction with the cystic duct to form the common bile duct. When the gallbladder and cystic duct are removed, this freeway allows bile to flow into the intestine permitting digestion to continue even after surgery.

When a greasy meal enters the intestine, it triggers the release of a hormone which causes the valve at the end of the common duct to open. When that occurs, the gallbladder contracts and sprays its concentrated bile on the food to be broken down. The bile contains detergents just like Dash. You've seen those pants with — miraculously — just one oily knee? The oil that begins to float away the minute it's dipped in the soap? Well, in much the same way the liver bile stored in the gallbladder attacks the fats we eat and forces them to dissolve in water — a process that extracts what nutritional value they have while washing away much of the cholesterol (that heart attack bugaboo) they contain.

Another interesting — if confusing — fact about the gallbladder is that we seem not to need it. People who have had theirs removed, as we mentioned before, get along very well without them, sometimes even eating and enjoying the fatty foods that gallbladders alone are supposed to help digest. Liver bile flows directly into the intestine in these surgically streamlined folks, and they can smile even after an occasional chili dog. In some animals with digestive systems very much like our own — the deer, for instance — the process of evolution has done away with the gallbladder entirely.

Which brings us to the confusing part of this business. The deer, of course, eats very little fatty food and so can easily dispense with his detergent-maker. Man, on the other hand, invented the french fry and would seem to need his, but most surgeons and all their successful gallbladder patients claim not. Why? As we said, gallbladder disease is the gout of our day. Most authorities agree that as man began to eat more, to eat richer foods, to grow fatter and to do less hard work, he began to have more and more trouble with his gallbladder. Frank Glenn, M.D., of New York Hospital and Cornell University Medical School, calls gallstones — the source of most gallbladder trouble — a "disease of overabundance." Demetrius Pertsemlidis, M.D., of the Mount Sinai School of Medicine, another leading researcher in the field, adds that studies in Japan have shown that the incidence of cholesterol gallstones has gone up tremendously since World War II, since the Japanese exchanged their ancient low-fat, vegetable-protein diets for modern food. When Mr. Donut came to the Land of the Rising Sun, he brought gallstones with him. Such troubles are also common in American Indians who have adopted the white man's ways, but rare among black Africans who have, in part, held on to their traditions. The Pima Indians of the American Southwest are chronic sufferers of gallbladder disease. The Masai tribe of East Africa, however, is not, though its members eat a diet — very high in fats and animal proteins — which is disastrous by gallbladder standards. The Masai stay lean and fit, it seems, because they cling to their traditional life of hard, physical labor. So, if gallstones follow civilization, and civilization brings greasy foods and lazy ways; if — to back up — the gallbladder's function is to handle these oily modern foods, how is it that man can do without a gallbladder? We don't think he can, and this chapter will outline the proper care and feeding that can help you keep yours. Man cannot hope for the gallbladder of an ox — which forms gallstones each winter and dissolves them each summer. He has to live with what Nature has given him; it's our advice that he take the best care of it he can.

Both the good and the bad news about the gallbladder are in the nature of the liver bile it processes. The bile itself is a thick fluid which may be yellow or orange in color. It is not green except in colloquial expressions and King Arthur stories. The fluid is mostly water, and of the 3 percent that is not, the most important ingredients are pigments from the liver (which give it its characteristic color), cholesterol (a waxy, crystalline substance), an oily compound called lecithin and various mineral compounds and acids, usually lumped together as either "bile acids" or "bile salts" for convenience. They'll be called "bile acids" here. The cholesterol is a fatlike substance, and the active ingredients of bile are fat emulsifiers or "detergents." They break down "the polar resistance of oil and water," which means that they mediate the unfriendliness between oil and water and thus allow the oily cholesterol to mix with the water in the bile, pass into the intestine, and be excreted. In simpler terms, they break large fat globules into smaller ones that can be worked on further by the fat-splitting enzymes of the bowel and pancreas.

Despite its nasty role in heart disease, cholesterol is necessary in humans. It's an ingredient of some important hormones, of cell membranes, and it is the raw material from which bile acids are produced. The trouble with cholesterol is that we don't have to eat any to satisfy our needs. We can make all we need right in our bodies. The cholesterol in the liver bile in the gallbladder is what's left *after* the liver has turned the body's domestic supply into bile acids. Under normal circumstances, some of this will be used in other important ways, and the residue will be flushed away with the waste products of digestion. But if there's no dietary *need* for cholesterol, there is apparently a dietary *taste* for the things that contain it. We like butter and eggs and sausage, and unfortunately, we like them together. The body, that faithful servant, tries to compensate for this peculiarity of the mind or taste buds by regulating its own production of cholesterol according to the amount eaten. The more sausage and eggs we eat, the less cholesterol we make. Give half a chance, our bodies will maintain this balance very carefully. However, once we get hooked on fatty foods, we stuff more cholesterol into our systems than they can handle. So much that it can't all be turned into bile acids or hormones or cell membranes or even excreted as waste. As a result, cholesterol piles up in the liver and gallbladder.

Bile acids, to get back to the good news, are the major fat-emulsifiers of the body. We maintain a fairly constant pool of them at all times. This pool circulates through the digestive system as food is processed while we eat — twice at each sitting, in fact. As acids are lost during the process, more are produced by the liver, thus more cholesterol is used up. Anything that permanently decreases the size of this bile acid pool — like an illness of the lower bowel which prevents it from being recycled — can cause gallbladder trouble.

The third major constituent of liver bile is lecithin, another fat-eating "detergent." It is not known exactly how important to human digestion lecithin is, but dogs have bile that is rich in lecithin and they have very few cholesterol-induced heart attacks and almost no gallstones.

Gallbladder disease and gallstones are problems of the liver bile, but the "dirty" conditions in the bile which lead to them are merely symptoms of things more generally wrong with the patient. Too much cholesterol in the bile means too much cholesterol every place; it's just that things often go wrong in the gallbladder first. There is an optimum balance between cholesterol, bile acids and lecithin in the bile, and that balance allows the 2 emulsifiers to hold cholesterol fat in solution until it can be whisked down the intestinal drain. Again, it works just the way detergent works in your washer. Cholesterol is like the "greasy dirt" in your kid's dungarees. Bile acids are like the detergent in the soap. And lecithin is like the water softener that most laundry products contain (to neutralize water minerals which block the action of detergents). If you have the right amount of detergent and the proper measure of water softener, the dirt your child grinds into his jeans doesn't stand a chance. If liver bile contains 3 cups bile acid and 1/4 cup lecithin to each 3/4 cup cholesterol, everything's fine. But when more cholesterol is added to the bile, or more dirt to the jeans, things start to go wrong, and the "grimy oil" doesn't come out in the wash. People with gallbladder disease — especially those with gallstones — have so much cholesterol in their systems, hence also in their liver bile, that these ideal proportions are knocked for a loop. Proportionately, the size of their bile acid pool, their measure of fat-splitting "detergent" is cut in half, and their bodies can't get rid of the excess fat, which clumps together to form gallstones. And they are capable of causing all kinds of trouble.

An Inside Look at a Gallstone Attack

Since it's been estimated that 15 million Americans have gallbladder troubles; since 800,000 unfortunates join their ranks every year; since 500,000 of them are hospitalized for their complaints with each yearly turn of the calendar; since most of these folks lose their gallbladders in the process; and since at least 90 percent of all these painful episodes involve gallstones, perhaps we'd better remain on the subject of gallstones a little longer. Folks *do* lose their gallbladders for other reasons, and we will talk about them too, but gallstones are the major problem. How major — as if the numbers above weren't enough of an indication — is easily stated. If each of the 500,000 hospitalized sufferers spends $2,000 on his stretch in the sheets and loses $1,000 in income while he's laid up, gallstones rob nearly $2 billion a year from our wallets. *That* major!

Gallbladders get pesky for a number of reasons. They can simply break down and fail to empty their bile when called upon to do so by the intestine. No one knows why this occurs, but such a mechanical malfunction causes the gallbladder to swell up with bile that cannot escape and to become infected from the pressure or actually to rupture. Gallbladders can become infected with bacteria from other illnesses in the body and cease to operate for that reason. In many cases these infections are not serious, but they do leave cellular debris in the organ, and cholesterol globules can cluster around these bits and pieces to form gallstones that *are* serious. "Gallstones," as one waggish authority puts it, "are the tombstones of infection." But the most common source of gallstones and the most frequent destroyer of gallbladders is a chemical one. When the liver bile stored in this sac becomes supersaturated with cholesterol; when the load exceeds the ability of the bile acids and lecithin to hold it in equilibrium, crystals of the waxy substance begin to precipitate out of the solution in the same way that clumps of dirt, oil and soap form in a washer when the water's too cold or too hard to dissolve them. These crystals, being sticky, bunch together to form larger bodies; they pick up cells shed by the gallbladder's lining, liver pigments from the bile itself and minute amounts of calcium, and finally grow like snowballs into large, round stones.

Some people think these often large, sometimes small, round stones are beautiful. Some make jewelry out of the gallstones they have had removed. We even came across a report of a stolen gallstone necklace. Most folks, however, have trouble relating to their gallstones in the same way they have trouble relating to their gallbladders. They compare them to fruits and vegetables. A gallbladder may contain a single stone, which might be the size of a plum or a hen's egg. It may contain several stones, which might resemble grapes or lima beans in size. Or it may be loaded with nearly a hundred stones, all the size of corn kernels or even millet seeds. In any event, there is *no* correlation between the size and number of stones and the amount of trouble they can cause. Like Moby Dick, gallstones are no one color. They are mottled with the shiny white of cholesterol, the flat white of calcium, the red of liver pigments and the yellow of body fat. Most of the stones found in American and Western European gallbladders are predominantly the glossy white of cholesterol, their chief component. Just under half of Japanese stones, on the other hand, are the dull white of calcium — the oriental diet contains a smaller percentage of animal fat and protein. None of these color combinations seems to put the stones in the semiprecious category.

How do these nasty little baubles actually raise Cain? Several ways. A gallbladder filled with many tiny stones can be sent into painful spasm and malfunction when the pressure created by the stones increases its size and thins out its walls. If one of the stones happens to be sharp edged and the pressure of the whole bunch is extreme, the gallbladder may be punctured and spill its caustic bile all over the patient's insides — causing intense burning pain and spreading infection. Both of these disasters are one-time and fairly rare affairs. More common are situations in which stones move out of the gallbladder and get temporarily or permanently lodged in the plumbing that leads away from it, the cystic and the common bile ducts. When a stone is temporarily stuck, most often in the cystic duct, the gallbladder swells with trapped bile, and digestion, suddenly stopped, turns into serious indigestion. Since they are floating freely in a thick liquid, stones get stuck and unstuck without warning or any real regularity as bile flows in and out of the gallbladder. The attacks caused by that start-and-stop, in-and-out process are called onslaughts of *chronic* gallbladder disease, because they occur repeatedly, end suddenly, and can't be controlled or predicted.

When a medium-sized stone moves out of the gallbladder with the tides of bile and gets *permanently* jammed in one of the ducts — usually the common duct that connects to the intestine — a complication of chronic gallbladder disease results called *acute* gallbladder disease. A medium-sized stone is most often involved, because large ones can't leave the gallbladder and small ones frequently pass unimpeded through to the duodenum. In an acute attack, the gallbladder and the entire duct system fill with bile which then begins to back up to the liver, its source. When that happens, liver pigments and other bile ingredients that normally escape through the gallbladder are forced into the bloodstream causing jaundice and its characteristic yellow staining of the body's soft tissues, the eyes and the skin of the face, neck and upper trunk. The huge pool of bile (as much as 64 ounces) dammed up by this unmoving obstruction causes the gallbladder to swell tremendously. The swelling causes inflammation of the walls and can cut off the organ's blood supply. When that happens, infection sets in, pus collects and the swelling grows. Then the worst may happen. The gallbladder ruptures, and its infection spreads throughout the body cavity. Needless to say, an acute gallbladder attack is a one-time-only complication of a chronic problem. Most acute attacks lead directly to surgery.

Who Gets Gallbladder Disease?

An awful lot of people have trouble with their gallbladders. More of them are women than men. But all of them get gallbladder disease for very specific reasons. Published estimates say that 10 percent of American men and 20 percent of American women between the ages of 55 and 60 have gallstones this very minute. These same figures, based on autopsy reports, claim that one-quarter of the women and one-tenth of the men of any age in this country will develop gallstones some time before they're 60. And a British study found that gallbladder victims are becoming younger and younger every year — at least in Canada. Scott Grundy, M.D., Ph.D., chief of the metabolic section at the Veterans Administration Medical Center in La Jolla, California, told us that conditions (such as obesity) which raise cholesterol production in the body or lower its bile acid pool, increase the risk of gallstone formation and gallbladder disease, but we were able to pin it down a bit more specifically. It used to be said that gallbladder patients were "fair, fat and forty," and while obesity and age remain the primary villains, there are some other evil-doers. Certain diseases can be implicated. Blacks are not prone to gallbladder disease, but it has been loosely tied to sickle cell anemia, an illness fairly common among blacks. Diabetes has also been identified as a simultaneous problem. Any malfunction or injury to the lower bowel can encourage gallbladder trouble by preventing the free circulation of bile acid "detergents." Eldon A. Shaffer, M.D., of the University of Calgary in Alberta, Canada, told us of one more cause — he says that gallstones in the slim and healthy may be the result of an inherited metabolic deficiency, an inability to manufacture enough bile acids or a failure to recirculate them properly. That may be one reason why American Indians have such troubles with the disease.

Women more frequently have gallstones than men probably because they bear children and produce the hormone estrogen. Of the women who suffer from gallstones, 3 out of 4 have been pregnant at some time in their lives. During pregnancy, a woman's body produces more cholesterol and her gallbladder empties more slowly, allowing that cholesterol to stand and crystals to form. The muscular gallbladder empties more slowly during pregnancy, because all smooth muscles in the body lose tone then, due to a rise in estrogen levels. The gallstones that form in the mother before a child is born are usually small and "silent"; that is, they cause no symptoms. But as the years go by and the woman puts on weight (or fails to lose the weight she gained during pregnancy), they grow in size and meddlesomeness. Dr. Frank Glenn, perhaps the dean of U.S. gallbladder specialists, says this syndrome is one reason to avoid gaining excess weight while carrying a child. Why, he asks, add to a situation that is already dangerous?

Many doctors have recently noticed a greater number of slim, childless women among their gallbladder patients. A group of physicians in New England conducted a survey of 24 Boston-area hospitals to find out why. They discovered that a woman's gallbladder becomes saturated with cholesterol during the normal menstrual cycle and that this saturation reaches dangerous levels when she is taking any kind of estrogen therapy — either an oral contraceptive or hormone supplements before menopause (*New England Journal of Medicine,* January 3, 1974). That saturation, of course, invites the formation of gallstones. In a parallel study at

New York's Mount Sinai Hospital, it was discovered that women who use birth control pills are 2 times more likely to develop gallstones than those who do not, and that women who take estrogen for menopausal symptoms are 2½ times more susceptible to them than those who deal with menopause without drugs. The role of estrogen and estrogen therapy in gallbladder disease accounts for the greater number of female victims. It probably also accounts for the decrease in the age of victims. Gallstone sufferers have become younger as the Pill has grown more popular.

It was discovered by the nationwide Coronary Drug Project Research Group that men with heart conditions taking the drug clofibrate (or Atromid S) to reduce their blood cholesterol levels had 54 percent more gallbladder trouble due to gallstones than men not taking the compound (*New England Journal of Medicine,* May 26, 1977). The irony of a cholesterol-reducer inciting cholesterol gallstones in its faithful was not properly appreciated in the medical community.

Unfortunately, all these identifiable, avoidable contributors to gallstone formation are mere fooling around compared to its major cause — fatness. Study after study has shown that fat people load their liver bile with far more cholesterol than do thin people. Even after the removal of a stone-loaded gallbladder and the resulting increase in bile acid production, a tubby patient's level of cholesterol will remain higher than his "detergents" can manage, because his fat-factory continues at full-steam. In the famous heart study of 5,000 people in Framingham, Massachusetts, it was learned that folks who weighed at least 20 percent more than the median average poundage for their height, frame and sex were *twice* as likely to get gallstones as were their normal neighbors. The Pima Indians of Phoenix, Arizona, are nearly all overweight, and they have become famous in gallbladder annals, because almost 70 percent of the tribe develops gallstones. A survey of deaths due to gallbladder complications in a Los Angeles VA hospital revealed that just about half of the dead were 20 or more pounds overweight. A person who weighs 300 pounds will produce *twice* as much cholesterol as a person who weighs 150 pounds. What's more, the National Institute of Arthritis, Metabolism, and Digestive Diseases says that this imbalance gets even crazier during the periods of weight fluctuation that chronic dieters undergo. The moral for everybody, according to the Institute, is: Get Thin, Stay Thin and Avoid Gallstones. But beware: the upper bowel bypass operation that's being touted as a way for many terminal tubbies to lose weight is *no* help. As Dr. Pertsemlidis of Mount Sinai tells it, the operation *may* help you lose weight, but it will probably also mess up the system that recycles the body's bile acids and therefore actually encourages the formation of gallstones.

Early and Advanced Symptoms of Gallbladder Disease

The symptoms of gallbladder disease may be categorized in a number of ways, the simplest of which is: early, late and awful. These somewhat unclear categories may be clarified a bit if we associate them with the kind of gallbladder trouble they represent. The early signs usually mean the growth of stones in the gallbladder, and they indicate that the nagging stomach distress of chronic gallbladder disease has come to stay. The early stage becomes the later stage when the signs show up more often, and that means the stones have grown larger and more numerous. The truly awful symptoms mean — invariably — that one of the stones has gotten stuck someplace (usually the cystic duct) and may never leave. If it doesn't, the patient suffers an acute attack. This symptom normally precipitates a medical, if not a surgical, emergency.

It used to be said that the first signs of gallbladder trouble were indigestion, heartburn and a too-full feeling brought on by greasy foods and certain gas-producing raw vegetables like cabbage and cauliflower. Lately, however, that conventional wisdom is being sharply questioned. Too many people with bum gallbladders simply never experience such discomforts. These things are signs of overeating, the labor pains of a fat person coming into being, and since fat people also tend to be people with gallbladder problems, perhaps the symptoms may be regarded as indirect and prehistoric signs of some gallbladder agony to come. A complaint that generally *can* be associated with gallbladder disease is a dull ache after a big or oily meal, an ache that begins just below the ribs on the right side of the abdomen and spreads to the chest and back. In severe attacks, the pain may seem to torment the whole upper body. This pain is caused by some obstruction in the plumbing that leads from the gallbladder. Perhaps a stone is pushed from the organ when it contracts to do battle with a bowl of chili and lodges somewhere, again, usually in the cystic duct. As we said before, once the obstruction occurs, the normal functioning of the gallbladder causes pressure to build up behind the block, and the pressure causes pain. The pain subsides when the food moves on through the intestine and no longer stimulates the gallbladder to dispatch its contents. If the patient is lucky, that letup in demand allows the stone to fall back into the gallbladder, and he is safe until his next taco. If he's not, and the stone is a monster, it will take up residence, and the pressure will continue to grow — his attack will become acute and his situation dire. The pain associated with the worst of gallbladder attacks is called "biliary colic," because it turns grown men into babies. It is an intense, knifelike pain which pulses in spasmodic bursts from the upper right abdomen to the shoulder and through to the back. It is completely debilitating and may last a few minutes or several hours. But we'll get to these straits in a minute. Nausea and vomiting sometimes accompany moderate gallbladder pain, and this vomiting is often self-induced as a way of relieving the pain. Vomiting is much more common in severe and acute attacks and usually does lessen pain.

The symptoms of individual attacks of chronic gallbladder disease differ very little from those of a one-time-only acute onslaught except, of course, in duration. The pain and debilitation of an acute attack usually do not stop without medical or surgical intervention. The pain of the acute phase begins like chronic pain but then persists and ceases to fluctuate — a sharp, steady pain which may last from 12 to 18 hours without relief. Chronic attacks usually pass in half an hour. The major signs that a bout of pain is not going to stop are also the signals of systemic infection — warnings that the gallbladder has become infected. The patient's temperature goes up; he complains of chills; his stomach is tender; and, when he goes to the hospital, a high white blood cell count is discovered. If, for some reason, nothing is done about the pain and the apparent infection, perforation of the gallbladder and the onset of gangrene can occur as soon as 3 days, but are more likely after 2 weeks — 2 weeks of terrible pain.

The worst form of gallbladder disease results when a stone gets caught in the common bile duct, because an obstruction there stops *all* drainage from the liver to the intestine. When just the cystic duct is blocked, there is still the hepatic duct (a branch of which bypasses the gallbladder) to help empty the liver of its bile. But when the common duct is stoppered, the entire bile system backs up, and incredible pressure and pain build up. As a result, infection sets in more quickly, and, in addition to the other symptoms of gallbladder attacks, jaundice and cirrhosis (or infection) of the liver soon become grave dangers. About 15 percent of people who have gallstones suffer a common duct stone eventually, and nearly 50 percent of those who suffer an acute attack because of it die — even with prompt surgery. As gallstone victims pass 60, the danger increases that a stone will make its way down to the common duct.

How Doctors Diagnose Gallbladder Disease

What with its miserable symptoms and sharp characteristic pain — a stab in the stomach that radiates to the right shoulder — gallbladder disease is not usually very hard to diagnose. The patient's history typically reveals chronic indigestion; that, coupled with the suggestive pain, causes the examining doctor to call for his most useful diagnostic tool — x-ray. Abdominal x-rays of the gallbladder region are done in 3 or 4 stages, and they are generally done 2 days in a row, because about 25 percent of the folks examined have a falsely negative result on the first go-round. Why, no one knows. On the *outside* chance that the ailing gallbladder holds stones containing lots of calcium, the first step is a plain series of pictures in the target area to pick up shadows of those white objects. If those portraits show nothing, the patient is given a pill containing a dye which makes the gallbladder and its cholesterol show up on the next series of x-rays. The pill is taken with a lightly fatty meal at night, and the exam takes place in the middle of the next morning. The fatty meal causes the gallbladder to empty, and this injects dye into the duct system, causing it to "visualize" on the x-rays.

Sometimes the gallbladder fails to show up on x-ray plates even with the staining material. That happens — or doesn't happen — for one of two reasons. If the patient's gallbladder is seriously diseased, the dye does not reach it, thus picture-taking is impossible. When two so-called oral exams in a row reveal nothing, the physician usually concludes that gallbladder is the source of the patient's problem. However, that positive conclusion cannot be drawn from definitely negative results when the patient is suffering from diarrhea or vomiting. Those symptoms also prevent the dye from entering the gallbladder and so ruin "oral" x-ray exams. When vomiting and diarrhea are factors, the staining material is injected into the patient's bloodstream and reaches the gallbladder by that route. Because the dye is circulating widely through the blood, the gallbladder's duct system is also flooded with it and does show up when x-rays are taken. In this way stones that are lodged in the organ's attendant plumbing are detected.

In recent years ultrasonic scanning has also been used to "read" the contents and condition of a troublesome gallbladder when plain films and "oral" x-rays reveal nothing. This ultrasounding produces a picture which is less sharp than the images from an intravenous x-ray, but the technique is far more comfortable for the patient. The sound scan is used as a halfway measure. If it discovers gallstones, then their host is subjected to the discomforts of the IV test.

X-rays are the standard diagnostic tool in gallbladder treatment. They offer true pictures of internal goings-on in 80 to 90 percent of the cases studied. The irony of the radiologist's role in the gallstone business, however, is that he often misses the worst cases. Fat people get more gallstones, and fat people are harder to photograph in the peculiar inside-out way that x-rays demand. Their layers of fat block or deflect the pentrating rays, and their bulk makes them harder to position on the examining table. And if a patient can't be positioned correctly, the x-rays can't visualize what the doctor wants to see. Fat people are also harder to palpate (to discover swelling in the organ); they often feel pain later than their thinner co-victims; and they make for more difficult operations (if it comes to that). Thus, a word to the fat should be sufficient.

Because the extreme symptoms of gallbladder disease usually mean that a gallstone has gotten stuck somewhere in the duct system, stones in the *common* bile duct are seldom seen in routine x-ray tests. The common bile duct is the last leg of the gallbladder's piping, and since trapped stones are most often found in the higher-up cystic duct, the dyes used in x-rays often do not reach the common duct and so cannot reveal stones that may be lodged there too. Consequently, during operations to remove the gallbladder, 2 procedures to discover common bile duct stones are done. If there are many small gallstones in the gallbladder itself, or if it is inflamed but empty, if jaundice has been a problem or if lumps can be seen or felt in any of the ducts, dye is injected directly into the ducts and an x-ray is taken on the operating table. An alternative method of inspection is the use of an endoscope, a flexible little telescope that is inserted through an incision in one of the ducts and then snaked around until all the passageways have been explored. When stones are discovered by either of those methods, the ducts must be opened — a ticklish business, so to speak — and their contents removed. But we're getting ahead of the story.

The only other tests involved in gallbladder diagnosis are certain blood analyses to determine what liver damage — if any — has been done by the disease.

There is a quirk of gallbladder diagnosis — and a serious medical squabble — we have to deal with. Gallstones which cause absolutely no symptoms are frequently found during examinations for other health complications. X-rays of suspected ulcers, appendicitis, broken ribs, lung congestion, even — of all things — hernias, often reveal these so-called "silent gallstones," and the problem is, what to do about them. Should their container be removed immediately before they can cause trouble or before the patient becomes old, sick and a poor risk for any kind of surgery? Or should sleeping stones be left to lie quietly until they wake up and demand attention? The standard advice has been to be governed by the patient's age. If he is under 60 and in good health, remove the gallbladder, symptoms or no symptoms. The patient is relatively young and strong, and the procedure will be a breeze. Why wait for an acute attack and an emergency? Statistics show that 50 percent of silent-stone carriers eventually develop uncomfortable symptoms and 30 percent of them will someday require surgery. On the other hand, if the patient is over 60, leave him alone. The risk of even elective surgery for these folks (no matter their health) is much greater than it is for younger people. If the 10 million Americans over 60 that statistical projections say have silent gallstones were opened up, the operation itself would kill 30,000 of them. The answer here seems obvious: follow the standard advice. But it's not all that simple.

The same calculations that say yank a silent but stone-laden gallbladder also say that stones usually float freely for 10 years before causing any trouble. Recent studies also suggest that gallbladder conditions do *not* deteriorate rapidly and that a wait-and-see attitude is safe for most people. Eugene Vayda, M.D., professor and chairman of the Department of Health Administration at the University of Toronto in Canada, is a wait-and-seer. He told us the conflict between operation and observation is in large measure, an argument between surgeons and internists. Surgeons, naturally, want to operate at the first sign of stones, while internists will generally hold off to see how symptoms develop. In an article in the *New England Journal of Medicine* in 1973, he presented an even more discouraging view of the problem. He compared the number of various surgical procedures — including gallbladder removal — in Canada and England. When he did, he found that the incidence of these surgeries was much higher in Canada than in England and guessed that 3 factors contributed to this discrepancy. There are more surgeons in Canada than in England (including Wales), more hospital beds and different methods of determining doctors' fees. Under the national health plan in effect in the British Isles, surgeons work for a set national salary. In Canada, they negotiate their prices individually and come out considerably ahead.

Of course, that still doesn't tell us what to do about silent gallstones, and perhaps nothing can. However, Dr. Vayda is conducting a study right now which may help. He's sending large numbers of hypothetical gallbladder case histories — both with and without symptoms — first to a group of surgeons and then to a group of internists and family doctors and comparing their recommendations. When he finally tabulates the combinations of circumstances under which surgery is chosen, he may have some definitive ideas for us. But that won't be for at least a year. Till then, Dr. Vayda and most doctors — surgeons and internists too — would probably agree that silent stones in diabetics should be operated on immediately, as should any stones that cause severe symptoms traceable to the gallbladder — no matter who the patient is. Diabetics become surgical risks at very young ages, and big stones can become big obstructions very quickly. A standard textbook of surgical diagnosis ends its comment on silent gallstones with the prescription that *any* gallbladder that fails to "visualize" on repeated x-rays should be surgically explored and possibly removed, because this hide-and-seek quality is normally a sure sign of advanced gallbladder disease. Perhaps the most telling contribution to this argument, however, comes from a story that was retold by nearly every authority we consulted. As *Medical World News* (March 29, 1974) had it:

> A few years ago, at an annual meeting of the American College of Surgeons, several thousand members of the specialty were arguing the pros and cons of cholecystectomy [surgical removal] for silent gallstones, recalls a California surgeon. When the discussion became stalemated, one of the

> panelists asked those present to stand up if they personally had undergone gallstone surgery. Out of an audience of about 10,000 adults in the 40 to 60 age range, one would expect at least 100 to 200 to have had their gallbladders removed. But only a handful of the surgeons rose to their feet. "Actions speak louder than words," says the Californian. "Surgeons do consider gallbladder surgery a very serious type of surgery indeed — one not to be thought of lightly. Don't let anyone tell you differently!"

Surgeons, it seems, are not as worried about silent gallstones as they want their bill-paying patients to be.

Even those doctors who are not anxious to remove gallbladders with silent stones expect these patients to be back someday for surgery. And nearly all physicians who treat gallbladders would suggest removal with even the moderate symptoms of a chronic condition. The reason this is true is that there is no effective medical — or nonsurgical — treatment for gallstones and gallbladder disease. No proven method, that is. The conventional wisdom always has been, avoid the foods that give you trouble: any fried or greasy foods, heavy sauces, turnips, cabbage, cauliflower, radishes and most raw fruits. Eat a bland, balanced diet with *no* large meals. How a balanced diet can avoid vegetables and raw fruit, of course, is never explained. And take these pills; they'll stop the pain in the gallbladder's plumbing and neutralize digestive acids. The trouble with following this venerable advice is that it works on symptoms and not causes. It won't stop the progress of gallbladder disease, and it won't clip its complications. Nevertheless, generations of kindly healers have given it, because there was no reason not to, no reason to look for something better or little reason to expect something better to turn up. Modern surgery has made gallbladder removal very safe. The death rate today is less than 0.3 perfect for people under 50, rising to about 3 percent for those over 60. The surgery is so safe that the American attitude toward gallbladder disease has become: Eat, Drink, and Be Fat, for Tomorrow You Can Always Ditch Your Gallbladder. Well, we believe there are alternatives to surgery in this case, and so — instead of going on to a description of a typical operation — we'll give you the lowdown on these alternatives. One of them we believe in, and one of them we don't. Neither has been proven down to the last statistical point, but one of them makes sense, and the other doesn't.

A "Miracle" That Doesn't Make Much Sense

Let's get rid of the nonsense first. For years medical alchemists have been looking for the magic that would turn cholesterol gallstones back into golden — well, greenish yellow — liver bile, a drug that could dissolve gallstones once they formed in the gallbladder. Fanfare. They've found it in a number of natural "detergents" isolated from the body's own bile acids. These drugs — the most studied of which is chenodeoxycholic acid or chenic acid (for short) or cheno (to its friends) — when taken orally *do* dissolve gallstones. Most people with stones have either a chronically short supply of bile acids to dissolve a normal amount of cholesterol or an abnormal amount of cholesterol to be washed away. As a result, Johnson L. Thistle, M.D., and Alan F. Hofmann, M.D., of the Mayo Clinic in Rochester, Minnesota, tried to augment the body's supply of bile acids pharmaceutically, and they gave chenic acid tablets to a test group of gallstone sufferers. It worked — in about half the cases. Their liver bile was quickly desaturated, and most of the gallstones were dissolved in periods of from 1 to 2 years. Unfortunately, the minute these guinea pigs stopped taking cheno, their stones returned — in less than a year. There were also certain unpleasant side effects to the treatment, like stomach cramps and diarrhea — and the possibility of liver damage, and the worry of fetal damage in women of child-bearing age. Further tests at the Clinic and elsewhere have shown that the liver damage cheno does to laboratory animals is *not* a factor in human subjects. The specter of birth defects, however, has not been exorcised. What's more, current projections indicate that a gallbladder patient will have to undergo chenic acid therapy for the rest of his life to beat gallstones in this chemical way. That means 3 to 4 pills a day for the first 2 years to dissolve the stones and then 1 pill a day to maintain clear bile. And if present dosage rates hold up, the patient will exchange his gallstones for diarrhea. The most effective dosage for stone dissolving is also the most productive of this nasty side effect. Still another — and more literal — price to be paid for the benefits of chenic acid is the $1 per day that must go to the corner druggist. Right now, a nationwide study of 1,000 test takers of cheno is underway. It may teach us things that will make the treatment seem more acceptable. But as far as we're concerned, swallowing a powerful mixed blessing every day for the rest of one's — possibly urgent — life is no solution to any problem. Especially when there's a natural alternative.

The reason the old standby attempts to control gallbladder disease through diet don't work is that they never go far enough. Americans and Western Europeans (and more and more, everybody else in the world who apes our way of life) have gallstones because they have lousy eating habits. The only surefire way of coping with gallstones — the ones, of course, which produce no or only moderate symptoms — is to change those rotten habits *completely.* If eating lots of fats, lots of animal protein, and getting too little bulk in one's diet and too little exercise in one's life can cause gallstones, then reversing that trend can help get rid of them, or can, at least, help control them. If being fat causes gallstones, then getting skinny can help get rid of them. And if these healthful ways are naturally your ways, then naturally you stand to avoid gallbladder hassles. Be forewarned, doctors don't all agree with this line of reasoning. Most of them accept gallstones as a fringe benefit of Western abundance, but they do not accept a more parsimonious life-style as a cure. Because, they say, these methods haven't been nailed down to the last decimal point in the laboratory. One of the reasons for that, again, is the doctors themselves. It's too simple, safe and profitable for them to yank an ailing gallbladder to devote much time to alternative research. And, we suppose, doctors don't relish telling their patients that their eating and exercise habits stink. That's the beauty, for them, of the oral "detergent," chenic acid. The patient doesn't have to be told to stop doing anything. He just has to take the magic pill. Anyway, we would like you to know that there is both common sense and some scientific evidence to suggest that gallstones can be avoided or controlled by natural, uncomplicated means.

The most obvious of these is the lowering of one's cholesterol intake by all the usual methods. A true low-fat, low-animal protein diet should be adopted. That does not mean giving up the occasional baconburger as it did under the old regimen. It means eating a great deal less red meat and going lightly even on chicken and fish. It means learning about vegetable proteins and the theories of complementary protein sources in books like Frances M. Lappé's *Diet for a Small Planet* (Ballantine Books, 1974). It means, above all, losing weight if you need to. Fat people suffer more gallbladder trouble than thin people, because they produce more cholesterol. It does no good to cut down on the fats your mouth puts into your liver bile if you don't also cut down on the cholesterol your body itself manufactures. One way to help a lot in lowering cholesterol is to get regular exercise. Vlado Simko, M.D., of the University of Cincinnati Medical Center and a leading researcher in the field of exercise and cholesterol reduction, sent us a thick packet of graphs and charts to document his claims and said, "Even mild exercise (walking 3 miles/hour) decreases in human volunteers cholesterol in the red blood cells and increases the output of cholesterol and bile acids in the bile. From several studies in rats we know that if mild exercise is regularly repeated, besides decreasing cholesterol in the red blood cells, it leads to less cholesterol in the bile. (Higher output of cholesterol into the intestine during exercise probably leads to higher losses of cholesterol in the stool.) Decreased cholesterol content of the bile means better solubility of cholesterol in the bile and lesser propensity to form cholesterol gallstones (which are very prevalent in the technological societies)."

Think what more than "mild exercise" could do!

Natural, no-chemical, nonsurgical control of gallstones also means — for reasons not yet clear — the addition of bran and other fiber-fill to the diet. Several studies in England, Canada and Australia — no doubt under the influence of fiber pioneer, Denis Burkitt — have concluded that since the superrefined, "semisynthetic" modern diet is one of the villains in gallbladder disease, the first step to fighting it should be a return to bulky old-fashioned fare. These experiments have shown — in a very sketchy way — that lots of fiber in the diet tends to lower cholesterol saturation in the liver bile.

Finally, there is some reason to believe that supplements of vitamin C and lecithin (which is, you'll remember, one of the "detergents" in liver bile) do help improve the bile's ability to hold cholesterol in solution and hence to get rid of it and gallstones. These experiments — at New York's Mount Sinai Hospital and at the Institute of Nutrition in Bratislava, Czechoslovakia — are extremely tentative, but they do suggest that there are ways of at least limiting the formation of gallstones which do not require the flooding of one's body with strange, powerful and relatively unknown substances.

We would like to think of gallbladder surgery as a last resort in most cases, but of course, if a patient is plagued with acute attacks, surgery is the only answer. The indications for immediate surgery are: frequent attacks of colicky pain, signs of an acute inflammation of the gallbladder (high temperature, pain, abdominal tenderness, elevated white blood cell count), x-ray evidence of large numbers of stones (especially small ones and those in the common duct) and the presence of jaundice. The standard operation for gallbladder trouble means removal of the organ. It is more complex than appendectomy and considerably more painful for the patient. There is also one very nasty element that is sometimes necessary. A soft rubber drain may be inserted into the abdominal cavity near the gallbladder to draw off the heavy flow of bile and blood that now and then follows surgery. The drain passes outside the body through its own incision and empties into a small plastic bag strapped to the patient's side. It is a slightly distasteful nuisance which is usually left in place for a few days or as long as it's needed. It's needed because liver bile is highly caustic, and any that might drip out of a fresh incision would cause painful damage to the body cavity. Fortunately, this is not a standard procedure and not frequently needed.

Preoperative care for gallbladder surgery is limited. If jaundice is a factor, the patient is given vitamin K, and all patients enter the operating room with empty stomachs. The type of anesthesia used varies from doctor to doctor, but most of the time it is some form of general anesthetic.

Most gallbladder operations take 60 to 90 minutes. A fairly large incision (5 to 7 inches long) is made just below the ribs and to the right of the navel. It may go straight up and down or straight across or slant along the line of the rib cage, depending on which type the surgeon feels offers the best exposure of the gallbladder. The removal process is quick. The blood vessels to and from the gallbladder are tied off and so is the cystic duct which carries bile away from the organ. Then the doctor simply snips the villain away. His largest difficulty comes from the close quarters and the anatomical peculiarities of individual patients. The gallbladder area is like a funnel; it gets narrower as the surgeon gets closer to his job. He may have trouble avoiding the things he wants to leave behind. And because everyone's bile plumbing is unique in some ways, rearrangement of its flow may present an anxious moment or two. After all this is sorted out, and if the doctor thinks he can *see* stones bulging through the common duct, he places a small catheter — or T tube — in it and takes an x-ray through the tube. If stones are present, he'll open the duct and remove them. That done, the wound is closed, and the patient is wheeled to the recovery room.

There is pain involved with a healing gallbladder incision, because the wound is very near where several large muscles attach to the ribs. These muscles allow the torso to twist and help in bending, and so those activities are painful for a few days. The muscles are also jostled during respiration, and deep breathing, coughing and laughing can be problems for a short time. Painkillers are generally needed. Nevertheless, most people get out of bed on the day of their surgery and are moving around well a day or two later. The average hospital stay following gallbladder surgery is somewhere between 5 days and a week but can stretch to

2 weeks if a T tube or an abdominal drain is involved. The volume of flow must be checked frequently. Heavy drainage from the T tube suggests that one of the ducts that were tied off is leaking or that a stone in the common bile duct was somehow overlooked. If one of these errors is suspected, *more* x-rays are taken through the tube. If a new stone is discovered, it can be washed out with a saltwater solution administered through the T tube or picked out with tiny surgical tweezers — which, again, are pushed in through the tube. Because of the large muscles near the incision, most people do not return to normal functioning for 3 to 4 weeks. The healing of the wound is not complete for 3 to 6 months. It is true, unfortunately, that gallstones can re-form in the remaining ducts if the patient does not change his diet and lower his cholesterol levels. So, gallbladder removal does not open the door to scot-free gluttony. It is true that stones are sometimes overlooked during surgery and that they cause much of the later trouble.

The only other gallbladder operation is a make-do measure used when a patient is judged too sick to undergo a complete removal — too sick either from the effects of an acute attack or from an unrelated illness. After his health has been stabilized as best it can be, his gallbladder and duct system are opened up and cleaned of stones, a tube is inserted in the gallbladder and he is buttoned up to recover completely. While he's convalescing, x-rays are taken through the tube (which is left in place) to get the jump on any ensuing attacks. Once the poor fellow is fully recovered — it sometimes takes 6 months — the removal of his gallbladder is scheduled.

Another reason to change one's eating habits even after gallbladder surgery is that 10 percent of all patients suffer some of their old symptoms *after* the operation. They have indigestion after eating greasy food and bouts of colicky pain. The reasons for this are unclear. Some doctors — generally not the ones who do the initial surgery — say that symptoms continue because gallbladder disease was a misdiagnosis in the first place. Others say that too long a remnant of the cystic duct was left in place and that *it* is causing the pain. Still others say that the trouble is yet another gallstone which has somehow eluded the gaze of all the x-rays before, during and after the operation. No one knows who's got the right answer. It is known, however, that a fairly high percentage of gallbladder folks suffer mild indigestion for a short time after surgery, sometimes for as long as 3 or 4 months. It is guessed that this discomfort occurs until the new ductwork gets broken in to its task.

Gallbladder removal is a messy business, and it is not a cure-all. It is successful, that is, it satisfactorily relieves a patient's symptoms, in most cases. But, if the poor devil doesn't change his eating habits, the ghost of his gallbladder can come back to haunt him. Gallstone management is possible, but it isn't a guaranteed enterprise either. The way to cope with gallbladder disease, then, is through prevention. You should coddle your gallbladder; the natural way of life — lots of exercise and unprocessed, fiber-rich foods — seems the best bet.

12
Ulcers

The many myths about ulcers and their treatment have been chronicled in both medical journals and popular chitchat. And now, just when treatment is finally becoming more effective and standardized, ulcer incidence is plummeting, independent of medical know-how.

Various treatments for ulcers have been bandied about over the years. Patients have coddled and cajoled the misfit sores in their stomachs with one thing or another—often a combination of rest, hospitalization, tranquilizers, antispasmodics, bland diets and frequent feedings of milk. Every one of those treatments has been studied more than once with contradictory results. Many times, pain and discomfort return after initial improvement.

In desperation after months or even years of treatment, many ulcer victims have undergone surgical removal of most of the stomach, quite often to find surgery followed by diarrhea, weakness and inability to gain weight or eat full meals.

The picture is much brighter now. A new drug called cimetidine has replaced less effective drugs, cut antacid use and enabled ulcer patients to eat more liberal diets. Fewer patients need surgery to relieve pain, and more meticulous surgical procedures with far fewer side effects have made surgery less unpleasant for those who must have it.

Still, about 140,000 peptic ulcer patients are operated on each year, and 6,000 Americans die each year from complications of the disease, the National Center for Health Statistics estimates. For the 14 million Americans who suffer ulcer distress, relief of any kind is heartily welcome.

To understand how an ulcer forms, let us first look at the digestive system itself.

Many people say they have a stomachache when they hurt anywhere from under the nipples to the pubic bone. Actually, the stomach is tucked into the abdomen at the lower rib line. When empty, it looks like a collapsed balloon. When full, it's top-heavy, like an upside-down pear.

Acting on an involuntary message from the brain, the vagus nerves, located along the esophagus and branching to all areas of the stomach, signal certain glands to release hydrochloric acid into the stomach. The combination of acid, water, digestive enzymes and some mucus from the stomach lining totals 1 to 2 quarts of gastric juice per day.

When food enters, the stomach begins a series of muscular contractions that combine gastric juice and food into a mixture about the consistency of cream soup. Gradually, that highly acidic mix is squirted through a valve called the pylorus into the upper part of the small intestine—the duodenum. There, further digestion is promoted by secretions from the duodenal glands and the liver. On signals from the duodenum and stomach, the pancreas also contributes enzymes and alkaline juices to help neutralize the acid and digest the meal.

The small intestine processes a meal in about 8 hours. Waste products are separated out and sent to the colon, or large intestine, which sends water and minerals back to the bloodstream. The semisolid residue is passed on to the colon, where it is stored and finally eliminated through rectum and anus.

What Is an Ulcer?

Any break in the surface of an organ or tissue, inflamed or not, is an ulcer. Those which occur in the stomach and duodenum are tagged peptic ulcers because the enzyme pepsin, which helps digest protein, is mixed with food in those organs.

Pepsin is activated by the natural presence of acid in gastric juices. Ulcers can occur anywhere that pepsin and acid intermingle, including the esophagus, but 99 percent of peptic ulcers occur either in the stomach itself (gastric ulcers) or in the upper part of the small intestine, just below the stomach (duodenal ulcers).

An ulcer looks a lot like a mouth ulcer or "cold sore." A whitish, craterlike hole surrounded by a reddish, shaggy rim develops in the glossy pink lining of the stomach or duodenum. Ulcers may be shallow or deep, and are, on the average, about the size of a penny, although they may be much larger or smaller.

Duodenal ulcers are about 4 times as common as gastric ulcers. Occasionally, both occur in the same person. This chapter will be concerned primarily with the more common duodenal ulcers, although gastric ulcers will also be discussed.

Normally, there is a balance between the aggressive action of acid and the protective capacity of the slippery mucous lining of the stomach and intestine. If such were not the case, everyone would have ulcers.

What exactly triggers an ulcer in that protective lining is not known. We do know that the balance of acid production and protection can be tipped in a number of ways: there may be an excessive number of acid-producing cells, more acid released by nerves and glands, a weak spot in the protective mucous lining and less inborn control over acid release in response to food. Those physiological factors may be either inherited or triggered by outside agents, such as aspirin—or both. Exactly how all those factors interrelate still bewilders "ulcerologists." Even more bewildering is the fact that for no clear reason, the ulcer rate has dropped dramatically over the past 25 years.

Why some people get ulcers and others don't is a big medical question mark. Most people have acid in their stomachs, even though it is no longer absolutely necessary for digestion in humans. Quite possibly it's a vestige of the physiology of our ancestors, who didn't find their dinners in boxes on the grocery shelf and ate more primitive foods which did need acid for digestion. Some of us, apparently, inherited more acid than others. There's a general tendency for people who produce more acid to get more ulcers. But not everyone who produces extra acid gets an ulcer.

Stress appears to stimulate acid secretion, and can instigate ulcer formation. Stress, living habits and personality are closely related, but while stress is a factor, personality is not.

"I don't think that an ulcer personality has ever been established, although the notion that it exists has often been advanced. I don't think the evidence for it even strongly suggests it," says Morton I. Grossman, M.D., Ph.D., director of a research program in Los Angeles which has studied almost every aspect of who gets peptic ulcers and why. The Center for Ulcer Research and Education, with the optimistic acronym CURE, has been in operation at the VA Wadsworth Hospital Center and UCLA-affiliated hospitals since 1974.

So ulcers, in fact, are not the distinct—and dubious—badges of success of hard-driving male executives, after all. Men victims still outnumber women, but the gap is narrowing. Why, no one knows. More and more college students, too, are turning up in infirmaries and doctors' offices with ulcer-generated complaints. Practicing physicians blame students' irregular hours, late-night partying and studying, heavy use of coffee, cola and aspirin, along with missed meals, for the marked increase in younger adults. One theory is that certain personalities and life-styles indirectly lead to ulcers because they carry a tendency to use agents which are known to either cause or aggravate ulcers. In addition to caffeine and aspirin, cigarettes and alcohol are two other known irritants.

The most common symptom of duodenal ulcer is a gnawing, rhythmic pain, usually well localized in the epigastrium (upper middle abdomen) and rarely felt below the navel. It's not the sort of pain you can't stand or feel you have to go to the emergency room for. Queasiness or exaggerated hunger sensations are less common but not unusual. What's most characteristic about duodenal ulcer distress is that it occurs day after day about the same time, usually up to 1 to 3 hours after a meal. Some people have pain after every meal, or just the noon meal, or it wakens them during the night. Symptoms may even subside without treatment. Many patients are delighted to be symptom-free for months and months, only to have the pains reappear with no warning.

Gastric ulcers don't stick to such a definite pattern. Some patients may have pain right after meals, or simply a feeling of fullness. Because the symptoms are not as clearcut, gastric ulcers are more difficult to detect and often not diagnosed immediately.

Then there are "silent ulcers" of either type, which produce no symptoms. One-third of the people who show peptic ulcers by x-ray or endoscopic exam have no prior inkling of their disease.

If you have no history of ulcers and start suffering stomach pain, don't jump to the conclusion that you have an ulcer. Stomach pains can be caused by a range of gastrointestinal and nongastrointestinal conditions, including hiatal hernia, kidney problems, psychological distress and others. Inflammation of the gallbladder or pancreas can also mimic an ulcer.

Even if it turns out that you do have an ulcer, thumbing through the Yellow Pages in search of a gastroenterologist is still not a good idea. In many areas of the U.S., gastroenterologists see new patients by referral only. Or, you may wait up to a month for an appointment, only to find that your problem is not an ulcer or even gastrointestinal at all. That's frustrating—for both you and the doctor. See your family doctor or internist first. Even if a gastroenterologist finds that you do have an ulcer, in the absence of serious complications or totally unmanageable symptoms, you will be returned to your own doctor for ongoing treatment.

Diagnosis must be based not only on your recital of symptoms, but on x-ray and endoscopy (or more specifically, upper gastrointestinal endoscopy or gastroscopy—painless insertion through the mouth and esophagus into the stomach of a flexible lighted tube about the size of a forefinger). Gastroscopy may be combined with biopsy and cytology (microscopic examination of tissue samples) to rule out stomach cancer. A small percentage of gastric ulcers are cancerous; duodenal ulcers almost never are.

If you have ulcers and start feeling weak, dizzy or faint, pass black or tarry stools, or vomit blood or a substance that looks like coffee grounds, call your doctor. You could be bleeding internally. He may tell you to start drinking milk or eating small snacks or soft foods every 1 to 2 hours until you get medical attention.

The Care and Feeding of an Ulcer

"The goals of ulcer therapy are fourfold: to relieve pain, to hasten ulcer healing, to prevent complications and to prevent recurrences," writes Jon I. Isenberg, M.D., gastroenterologist at the UCLA School of Medicine in Los Angeles (*Annals of Internal Medicine,* January, 1976). Most doctors—and patients—would agree.

But a patient may be told by one doctor to eat 6 or 7 small bland meals a day, downing antacids with each one. He may be told to quit his high-pressure job or at least pare down his working hours. Tranquilizers may even be prescribed for him. If he switches doctors after weeks of strict adherence to his regimen with no improvement, the second doctor may tell him his occupation and life-style have nothing to do with his ailment. He may be given *carte blanche* to eat anything he likes as long as he takes daily doses of a drug called cimetidine.

Because the stomach is the body's food processor, ulcer victims have traditionally journeyed to their doctors in quest of the ultimate ulcer diet, when in truth no such diet exists. From the hourly feedings of milk and cream, pioneered by a man appropriately named Sippy, to spartan diets of bland food, patients have been willing to try almost anything.

Those diets did seem to heal ulcers at first. Eventually, the ulcers always recurred. What was actually taking place was the natural ebb and flow of healing and recurrence, healing and recurrence that is so characteristic of duodenal ulcers, *with or without a special diet.* Hourly milk is now reserved for the immediate and acute stage of healing only, especially if there is bleeding.

Nowadays, most doctors feel that a modified ulcer diet, consisting of 3 small meals and antacids or snacks in between, is an important part of an ulcer regimen. Many tell their patients that they may eat a fairly normal, wholesome diet, using antacids instead of between-meal snacks if weight control is a problem. Spicy foods may or may not be irritating. Spices like horseradish used to be strictly prohibited, but since some patients can tolerate them, they may use moderate amounts.

Not eating at all is worse than eating the wrong foods. While there is still some debate over whether a patient should eat 6 small meals or 3 regular meals, there is no question that 1 of those meals should be breakfast. Skipping breakfast, as a matter of fact, is about the worst thing an ulcer-prone individual can do if he wants to avoid recurrences.

"It's astonishing how many duodenal ulcer patients skip breakfast. That's how they get into trouble," a leading gastroenterologist told us. "In a normal person, the stomach secretes acid in response to food, then the acid stops. Ulcer patients, however, tend to produce acid 'round the clock, including during the overnight fast. With no food to neutralize the acid, the damage is promoted. If you skip breakfast, you extend that unprotected period by another few hours. The most important aspect of treatment is diet, and that includes breakfast."

Protein content of the diet has been a controversial area. Foods which contain a high proportion of protein reduce the acidity of the stomach contents longer than do foods which contain low protein. Yet those same high-protein foods also stimulate a rebound of acid secretion after the initial buffering effect wears off. Advice on protein intake, then, depends on whether the physician thinks it's more important to eat food that will buffer acid immediately after a meal or to avoid food that will stimulate it later. Physicians we spoke to urged a moderate and reasonable intake of protein rather than a high- or low-protein diet. One advised that red meat be avoided during the acute healing stage because it probably stimulates more acid than fish or poultry. Still others said that antacids, not food, should be used to buffer acid.

When you do sit down to a meal, don't gobble your food. Gobbling might be a survival mechanism for some animals in the wild who have to eat their catch before it's stolen by wolves, but the practice is outmoded in humans. Research indicates that food which is not chewed thoroughly has little time to mix properly with a substance called urogastrone from the salivary glands. Urogastrone protects the intestinal lining from erosion in experimental animals, so chewing food thoroughly may be another major safeguard against ulcers. It becomes not only a matter of what you eat, but how you eat, says Dr. Isenberg, who conducted the research at the VA Wadsworth Hospital Center, associated with UCLA.

Most ulcer patients are better off avoiding alcohol, coffee (even decaffeinated coffee), cola and strong tea, which are known to provoke ulcers. If used at all, they should be taken with meals, as food helps to buffer their irritating effects.

Avoid aspirin and aspirin-containing anti-inflammatory drugs. Aspirin causes gastric ulcers outright, evidently by corroding the stomach lining, and aggravates duodenal ulcers. You may not be aware that aspirin is an ingredient of over 200 drugstore items, including Alka-Seltzer, Anacin, Bufferin, Coricidin, Darvon, Empirin and Excedrin. Anti-inflammatory drugs like corticosteroids and phenylbutazone also aggravate ulcers.

Cigarette smokers are twice as likely to develop ulcers as are nonsmokers. Besides reducing the effects of antacids and impairing healing, cigarettes are thought to suppress pancreatic release of the alkaline juices that neutralize acid dumped into the duodenum by the stomach. Cigars and pipes are no better.

All about antacids. Antacids have been used to treat peptic ulcers since the first century A.D. The rationale for their use today is that ulcers almost never occur in the absence of acid. Since antacids neutralize acid, they theoretically cut its effects. That rationale is backed up by experiments confirming that ulcer formation is slowed down by antacids and by the effectiveness of acid-reducing surgery. Other studies indicate that antacids have only a placebo effect (the power of suggestion) in healing and pain relief. But doctors and patients alike swear by them, and they are widely prescribed.

Just how much antacid is needed varies from one patient to the next. Doses of the white, chalky liquids customarily prescribed range from 1 to 4 tablespoons, depending on strength of the antacids and how much acid you secrete. They seem to be most effective taken 1 to 3 hours after eating. Tablets are more convenient than liquids, but slightly less effective and must be chewed thoroughly for full benefit.

Calcium-containing antacids were once considered to be the ideal type of antacid, but they put patients at risk of kidney stones or partial kidney failure. Magnesium and aluminum hydroxides have replaced calcium-containing antacids. Magnesium in high dosages may cause diarrhea and aluminum may cause constipation. Doses prescribed are adjusted to minimize those side effects.

Antacid use is often coordinated with diet and cimetidine (a drug we'll discuss later) for optimum effects.

Anticholinergics (or antispasmodics) block nerve impulses to the stomach, quelling muscle spasms and relieving pain. (Belladonna is an example.) Those drugs inhibit food-stimulated acid secretion by up to 50 percent when taken 30 minutes before a meal. The effect lasts about 4 to 5 hours, so they are sometimes used to relieve overnight pain. Their actual healing power, however, is very doubtful. Side effects including dry mouth, blurred vision or urinary retention, can be somewhat controlled by manipulating the prescribed dosage. Anticholinergics cannot be used by patients with glaucoma, prostate disease, chronic lung disease, hiatal hernia or serious heart disease. With the advent of cimetidine, those drugs are used much less frequently for ulcers.

Baking soda, or sodium bicarbonate, is an old-time remedy for stomach woes that is neither safe nor natural. While baking soda may neutralize acid, the sodium raises blood pressure, damaging the kidneys and causing a risk of heart failure. It's clearly out of the question as an ulcer remedy.

Natural remedies for ulcers. Aside from drugs, a few foods seem to lessen ulcer symptoms in some patients. While their actual healing powers have yet to be scientifically confirmed by the medical establishment, patients have reported that both raw cabbage juice and raw potato juice have helped to relieve ulcer symptoms, without the side effects of drugs.

From the 1920s to the 1950s, Garnett Cheney, M.D., a San Francisco gastroenterologist, did a series of experiments testing the effect of cabbage juice on ulcers in both animals and humans. He concluded that it was an effective treatment. In a study published in *California Medicine,* January, 1965, Dr. Cheney reported 24 of 26 ulcer patients receiving cabbage juice during a 3-week treatment period were healed. Only 6 of 19 patients who received a placebo were healed, and 10 who had not been healed with a placebo were healed later with a 3-week treatment of cabbage juice. Since then, researchers at a London university have found that raw cabbage protects experimental animals against ulcers, but that cooked cabbage has no effect (*Postgraduate Medical Journal,* June, 1975).

Even acupuncture has been tried. A doctor in Czechoslovakia reports he has had success treating both duodenal and gastric ulcer patients with acupuncture. Vaclav Kajdos, M.D., treated 71 patients at the National Institute of Health in Prague and summarized his results in a published report:

> Out of 71 patients treated with acupuncture, a surprising number of 45 patients lost their subjective complaints of pain, nausea, vomiting or anorexia entirely (63 percent). In some of them there were occasional relapses after months or years of having been free of all symptoms which, however, could be promptly eliminated by repeat acupuncture sessions. In the second group of 20 patients, spastic pains vanished but the feeling of pressure and occasional nausea remained. In both groups, however, the patients were able to either drop their diet entirely or widen it substantially. In only six instances did acupuncture fail to have any beneficial effects (*American Journal of Acupuncture,* July–September, 1977).

Those promising preliminary studies were heartily rejected as unscientific and invalid by most prominent gastroenterologists, and no one has been inclined to reassess them more extensively. Lack of research funds could be one reason. Another may be a tendency to attribute the success of unconventional treatments to the disease's own periodic healing pattern, which was apparently behind the success of the traditional Sippy diet.

No particular vitamins or supplements have been recommended for the treatment of duodenal ulcers in the literature we've seen. Several preliminary studies have shown that zinc may hasten the healing of gastric ulcers, but the results haven't been conclusive, and no link to duodenal ulcers has been established.

The herbal approach is another unconventional—and not widely accepted—tactic. A nutrition-oriented physician in Merion, Pennsylvania, Howard Posner, M.D., described his drugless regimen for ulcer patients:

"I generally take the patient off all meat, tobacco, alcohol, coffee, tea, chocolate and strong spices. I ask them to eliminate fried foods and avoid acidic foods like vinegar. During the acute phase of the disease, I ask them not to eat raw fruit or vegetables. They should chew very well so the food is less irritating to the stomach.

"In the very, very acute stage," continues Dr. Posner, "I have patients eliminate whole grains and nuts. They can have well-cooked white rice. I also recommend frequent sips of goats' milk and soured milk products like yogurt.

"In addition, I find patients do very well with a slippery elm drink, which coats the stomach and intestine. They combine warm milk and honey in a blender, then add 1 to 2 teaspoons of powdered slippery elm bark once the blender is turned on."

Dr. Posner worked as chief of the Infectious Disease Division at Lincoln Hospital and as assistant professor of Internal Medicine at Albert Einstein Medical School, both in New York City, before going into private practice. He believes that ulcers have an emotional component that requires serious attention. Drug regimens and surgery can both be avoided, he believes, if the psychological or emotional problem can be solved.

While other doctors say that the emotional factor in ulcer disease has been overemphasized, sedatives such as Librium and phenobarbitol are nevertheless frequently offered to ulcer patients who appear nervous. Not only do tranquilizing drugs carry with them a myriad of symptoms including nausea and dizziness, they tend to be habit forming. If the disease is really aggravated by emotional or psychological stress, sedatives don't get to the root of the problem. Natural methods of relaxation like meditation, yoga and exercise are just as effective—and much safer.

Cutting down on stress is by far the most difficult advice for many ulcer patients to follow. Much stress simply cannot be avoided. How a person handles stress, though, is what makes the difference.

A person caught in a traffic jam at rush hour, for instance, is likely to fuss and fume, directing his anger at the poor soul up ahead whose broken-down pickup truck is blocking the highway. That stress response sparks a gush of acid, ripening the stomach for an ulcer. If instead the motorist checks the backseat of his car for that copy of *Newsweek* he's been meaning to read, he'll save himself a lot of harmful aggravation and perhaps learn something new.

So much for unexpected stress. What about day-to-day stress at home or in the office? A well-paying job is likely to carry the strain of heavy responsibility. Do you forfeit the job—and a nice paycheck—to rid yourself of the strain? Not necessarily. If there's an element of satisfaction, stress may be healthful.

Should you find yourself getting worked up over nothing, day after day, at home or at work, you are ripe for an ulcer. When you feel jumpy, slow down. Organize your time more efficiently. Delegate some chores to others. Make only those decisions today that must be made today, and don't worry over the ones you may never have to make at all. Don't try to solve all your problems today. If you have a salary review in 2 months, do you have to begin worrying about it now? Do you have to do the grocery shopping and laundry all in one evening?

Unrelenting stress will wear a hole in your stomach. Break that stress. Take a nap. Go to bed early one night a week. Exercise. Play golf if you like.

Be wary of competitive exercise, like squash. If you come out of a game feeling relaxed, fine. If you get all worked up, you've only substituted one form of aggression for another. If you are aggressive by nature, exercises such as walking, jogging or biking may be more helpful.

Cimetidine — A New Drug Approach

Marketed under the trade name Tagamet, cimetidine is being hailed as a breakthrough in ulcer management. The drug began as the brainchild of a British researcher and was then developed by Smith Kline and French Laboratories. In some patients, the original drug had disastrous effects. Over 700 compounds were then tested before the present form of the drug was approved by the FDA for both safety and effectiveness in treating duodenal ulcers. In gastric ulcers, it is somewhat less effective—not effective enough to meet FDA standards, but as safe as it is for duodenal ulcers should a physician wish to try it.

At first, cimetidine was approved for 8 weeks' use only. Ninety-nine percent of duodenal ulcer patients treated with cimetidine in tests healed during that time, but most recurred within 6 to 9 months after treatment was stopped. What many doctors do now, with the FDA's go-ahead, is taper the dose after the initial 8-week healing period and continue indefinitely with maintenance doses of 1 or 2 tablets daily. Nearly all duodenal ulcers will stay healed under that regimen.

Here's how the drug works:

There are 2 kinds of cells in the body with receptors for a substance called histamine. H1 (H one) cells, in the nasal passages and elsewhere in the respiratory tract, react to histamine by constricting bronchial muscles. Conventional antihistamines bring relief to hay fever patients but they don't work on the other set of histamine receptors in the lower stomach. When those H2 receptors are stimulated by histamines, they secrete acid. Acid aggravates the ulcer. Cimetidine blocks off those H2 receptors, and the ulcer heals.

No one claims that cimetidine cures ulcers. Once the drug is withdrawn, no matter how long you've taken it, the ulcer will tend to recur. Cimetidine is acclaimed because of its effect on both surgical and nonsurgical management of ulcers.

While cimetidine has not made antacids obsolete, its cutback of acid secretion means that smaller doses of antacids are needed to neutralize whatever acid does leak out into the stomach. Diets, too, can be more liberal.

Ulcer surgery was rapidly diminishing even before the advent of cimetidine. Now that decrease is accelerating. In some people, ulcers will recur no matter how they're treated; but as far as surgery goes, long-term maintenance on cimetidine keeps ulcers healed and patients off the operating table. For patients who choose surgery for clearly unmanageable ulcers, that 1 to 5 percent that recur seem to come back with a vengeance, far more severe than the primary ulcer. Cimetidine makes it possible to becalm many of those relentless ulcers, when previously, reoperation had been the standard recourse.

As drugs go, cimetidine has stirred up fewer side effects than would be expected, at least on a short-term basis. The major problems are central nervous system effects—confusion, dizziness and hallucinations, primarily in older people. Some people lapse into unconsciousness. Alarming as those side effects sound, doctors say they are reversible and managed by cutting the dose.

Long-term side effects are not yet known. A preliminary report from England got much publicity because it linked cimetidine to gastric cancer. J. B. Elder, of the Royal Infirmary in Manchester, raised the possibility that cimetidine, in the presence of gastric acid and dietary nitrites, might form cancer-causing nitrosamines in the stomach (*Lancet,* May 12, 1979). The study was immediately scrutinized by both the drug's manufacturer, Smith Kline and French, and an independent cimetidine researcher. Both seriously questioned the validity of the study. Elder's speculation, however, is worth checking out and is being investigated further.

Another promising drug, ranitidine, is in the early stages of testing and development. Stronger than cimetidine, ranitidine has 5 times the capability to suppress acid secretion. Toxicity may even be lower.

An avalanche of ulcer drugs may follow cimetidine, which so far appears to be the most effective way of avoiding surgery. Taking it may be worth its theoretical risks, since even elective surgery carries *known* risks.

The Surprising Decline in Ulcer Surgery

If you develop certain complications and they are severe enough, surgery is urgent. Those complications include bleeding, perforation and obstruction.

Bleeding results when the ulcer erodes the wall of a vein or an artery. Venous bleeding is not an immediate danger and may be treated medically. Untreated, it can cause anemia and weakness. In arterial bleeding, blood spurts out more forcefully, like water from a hole in a pipe: surgery is mandatory.

Should the ulcer erode deeply enough, it can perforate the stomach or duodenal wall. The contents of the stomach spill out like garbage from a hole in a trash bag, irritating the sensitive surrounding tissues. The result is peritonitis—a serious condition that can lead to infection and death. Usually, the perforation is merely closed off surgically as an emergency measure. However, patients in whom perforation occurs again and again may undergo more definitive, or corrective, surgery to prevent future perforation.

Every ulcer, whether healing occurs spontaneously or is medically achieved, produces some scar tissue. Obstruction occurs when the ulcer inflames, swells and builds up so much stiff scar tissue that digestion is thwarted. Vomiting, pain and dehydration result. Although not quite as immediate a threat as bleeding or perforation, obstruction calls for surgery.

In the absence of such serious complications, ulcer surgery can be undertaken on an elective basis at the patient's convenience. The major indication for elective surgery is an intractable ulcer; that is, one that refuses to respond to any other kind of treatment. Although elective ulcer surgery has been refined to the point where mortality is less than 1 percent, any time you undergo general anesthesia there are risks, and no mortality rate is entirely acceptable. Freedom from ulcer recurrence is not guaranteed through surgery, either.

"The patient should have a choice," says J. H. Baron, consultant at the Royal Postgraduate Medical School and Hammersmith Hospital in London. "We reckon that a percentage of all patients who have stomach operations, whether it's vagotomy or whatever, have some recurrent ulceration—and I think it's fair to tell the patient of that possibility before they agree to surgery. Some patients say they couldn't possibly go on taking tablets for the rest of their lives; others are only too willing to do so" (*British Medical Journal,* January 20, 1979).

Elective surgery for ulcer patients—like drugs or diet—is aimed at reducing excess acid secretion. We say "reduce excess acid" because the only way to eliminate acid completely would be to remove the entire stomach.

One form of surgery, no longer used for ulcers, did in fact remove up to three-quarters of the stomach. The results were often disastrous. Dumping syndrome was the most common and unpleasant side effect—after that operation, food passes much more quickly from the stomach to the intestines. The patient feels warm, weak, nauseated and sweaty and has diarrhea. Fainting and weight loss often follow.

On the other hand, surgery which only cuts out the ulcer is inadequate, because unremitting acid secretion will form still another ulcer in a nearby area.

The most widely used procedures today are vagotomy with either pyloroplasty or antrectomy. The results are much more satisfactory than the simple removal of an ulcer or of most of the stomach.

Because it is the vagus nerves, coming down along the esophagus, which control acid secretion in the stomach, cutting them blocks the nerve impulses to acid-secreting cells. But since some of those vagus nerves also control emptying of the stomach, a surgeon doing vagotomy has to provide for that function. That can be done by enlarging the pylorus, which is the opening between the stomach and the duodenum. People who have a vagotomy combined with pyloroplasty still have about a 10 to 15 percent chance of developing the same ulcer trouble later. Mortality—the chance of dying during the operation—is considered low, about 1 percent or less.

Vagotomy may be combined with either of 2 other drainage procedures. One is an infrequent procedure called gastro-jejunostomy. But more commonly, a less extensive removal of the lower half of the stomach, the antrum, is done. The ulcer recurrence rate for vagotomy with antrectomy is more favorable—about 1 percent—compared to 10 to 15 percent for vagotomy and pyloroplasty. Side effects for both operations are few.

The newest variation of ulcer surgery is superselective vagotomy (also called proximal gastric vagotomy, highly selective vagotomy or parietal cell vagotomy). Only those vagus nerves going to the acid-secreting portions of the stomach are cut; the ones going to the pylorus and antrum are left intact, so the stomach can empty itself. Diarrhea and the dumping syndrome are virtually abolished. Long-term digestive side effects seem to be about 10 percent. A mortality rate of practically zero makes it a very attractive option, but it is a more technical operation than the others. Doctors interviewed said superselective vagotomy should be done only by surgeons who perform it often. As yet, it is not widely used.

The type of surgery chosen is geared to the patient's age, location of the ulcer, amount of acid the patient secretes and sometimes the surgeon's preference for one procedure over another. Only about 1 in 10 duodenal ulcer patients requires surgery. The choice for these patients is usually vagotomy and antrectomy. For gastric ulcer patients, the acid pattern varies a great deal according to level and location. Surgeons may choose vagotomy and antrectomy, or antrectomy alone. About 1 in 4 gastric ulcer patients ends up with surgery.

Your surgeon will probably explain what type of surgery he recommends for you with a simple diagram of the stomach. If he doesn't, ask him to.

Hospitalization for routine ulcer operations, with no complications, is much shorter than it used to be—about 10 to 12 days now, sometimes even less. Side effects vary not only with the operation but also the patient's condition and the surgeon's skill. Diarrhea, gas and other digestive problems are not nearly as much of a problem as they were years ago. Some patients still have dietary restrictions and many continue to take antacids or cimetidine or both to keep new ulcers from forming.

An ulcer is considered healed after 2 or 3 months of freedom from ulcer distress, whether the treatment is surgery, drugs, diet or something else. Recurrences may be symptomless, discovered only by endoscopy. Return to the same dietary habits or stressful living that brought on the ulcer in the first place, and you can expect the ulcer to return sooner or later. Skip meals, eat fast, gulp down lots of coffee, aspirin and alcohol, smoke a lot of cigarettes, and it will more likely be sooner than later.

No need to lead the life of a monk. Just remember that all your treatment has done is turn back the clock.

While rates of surgery in general have risen in recent years, the rate of ulcer surgery has dropped. A study in 3 Seattle hospitals showed a 35 percent drop in ulcer surgery from 1971 to 1975 as compared to 1966 to 1970 (*Journal of the American Medical Association,* March 7, 1977). Part of that decrease may be due to improved medical treatment. Much of it simply follows the unexplained drop in ulcer incidence.

13
Hemorrhoids

"Nine out of every ten men have piles."
(ancient Chinese proverb)

"Women during the state of pregnancy, and just after the menses have finally left them, are peculiarly subject to the piles."
William Heberden (1710–1801), *Commentaries on the History and Cure of Diseases*

The Chinese, it seems, were guilty of statistical sloppiness and male chauvinism. But Dr. Heberden was right about women and hemorrhoids. A proctologist we talked to said hemorrhoids turned up in *only* 72 percent of the 2,000 rectal exams he had recently gone back to reconsider. And it's fairly common medical knowledge that women who have had children are as likely to develop hemorrhoids as men. In fact, pregnancy is the largest cause of the condition in young women, that is, women before the age of roughly 40 to 60 when the ravages of gravity and walking erect and plain old time take over to produce it. These causes, of course, also attack middle-aged men, and so in the elderly, hemorrhoids affect men and women about equally. But we're getting ahead of ourselves here. We've got some explaining to do before we can go on.

This chapter is going to be a little different from the others in the book, because hemorrhoids are not like the other surgical conditions we are considering. For one thing, they're the least serious problem covered, and for another, they're one of the least *treated* conditions on the list of common surgical complications. There were just under 200,000 operations to correct hemorrhoids in the U.S. last year, compared to nearly 800,000 hernia repairs and 500,000 gallbladder removals. So paltry were the hemorrhoid figures that the operation didn't even make the American College of Surgeons' Ten Most Frequent list, a distinction it last earned in 1968. This does not mean that a foolproof, nonsurgical means for the prevention and treatment of hemorrhoids has been developed, although *great* strides have been made. Nor does it mean that there are any fewer cases of hemorrhoids around lately. What it means is that hemorrhoids, being less dangerous and painful than, say, an obstructed bowel (at least in the early stages), are the most *ignored* of the major surgical problems. Ignored, because hemorrhoid exams can be embarrassing, and recovery from hemorrhoid surgery can be inconvenient and unpleasant. As a result, hemorrhoids are a structural failure whose consequences people often decide they can live with.

Because so many make that decision, for better or for worse, we're going to handle this chapter a little differently. Instead of taking you from the symptomatic beginnings of hemorrhoidal discomfort to its surgical conclusion in an informal but fairly technical essay, we're going to tell you a story—based on several case histories—which is centered around a step-by-step reconstruction of the complex set of experiences the patient goes through with the nuisance of hemorrhoids. We've decided to do things this way, because—in addition to warning you about the serious consequences of ignoring your condition—we want you to know that, no matter how embarrassing the examination looks to be, no matter how uncomfortable the convalescence promises to be, at least the 6 folks whose cases contributed to our story lived through them with their health, dignity and self-respect intact.

Another thing this story will do is help to introduce the hospital routines that are part of *each one* of the operations described in this book. Many of the things that befall and frustrate our hemorrhoid heroine have more to do with the state of hospitalization these days than with her particular medical problem. Things like the battery of defensive admissions tests she undergoes, the bookkeeping red tape, the insurance grillings, her hassles with overworked staff members and her ignorance of exactly how she's doing are, unfortunately, all part of being sick today, and we think you should be prepared for them. The huge plants and intricate processes that make up modern hospitals can overwhelm patients and drive the questions they should ask about their treatment right out of their heads. As a result, we'll try to gird you for the assault on your wits in this chapter and fortify you with batteries of ready-to-use questions about specific procedures in the others.

Once upon a time there was a woman named Eloise Williams. She had been seeing blood on the toilet tissue for several weeks and trying to ignore it. But there it was again, and somehow it concerned her more this morning. She was a practical woman who didn't baby herself, but she kept thinking about the faded list of cancer warning signals she had tacked on the inside of the medicine cabinet years ago. The blood and mild pain were probably nothing—hemorrhoids at worst—but she supposed she had better call her gynecologist. After she had started her family 30 years before, it had seemed easiest to continue consulting her gynecologist for her checkups and routine medical care.

"Well," Eloise began. She felt embarrassed to divulge such an unlovely complaint to the nurse but forged ahead. "The toilet paper has been bloody when I use the bathroom lately."

"What color is the blood?"

"Bright red."

"Are you having pain with defecation?"

Eloise had to think for a minute what defecation was. "Oh, yes, a little. But it's probably nothing."

"That's for the doctor to decide. I'll tell him and get back to you."

The nurse called later to say the doctor thought Mrs. Williams should see a colon and rectal specialist, a proctologist, right away. He suggested she call either of two offices; one was run by an individual doctor and the other by a group of doctors. She looked them both up in the phone book, deciding on the group practice because it was located much closer to her house. Besides, she decided, with several doctors working together she could probably get in sooner. On the day of her appointment, she signed her name to a stenographer's pad on a ledge outside the window that separated the office workers from the patients.

"Mrs. Williams," a receptionist called after Eloise had read halfway through a magazine article on decorating a nursery. Eloise was 49 and had delivered her last baby 23 years before, but she was expecting her first grandchild in April, several months hence.

"Sit here," barked a young woman in white who led her into an office and pointed to a chair across the desk from a slight and ancient man. This was Dr. Russell, she deduced from the gold nameplate on his desk.

"Hello, Mrs. Williams. My record here shows you have some pain and bright red bleeding. How long has this been going on?"

"Just the last few days," Eloise shortened it by several weeks, embarrassed that she had ignored the symptom for so long.

"Does it hurt just when you have a bowel movement, or for several hours afterward?" he asked in a gentle tone.

"Well, both, I think, although it doesn't hurt too much." Eloise, who never took novacaine for dental work and rarely took a pill of any kind, had what's known as a high pain threshold—even labor and an arm broken in several places hadn't bothered her much.

"How often do you move your bowels?"

"Oh, 3 or 4 times a week, I guess."

"Have you ever had any bowel trouble?"

"Not really, I guess I was a little constipated when I was carrying my kids, but that's been so long ago."

"Do your stools seem hard?"

"Well, lately, I guess they have been."

Eloise was relieved when the doctor dropped the subject of her bowels and went on to her personal health history. He quizzed her on the number of children she had had, her age, former surgery she had undergone, previous hospitalizations and the past and present ailments of herself and her family.

"That's all for right now," he concluded, pushing a button on his phone.

The young woman reappeared and ushered Eloise into an examining room.

Before we follow Mrs. Williams into the examining room, something needs to be said about her symptoms. They indicate that her hemorrhoids are not serious—yet. The bright red blood she's been noticing on the toilet tissue is usually the first—and often the only—sign that something is wrong. The doctor asked about bowel habits, because a change in them is normally the second warning. Hemorrhoids are varicose veins of the anal and rectal canal. Veins become varicose when unnatural swellings and knots develop in a vessel, obstructing the blood flow. Those blockages are caused by faulty valves or some other hindrance to proper circulation. Veins carry blood *back* to the heart after it's done its work around the body. Blood is pushed along the system by the massaging action of the muscles which surround each vein. It is prevented from flowing backward by flaplike valves located at regular intervals in the body's plumbing. If one of the valves should fail, or if some other blockage causes the blood flow to reverse, a varicosity or swelling or knot occurs when the weight of the pooling blood causes the vein wall to lose elasticity and bulge. A more common cause of such a failure, however, is a perfectly natural impediment to the blood's return to the heart. Many men and women with desk jobs develop varicose veins of the leg, because sitting for long hours produces physical obstructions at the knee and buttocks that prevent blood from leaving the lower extremities and returning to the heart. In Mrs. Williams' case—as it is with most women—varicose veins of the rectum occurred with pregnancy. During pregnancy, much more muscle force than normal is required to recycle blood from lower body areas to the chest, because the swollen uterus presses against the transporting veins and restricts their flow. The doctor asked Eloise about her deliveries, because he suspected they were the cause of her hemorrhoids.

When hemorrhoids develop—for whatever reason—they usually cause little trouble immediately. The veins involved may actually swell only during defecation—when straining further shuts down the blood flow—and then return to near normal afterward. The bleeding Eloise noticed is triggered when a varicose vein is forced through the membrane covering the rectal canal by the pressure of a bowel movement. As time passes, the vein wall becomes weaker and weaker and eventually will not return to its normal position after elimination. When this happens, the bleeding increases, and anemia can result. However, many people avoid treatment at even this late stage by learning to replace the bulging vein with their fingers and somehow convincing themselves that nothing serious is wrong. This is quite a project, because as the hemorrhoidal veins protrude for longer and longer periods, their covering is subjected to more and more irritation. As wastes are eliminated, they must squeeze past obstructing veins, and nagging trouble results. First, there is simple pain. Then the membrane begins to secrete a lubricating mucus in self-defense, and the patient complains of a "wet bottom." Finally nothing works—the constant abuse causes deep cuts in the anal passage which can become infected, and that produces an emergency. The worst thing that can happen to a hemorrhoid condition is the strangulation of permanently bulging veins. Swollen veins may be pulled so far out of their normal path by the strain and pull of defecation that they are bent double and their blood supply is cut off. When that occurs, an emergency situation definitely results.

Mrs. Williams's answers to her doctor's questions suggest that she's gone about halfway through these symptoms. She's had pain after moving her bowels, indicating that her varicose veins are not returning to normal after straining. That permanent swelling has resulted in irritation of the rectal wall. On the other hand, she has reported no trouble with elimination, and we can guess that the affected veins have not completely obstructed the passageway or strangulated.

Now, let's follow what happened during the rest of her examination.

"Kneel here," the nurse instructed, pointing to an examining table with what looked like a church kneeler attached on the end, a foot or two from the floor.

"Pull your dress up and everything else down."

Eloise sighed a little and complied. She felt the young woman cover her bottom with a drape before she left. She remained in that position, her dignity compromised, for what seemed like a half hour, but was probably 5 minutes. She had urinated before she left home, but by the time she had plowed through the traffic, parked, waited for her appointment and talked with the doctor, she had to go again. Pelvic exams, she knew, were uncomfortable if not impossible with a full bladder, but she wasn't sure if the same was true of a rectal exam. Anyway, she didn't know whom to ask where the bathroom was, and if the doctor came while she was gone, she would have to wait who knows how much longer with her behind up in the air.

She heard the door open again; Dr. Russell stood in the doorway, and summoned a passing nurse. Eloise hoped there were no curious passersby peeking in from the hall. Then Dr. Russell's dry, elderly voice was saying, "This may be uncomfortable, Mrs. Williams, but it shouldn't hurt."

The nurse pushed a button and the part of the table with Eloise's torso on it went slowly toward the floor. Her bottom was pushed up high and wide, if not handsome. Eloise felt like a beached whale.

"Ahh, ummm, yes," the voice continued as Dr. Russell probed with what Eloise was sure was a cactus. She gripped the sides of the table and was surprised to find herself blushing. After 3 children and myriad gynecological exams, she didn't think there was a blush left in her. The fullness in her rectum gave her the panicky feeling that her bowels were going to move. She tried to take her mind off the sensation by picturing the ducks she fed each morning in the park near her home.

"There now." Dr. Russell withdrew the fiendish instrument, an anoscope, rapidly. "You can dress and come in my office." Eloise dressed and hurried back to the chair she had sat in before.

"You must have been in pain for some time. You have hemorrhoids—several bad ones—and deep fissures, or cracks in the anal wall. Your operation will keep you in the hospital for about 3 days. In a week you can go back to work—do you work, by the way? Oh, well, in that case, you can start light housekeeping chores as soon as you're up to it. If it's painful to defecate, you can drink about 20 ounces of prune juice a day in the meantime. Drink less if your stools get too loose, or they will hurt as much as the hard ones do. My nurse will schedule the operation at Wardville Hospital Center—that's where my partners and I like to do this procedure. As you may have heard, recuperation from this operation used to be very painful. Of course, there will be some discomfort at first. But now techniques are improved. Your anesthetic will be local instead of general, which will help you recuperate faster. Any questions?"

Eloise's mind had gone blank as soon as she had heard the word "operation." She knew she would have questions later, but she couldn't think of any now.

Perhaps a look of our own at what Dr. Russell has seen will make clearer what's happened to Mrs. Williams and help us to understand what must be done to correct her condition. There are 3 large groups of veins—plus 2 smaller ones—in the rectal canal, but it is the larger collections that usually cause trouble. One large batch runs along the *top* of the canal and the other 2 come down either side. The smaller collections run between the larger veins on the lefthand side of the rectum. For purposes of identification, varicose veins *above* the anal sphincter—the muscular valve that closes the rectum—are called internal hemorrhoids, and varicosities *below* the sphincter are called external hemorrhoids. Frequently, hemorrhoids of the large vein clusters are accompanied by problems in the smaller groupings.

Hemorrhoids are further classified by their severity, that is, by the size of the varicose swelling and its position in the canal. In most cases, the longer the time a vein has been damaged and gone untreated, the more severe the hemorrhoidal condition is found to be when it *is* treated. If the vein swelling is fairly small and has never protruded below the sphincter line—and *will* not even when the patient is asked to strain during a doctor's examination—the internal hemorrhoidal condition is said to be of *first degree* severity. There may be no symptoms in these cases (a little bleeding is the most that can be observed), and frequently the person is totally unaware of such problems. *Second degree* internal hemorrhoids may be no larger than those of first degree severity, but they are usually older. The thin lining of the rectum is no longer strong enough to hold the swellings in place during defecation or other straining, and they drop down into the anal canal. However, after the strain, the lining is still resilient enough to return them to their normal position. *Third degree* vein damage means that the passage of feces has so weakened the rectal lining that it cannot snap hemorrhoids back into place after a bowel movement. That is the stage at which people must learn to replace them manually and to ignore the blood that usually appears on the toilet tissue—or seek treatment. Third degree hemorrhoids differ from *fourth degree* problems in that they remain in place between bowel movements. When the fourth degree is reached, the rectal lining has become so stretched (or, in fact, torn) that the varicose veins cannot be replaced manually. They become—in clinical language—"chronically prolapsed internal hemorrhoids." In plain language, they become such painful nuisances that they cannot be ignored. They cause serious bleeding, partial blocking of the anal canal, trouble with defecation and great difficulty in cleaning up afterward. Treatment must be sought.

External hemorrhoids—that is, those that *start off* below the sphincter valve—are not usually classified in this way, because they are detected and treated sooner. They don't normally have a chance to earn more than one degree.

But to return to our story.

Eloise had guessed she might have hemorrhoids but had hoped they would go away. She dreaded having to be like the postoperative hemorrhoidectomy patients she had seen, plopping pillows that looked like rubber life preservers on their chairs before they gingerly sat down. Finally, she gathered her wits enough to inquire, "What will happen if I don't have this operation?"

"You'll get worse," the doctor predicted. "It won't go away."

"I've got my kids coming next week for Christmas. Can I wait until January?"

"If you wish. It's probably a good idea for you to lose a few pounds before the operation; you're a little overweight. Call my nurse a week or two before you're ready to be admitted."

Dr. Russell directed Eloise to a smiling office helper who gave her a surgical slip to sign. "If you sign this now, you won't have to come in later to do it," she explained.

Eloise eyed it doubtfully, as it gave the doctor *carte blanche* to perform whatever surgical procedures he deemed necessary. She would rather have given permission only for the problems he had diagnosed. The office helper noticed her hesitation and laughed.

"Mrs. Williams, it's going to be done under local anesthetic. If they start to amputate your leg, you'll know it."

Eloise chuckled, too. After striking the section giving permission for the procedure to be photographed for a medical journal (and noting it was probably silly to think a medical journal would be interested in her hemorrhoids anyway), she signed on the dotted line.

"Just telephone when you're ready to go into the hospital," the girl said. Eloise hesitated a minute, feeling there was something else she wanted to know. When the girl said, "Bye now," she gathered up her things and left.

Harry, Eloise's husband, was sympathetic and a little concerned about the upcoming surgery when he came home from work.

"Would you like to have the other specialist Dr. Baxter recommended have a look? I've been reading a lot about unnecessary surgery lately. It wouldn't hurt to get another guy's opinion."

Eleanor sighed. "I would, Harry, but I just don't want to go through that awful exam any more than I have to.

Anyway, the problem seems pretty straightforward, and I don't think Dr. Baxter would refer me to a quack."

"That makes sense," her husband quickly agreed, sensing Eloise was more nervous about it than she was letting on.

"Do me a favor, Harry, don't tell anybody that I'm going in the hospital, not even the kids," Eloise begged her husband at dinner later.

"Are you sure? It might be nice to get some flowers and get-well cards." Harry, who complained vociferously about his rare stomachaches or head colds to anyone who would listen, had never been able to understand Eloise's silence about health problems.

"Well, it's minor, and I don't want to worry anybody. I won't be in the hospital long. Besides, it's such an icky thing, and I don't think I can stand a lot of jokes about the surgery being a pain in the rear. I just know Alice Jones would ask me at bridge the next week if everything came out all right."

"You've got a point there. My lips are sealed."

During the holidays, Eloise was so busy cooking, cleaning, wrapping presents and entertaining her family that she didn't think much about the surgery. Her mind strayed to it occasionally, much as a tongue explores the slightly tender site of a cold sore or pulled tooth. After Christmas, though, she called Dr. Russell's office and learned that elective surgery could not be scheduled at Wardville Hospital for at least 2 weeks. There had been an ice and snow storm in Wardville, and the beds were full of heart attack survivors who had shoveled too zealously, people who had broken bones in falls and victims of auto wrecks. Eloise was disappointed at the delay since she had wanted to get it over with. She wondered if Dr. Russell operated anywhere else, but she knew her case wasn't urgent, and she didn't want to seem pushy. An image of herself strapped face down and helpless on an operating table kept coming to her during the next 2 weeks, but by keeping busy with church work, bridge, shopping and entertaining, she pushed those thoughts away with some success.

On Monday, the hospital called to confirm that she would be admitted on Tuesday as scheduled. The admissions office asked her about her insurance coverage and told her to bring her Blue Cross-Blue Shield card. After learning that her husband was vice-president of Reliable Accounting, a large and respected firm in town, the officer asked her if she wanted a private or semiprivate room. Although the officer didn't indicate the difference in price, Eloise thought it would be considerable. She liked privacy, but her habit of frugality died hard, and as the operation wasn't very serious she said semiprivate would be just fine. The officer quickly hung up before Eloise was able to ask whether she should bring her own gown and robe, whether she would need cash, whether she would be allowed to bring the vitamins she customarily took and what time she would be operated on on Wednesday.

She had purposely planned a dinner party the night before her admission, correctly suspecting that it would keep her mind off the upcoming surgery. In fact, at 11:00 P.M. when the guests went home and she surveyed the wreckage of plates crusted with Veal Cordon Bleu, her hemorrhoidectomy was the furthest thing from her mind.

When Harry came home at noon the next day, he took Eloise to the hospital. Eloise followed the arrows in the lobby pointing to admissions, where a receptionist took her name and told her to sit down. Harry insisted on staying at the hospital until she was settled in her room. He tried to make conversation about the trip to England they were tentatively planning for spring, but Eloise was unusually quiet, and he gave up. The wait stretched into an hour, and Eloise was glad she had brought a book. Harry went to the snack bar for lunch, and Eloise lied that she had already eaten. In truth, she was too nervous to eat. And because no one had told her different, she thought perhaps food would affect her preadmissions tests. A cheerful volunteer in a salmon-colored smock brought her menus for the next 3 days while she waited.

"Well, I'm sure I won't be eating tomorrow before the surgery and probably I won't feel like it after. But I don't know when I'll be operated on, so I don't know what meals to check," Eloise debated.

"Just go ahead and check off what you would want if you were eating all the meals," the volunteer chirped.

Eloise frowned. It pained her to see food wasted, especially when hospitalization was so expensive. Harry assured her later that he would eat what she couldn't if meals were served when he was visiting.

The admissions officer noted their occupations (hers housewife, his accountant), place of employment and insurance policy number before slipping a printed plastic identification bracelet on Eloise's arm.

"Do you want a television?" she asked.

"No, thank you," answered Eloise, who would rather read than watch TV. She fervently hoped her roommate wouldn't be a game show fan.

"How about a telephone?"

"Give her one," Harry answered for her when she hesitated. "I'll probably call."

"Now, Mr. Williams, you can wait in Mrs. Williams's room, B4808, while she has her tests."

The admissions officer led Eloise to a chilly room where a harried receptionist tossed her a gown and pointed to a dressing room.

"Take everything but your underwear off and put this on," she directed.

When Eloise came back out holding her clothes, the receptionist wadded them up on a shelf. "You have your gown on backwards," she observed.

"Does it matter?" Eloise asked.

"I guess not. Sit down."

She gestured to folding chairs in front of her desk arranged as if for a piano recital. About 20 patients of both sexes and all ages, each dressed in a wrinkled yellow gown like Eloise's, waited for pre-admission tests.

In half an hour, Eloise's name was called. A silent lab technician with teased hair like cotton candy started drawing blood from a vein on the inside of Eloise's elbow into 3 tubes. Eloise watched in hideous fascination.

"What are you testing for?" asked Eloise, more for conversation than curiosity.

"Oh, lots of things," the technician replied. After the bloodletting, the technician gave her a Band-Aid and sent her back to her folding chair.

A few moments later, she was called for a chest x-ray. A friendly technician positioned her in front of the machine and got ready to take her picture. "Oh, I almost forgot," she gasped. "Any chance you could be pregnant?"

"At my age, it would make medical history. But I suppose there could be a chance in a million," replied Eloise, who used reasonable birth control but was still having menstrual periods and frequent sex.

"Then you'd better wear this," the technician said, tying a heavy leather apron around Eloise's ample waist.

"This would protect the fetus from radiation, just in case."

"Inhale . . . exhale," she called from in back of the machine. "Great, just one more now."

After the chest x-rays, Eloise waited another 10 minutes for an EKG. She had never had one before and was surprised at how quick, easy and painless it was. The technician attached tiny suction cups to her chest, hips and legs with greasy, white jelly. It was over momentarily.

"I thought you had to ride a bike or something," she said when the technician told her she could leave.

"Oh no, you're thinking of a stress EKG. It's for people with suspected problems. You just had a resting EKG. We give them to all our older—er—I mean, our patients over 40," the technician explained.

The receptionist told Eloise she could put her clothes back on. A volunteer was waiting outside her dressing room to take her to her room. It looked out unpleasantly on heating ducts and the roof of a wing below, but it was a light, clean room, reasonably free of hospital odors.

When Harry stopped by at 7:30 (he had left earlier in the afternoon) a half-hour before visiting hours were over, she still hadn't been told when her operation was scheduled.

"Did you ever find out when my surgery will be?" Eloise inquired of a nurse who came to take her blood pressure.

"Oops, I'm sorry. I forgot. I'll be right back," she dashed out.

"It's 8:00 A.M.," she said when she hurried back in. "I'm going to give you a Fleet's enema—it's just a little one. I want you to try to hold this about 10 or 15 minutes, as long as you can. And please don't flush. I'm going to check the returns."

Eleanor gasped a little when the enema was inserted, and the nurse apologized.

"I know it's not your fault," Eloise said. "It just hurts."

Almost immediately, she felt the urge to go to the bathroom. She called Harry to keep from thinking about it.

"Did Dr. Russell come and visit you?" he asked.

"No. I guess it's because it's so minor. I did want to ask him if I'd have any tubing or anything afterward, though. And I wondered if they'll keep me fairly doped-up so I won't know what's going on. I'm glad they're not going to knock me clear out, but it's funny to think about being operated on awake."

"I'm sure it will all be fine. You'll feel much better afterward. What time is the surgery?"

"Eight A.M. But don't bother to come, Harry. I'll have a nurse call you at the office. I don't know if they even allow visitors that early."

"Don't be silly. I'll be there. And you stop reading and turn off your light now. Sleep tight."

"Goodnight," Eloise hung up and made a dash for the toilet.

In the early hours of the morning, Eloise had another uncomfortable enema. The nurse took her bedside water pitcher and warned, "Don't drink anything now until after the surgery. You won't be able to wear makeup, fingernail polish or any jewelry to the operating room. Do you have any nail polish on? Good. Now I'm going to give you some pills. They'll make you sleepy. And later, you'll have a shot."

The next thing Eloise knew, Harry was at her side eating breakfast from a tray.

"What time is it?" Eloise asked him after glancing from habit at her now naked wrist.

"About 7:30."

Soon a nurse arrived and gave Eloise a painful but quick shot in her right buttock. For a few minutes, it continued to throb. Then a high, wide table with a mattress on it was wheeled alongside her bed. The pretty young woman who had pushed it in slipped a cap on Eloise's head.

"You might feel dizzy but I'm holding on to you. Can you just scoot over onto this bed?" Scooting took enormous effort, like running through a swimming pool full of water. How could a prone, drugged, 150-pound woman scoot? Eloise thought she might get the giggles.

"Say, Miss, can you call me as soon as she's in recovery?" Harry asked when they were on their way out.

"You bet," the nurse smiled and looked down at Eloise. "I don't think he wants to let you go."

"See you soon, Honey," Harry kissed Eloise's cheek and she smiled goodbye. She wanted to say something brave and clever but she couldn't think and her tongue wouldn't move.

On the way to the operating room, the corridors seemed to be sliding, so she gripped the sides of the table and closed her eyes. Her mouth was very dry. First she was taken to an enormous white room with beds on wheels, like hers, lining the walls. Many of them were occupied by forms she could barely distinguish. She was wheeled past a partly naked man. He called for the nurse to cover him.

"Hello, Mrs. Williams," a woman in green greeted her, checking Eloise's I.D. bracelet. Eloise wanted to answer, but her tongue felt huge and sandpapery, as though it were filling her mouth to the roof.

"I'll just check your blood pressure and temperature. Your turn in the operating room is coming up soon."

Then the bed was moving again. A bearded young man in a green scrub suit and mask greeted Eloise at the operating room door. He, too, checked her bracelet.

"Are you Eloise Williams?" he asked. She nodded, wondering if she could get out of the surgery if she lied. Dr. Russell was nowhere in sight. She wanted to ask for him, but the words wouldn't come out of her mouth. She heard a moan and looked around. There were no other patients in the room, so the moan must have been her own.

"You're fine, dear," whispered a reassuring nurse who saw her trying to speak. The dark-eyed nurse looked like a veiled Moslem with her green mask covering the lower half of her face. She helped Eloise roll onto her stomach on the operating table. Someone untied Eloise's hospital gown in the back and covered her with a heavy green drape that reminded her of a Girl Scout tent. She felt her arms being arranged around a pillow covered in the same heavy green cotton. She could feel chilly air on her bottom, the only part of her that was exposed besides her head and shoulders. Someone taped her bottom apart, and she was aware of several quick stinging sensations, like minature beestings, in her rectum. Her instinct was to jump but her body felt so heavy she couldn't move. She moaned, "Oh no, oh no."

We're nearly to the end of things here. Eloise has been given a local anesthetic, because many doctors feel that it leads to better results than general anesthesia. Her surgeon has decided that surgery is the only solution to her problems—there are other solutions to other problems, and we'll get to them in a minute.

The secret to successful hemorrhoid surgery is knowing what to cut and what not to cut. Unlike a varicose vein of the leg, where the entire damaged vessel is removed, only the bunched-up, bulbous section of a varicose vein of the rectum is removed. That means the surgeon must know just how much of the vein to remove and just how much of the surrounding tissue to take with it. The right decision in both cases means fewer complications after the operation. And the right decision is easier to make—many surgeons believe—with a local anesthetic. The end of the intestine which forms the anorectal canal retains its normal condition and shape with a local—it doesn't sag as it does under general anesthesia. Physical "landmarks" remain in place. Surgeons can maintain their bearings properly, and their work is more precise. And, of course, with this greater precision comes a greater chance that the anal canal will return to its normal circularity and diameter after the operation. And with *that* comes a decreased chance of your hemorrhoids recurring.

Eloise's body felt as if it were sliding slowly off the table. The brown-eyed nurse offered Eloise her hand and Eloise gripped it gratefully. She was dimly aware of the hum of voices and machinery and of pressure in her rectum, but there was no pain. Behind her there were clinking noises which she identified as the sound of used instruments falling into a metal tray.

She had lost all track of time. It didn't seem long before the bearded young man patted her shoulder and said, "It's all over now, Mrs. Williams. If you can help us a little, we'll roll you back onto the bed and take you to the recovery room."

Is Surgery the Only Answer to Hemorrhoids?

Now that surgery's all over for Eloise, let's go back and describe what was done to her, so *you'll* know what to expect if and when it befalls you. Remember the distinction we made between internal and external hemorrhoids? Well, it's important here. In certain cases, the internal type (those *above* the sphincter line) can be injected with an irritating liquid that eventually obliterates the swelling with scar tissue, or can be strangled with rubberbands. Injection and rubberbanding, however, are most successful when used in relatively mild, quickly detected cases. The external type of hemorrhoids (those *below* the sphincter line) usually cannot be managed by either injection or rubberbanding. The distinctions we made between first, second, third, and fourth degree hemorrhoids are also crucial here: they tell us when surgery is necessary and when it can be avoided by such means as changes in diet or exercise habits. Patients whose first or second degree hemorrhoids are discovered by accident will probably be told about good bowel habits and anal hygiene by their doctors and put on a program designed to postpone or prevent the worsening of their symptoms. That program will be either vague or clear depending on the physician, but it should include the recommendation of a high-fiber diet, which, by softening the stool, will decrease its irritation of the hemorrhoidal swellings. Stay tuned until the end of the chapter for the rest of our diet recommendations. If bleeding is the only symptom reported by the patient and his hemorrhoids appear to be first degree in size, doctors will usually examine the entire rectum and lower colon (with a proctosigmoidoscope, a tiny, flexible, lighted telescope) to make sure that the blood is not coming from a cancer, polyps or some other inflammatory disease. When bleeding is a factor with early-stage hemorrhoids, doctors normally augment their lecture on bowel movements with prescriptions for a bulk-type laxative to soften the stool, and chemical suppositories to reduce swelling. A high-fiber diet, however, does better than the foul-tasting laxatives, and most suppositories aren't worth what they cost and can be replaced with cold compresses of witch hazel and warm sitz baths. Witch hazel, an astringent, tends to reduce hemorrhoidal swelling as effectively as the more exotic preparations.

If these conservative means control the bleeding of early hemorrhoids but do not check their growth, there are few things doctors can try before resigning themselves and their patients to surgery. If the varicose swellings of first or second degree hemorrhoids are reducible—that is, can be put back in place with the fingers—most physicians will teach their patients to do this tidying up. The process is managed lying down and should be followed by firm compresses and at least a few hours of bed rest. A word to the wise, though: some people require a few *days* off their feet after the feat, and many need a pain-killer to accomplish it.

If bleeding becomes heavier despite these medical efforts, injection therapy is usually the answer for internal hemorrhoids of the first and sometimes the second degree. It can also be used to give temporary relief to an old or very sick patient who cannot undergo surgery. The reason that injection was not a possibility for Mrs. Williams is that her hemorrhoids had advanced beyond the second degree in size, and their presence had caused what Dr. Russell called "fissures"—cracks—in the anal canal. The existence of such cracks always nixes that technique. Injection, for those cases it can help, involves the introduction of an irritating chemical directly into the hemorrhoidal swelling. The scarring that results from this unsocial introduction can erase or at least confine the swelling, but published results claim success in no more than 50 percent of all applications. A rule of thumb says that the younger and more uncomplicated hemorrhoids are, the more effectively they can be helped by injection. The technique is usually done in a doctor's office or on an outpatient basis. If the swellings are large, one is injected on each visit and separated from the next treatment by 3 or 4 days.

With second degree hemorrhoids of a little greater size and age, the inelegantly but aptly named "rubberband method" of treatment is sometimes used as a means of staving off—at least for a time—full-scale surgery. In effect, this method causes a varicose vein to age unnaturally and die by strangling it with a rubberband. Again, it's suitable for use only with internal hemorrhoids. What happens here is that a rubberband is shot around a swollen vein with a specially constructed gun, and this band pinches the vein, cuts off its blood supply and causes it to shrivel and fall away in 8 to 10 days. It's one case when gangrene works in the patient's favor. When done by a practiced hand, this peculiar kind of target-shooting is an office procedure, requires no anesthetic and produces little pain. When going properly, the work of the rubberband proceeds without discomfort to the patient. However, it's best to treat each large batch of veins separately, and each varicose vein may require more than one rubberband strangulation before succumbing. Such treatments usually are administered 2 or 3 weeks apart. Unfortunately, this method (like injection) more often attacks the symptoms of the problem than the difficulty itself and so cannot be counted on to eliminate the possibility of later, more elaborate surgery. It does best with small to medium-sized second degree hemorrhoids and with patients who are not strong enough to have more complete operations. In fact, one standard medical reference book is positively snooty about the whole idea. It concludes, "This method has limited popularity."

You've already seen the indignities Eloise went through. Now we need to get behind the scenes. Her hemorrhoid surgery was complete—*all* of the varicose veins involved were removed—by a process which is called "closed hemorrhoidectomy." The operation is done under one of the common local anesthetics—a chemical freezing agent, a spinal or a caudal block—and involves cutting away the damaged or incompetent veins that form the hemorrhoids. It is a job that requires a sharp knife, a great deal of experience and a thorough knowledge of the anatomy involved. For this reason, when choosing a surgeon, you should probably select a doctor who does a lot of hemorrhoid operations over a well-recommended general surgeon. All this care is necessary on your part and the doctor's, because there's a crucial decision to be made about halfway through the whole business. When the varicose veins are snipped away, some of the rectal lining and its underlying tissue must go with it. The trick is knowing how much, knowing how to free the hemorrhoids without ruining their neighborhood, without narrowing the rectal canal and turning it into a bottleneck. So difficult are these decisions that some doctors do not sew closed the areas which are cut during the operation, because to do so would be to mess up their calculations. The pulling together of the sutures (which is just like drawing closed a duffel bag) might produce a narrowing of the canal. Even leaving the areas open and allowing them to scar over shrinks the canal a bit, because scar tissue decreases in size as time goes by and thus tends to pull the canal's drawstrings too. To counteract this inevitable crowding, some fibers of the muscles which form the anal sphincter are cut to relax and enlarge it. No harm comes of this, because the muscle heals as the rest of the tissues do, but the canal opening is larger as a result. And a great deal of harm could come from not doing it. If too much of the circumference of the anorectal canal is lost, defecation becomes a painful proposition, and, in some very extreme cases, next to impossible.

The operation is a slow and careful process of dissection and blood control. The damaged veins are gingerly freed from the lining and tissues of the anal canal, and as each of their supplying blood vessels is uncovered, it is tied off with sutures to stop it from bleeding. Because the skill with which this is done determines the success of the patient's recovery, we say again that you should seek out an experienced hemorrhoid surgeon rather than a jack-of-all-trades for your repair. That advice is especially important if the hemorrhoids cross or start or stop around the anal sphincter.

It is absolutely imperative that the varicosities be liberated from the sphincter without damaging it. Slight damage to this valve now can result in big trouble later. After completing these procedures, some doctors dress the wound with a flexible surgical foam and others merely apply a liberal amount of antiseptic cream before releasing the patient to the recovery room.

The procedures we've talked about here are pretty much the whole picture in the U.S. There are, however, 2 quite simple operations which are being done with increasing frequency in Europe, operations that promise instant relief for the hemorrhoid sufferer with very little of the pain that Eloise experienced after her conventional surgery. Both are being used in place of traditional and complete hemorrhoidectomies. One is called "Lord's dilatation" after its inventor, Peter H. Lord, a British surgeon, and the other has been dubbed an "internal sphincterotomy" by its devisor, a Swiss doctor named Allgower.

Neither of these pioneers accepts in whole cloth the theory that hemorrhoids are caused by a circulation problem, and both would rather relate the disease to a peculiar kind of constipation. Each man maintains that abnormal tissue bands exist around the anal canal of the hemorrhoid victim and strangle it, constrict it to such a degree that normal defecation gradually becomes impossible. These bands force the patient to strain so hard when defecating that great pressures are built up which actually dam up the blood in anorectal veins and cause them to fail, to become varicose. Both doctors say that conventional surgical treatments of varicose anal veins attack their symptoms without touching their source, these bands, which both term a "vicious circle" around the anus. Here, however, their agreement ends.

Lord says he doesn't know where the bands are apt to turn up in a given patient. They can grow at any point in the anal canal and must be located by touch. Once the culprits are found, they are stretched—again by hand (or rather finger)—and broken, thus enlarging and relaxing the anal canal. Dr. Allgower says he knows exactly where the offending bands are in every patient; they *always* grow in or around the anal sphincter, he says, and can be treated by snipping that valve a bit, a kindly cut that serves the same purpose as Lord's manipulation and dilatation. That increases the size of the canal, ends an unnatural constriction and relieves the artificial constipation that has plagued the patient and produced his hemorrhoids.

The advantages of both procedures are that they take very little time—a matter of minutes, really—and require very light anesthesia. Patients undergoing the procedures recover quickly, and the surgeries can be done on an outpatient basis. All except those whose work is very hard labor can return to the job a day or two after treatment. Best of all, neither operation causes much pain. Even the first bowel movement after surgery is no problem.

The disadvantages of each procedure are similar, too. The procedures can be sabotaged by an overzealous surgeon. If a Lordsman stretches the canal too much, or if an Allgower disciple snips a bit too generously, their patients may have trouble controlling their bowels. In truth, there is more danger of too much of a good thing with the Allgower process, and Lords-patients frequently suffer the opposite complication. Their anal canals shrink after a time and problems of constriction and hemorrhoids return. For this situation, Lord has invented a bullet-shaped appliance which the patient can use whenever it's necessary to redo the work of the stretching.

Neither of these innovations has been around very long, and neither has been thoroughly tested. Lord keeps talking about the same 100 patients in descriptions of his process, and Dr. Allgower doesn't mention numbers at all. Most surgeons we talked to are intrigued by the new developments but are content to wait and see how their originators' experience shapes up in wider practice. So are we, although we'd say now that at least the theory behind these practices looks good.

The recovery room nurse gave Eloise a shot that made her even sleepier.

"That is for pain," she whispered. "You don't feel any, but we don't want you to wake up hurting when you're back in your room."

With her eyes closed Eloise felt someone lift her arm and constrict it with what felt like a giant rubberband. Then she drifted into uneasy sleep, waking momentarily and trying to read the clock on the wall. She gave up, unable to remember whether the big hand indicates the hour or the minutes. Once when she awoke, she noticed gratefully that there were no tubes trailing from her.

"Can you wiggle your toes, Mrs. Williams? Can you open your eyes? Can you open and close your fists?" someone was asking.

"She seems fully reactive," a different voice observed.

The bed was moving again in what Eloise thought was a circle with her body in the middle. The twirling stopped when she came to an elevator. A curious little boy stared down at her with a face like a bobbing balloon. She closed her eyes.

"I was beginning to wonder," Harry exclaimed softly after she was settled in bed. "It's 10:30 now and no one ever told me you were in the recovery room. How do you feel?"

Unable to concentrate, she stared at him and drifted off to sleep, with him holding her hand. When she woke up, it was 3:30. Harry had left a note saying he would be back during evening visiting hours.

She looked around the room. There were carnations in a wicker basket on the window ledge, bless Harry's heart. Eloise drifted in and out of a fitful sleep, frequently jerking with panic, afraid she was falling out of bed. When Harry returned, she felt more awake than she had since the night before. Too awake, in fact. She was nauseated and grumpy, and her bottom was very sore. She wasn't in deep pain, but the skin in her rectum felt raw and scraped, as the heel of her hand had felt when she fell and scraped it on a rough cement sidewalk. She tried to lie on her stomach but it hurt too much to turn.

"May I have a shot for pain?" Eloise asked when a nurse came in and took her blood pressure.

"I'm afraid not. Your blood pressure's a little low. But I'll call your doctor and see if I can get you some pills. Have you urinated yet?"

"No."

"Try running some water over your fingers. I have an order to catheterize you if you can't go."

Eloise lurched to the bathroom with Harry's help and eked out a drop of urine.

"There now," she smiled at her husband for the first time that afternoon. "No catheter for me."

The nurse did not return for 2 hours. Eloise felt like crying. It felt like someone was holding a lighted match to her behind. Harry was getting angry.

"Maybe you should have gone to the old hospital, " he muttered. "It doesn't matter how modern the place is if they can't keep you from hurting."

Easing through Postop Discomforts

Eloise has gotten by the most serious postoperative complication of hemorrhoidal surgery (the retention of urine), but she still must face the most uncomfortable one—her first postoperative bowel movement. Trouble voiding the bladder is not uncommon with general or local anesthetics used in the lower abdomen or pelvis. The effects of the anesthesia linger in the bladder and urethral sphincter and can cause real discomfort if the patient is allowed too much to drink just before surgery or during the first day of recovery. Problems with retention can also come from the anxiety that surgery naturally brings, overzealous sedation against pain and obstruction of the prostate (in men) caused by swelling. Whatever the cause of the blockage, simple measures normally eliminate it. As you've seen, warm water over the fingers, a warm compress on the tummy, even a sitz bath will often bribe or trick the urinary system into working. Only rarely are drugs or catheterization required.

Trouble with the elimination of solid wastes is also encountered in a fair number of hemorrhoid surgery patients. In some hospitals hemorrhoidectomy patients are routinely given mineral oil to avoid this difficulty until their first bowel movement and a bulk laxative after it until their release from the hospital. Sometimes, however, the problem stems from a surgical miscalculation. Too much tissue was removed along with the varicose veins, and the anal canal has become too narrow to do its job. In these cases, doctors try to stretch the canal with their fingers (using a local anesthetic), but if that doesn't work, they must widen it surgically. Sometimes the preventive measures backfire. Too many laxatives are given; the patient's stool come out unformed, and the canal shrinks to a dangerous narrowness, because it is not stretched by the waste it passes.

Sometimes the cause of this constipation is psychological. The patient fears that a bowel movement will be painful and refuses to test the theory for himself. The pain of the first few bowel movements after a hemorrhoid operation—to be very honest—is no laughing matter. One doctor we consulted—a man whose descriptive powers exceeded his sense of decorum—likened the experience "to having barbed wire pulled through the rectum." But it is an unpleasant experience that must be risked.

The result of any of these causes of constipation can be impaction of the stool, and that may require (on the rare occasions that it occurs) an enema or even the doctor's fingers to correct—a painful procedure requiring light anesthesia.

The only other common complication of hemorrhoidal surgery is bleeding. Bleeding right after the operation usually means that one of the veins was improperly tied off and is leaking. It must be retied under anesthesia. Bleeding a week or so after the surgery often means that the wound has pulled from one of the vein ends and loosened its suture. Again, the knot must be redone.

When everything goes as it should, a person who has had hemorrhoid surgery is allowed to leave the hospital 3 to 5 days after the operation, and they recover without a hitch in fairly short order. Two weeks after the operation, the doctor will probably want to check his handiwork to make sure there hasn't been a serious narrowing of the anorectal canal, and the patient should be back to work (or doing whatever he normally does) within a few days to a week after his release from the hospital.

Finally the nurse from whom she had requested pain pills came in. The nurse promised Eloise she could have the medication as soon as her temperature was taken and her dressing (which was like a miniature sanitary napkin), was checked. Since Eloise's temperature was over 100°, the nurse insisted Eloise try some cold ginger ale after she took the pills. The smell of food repelled Eloise, but the soft drink tasted surprisingly good. The pills took much longer to go into effect than the shots she had received earlier in the day. She was still hurting when Harry kissed her goodnight and pulled the curtain separating her bed from her roommate's on his way out.

The oblivious roommate soon pushed the curtain aside and offered to turn up the color TV so both of them could watch the comedy special that was making her shout with laughter. Eloise declined, and the roommate mercifully turned off her lights and television when the show was over at 10:00 P.M. The pills were finally bringing Eloise some relief, but she didn't sleep well that night. Her blood pressure and temperature were taken several times, and twice she was offered pain pills, which she gratefully accepted.

By morning, her bottom still hurt, but Eloise felt much better. She choked down half a piece of cold toast and a cup of tepid coffee. A nurse she had not seen before took her blood pressure, and Eloise asked permission to take a shower.

"I don't see why not. Just ring if you need some help. There's a call bell in the bathroom. Turn around and run some warm water over your bottom when you shower—I've had this surgery myself and I remember that helped," she advised.

The shower relieved the soreness, especially when she followed the nurse's helpful suggestion, but the exertion made Eloise feel heavy limbed and tired. Still dizzy, sweating and slightly nauseated, she was a little afraid she might fall. She made it to a chair and rested a few minutes before hauling herself back to bed. Eloise was happy to note that while she was in the shower, her roommate—who had not been significantly silenced by preoperative medication—had been taken to the operating room. She put on some makeup, combed her hair and began to feel much stronger. Just as she picked up the book she had felt too ill to read the day before, the bearded young man from the operating room appeared and sat down in the chair near her bed.

"How do you feel?"

"Fine," Eloise answered with automatic courtesy. Although she felt much better, she was still considerably less than fine. "Who are you?"

"Dr. Jacobs."

"Are you the one that did the surgery?"

"Yes. It was routine and easy. It went very well."

"Do you work with Dr. Russell?"

"Yes. We're in group practice together."

Eloise was stunned. Since Dr. Russell was the only one who had spoken to her or examined her, she had expected him to perform the operation. But she realized it wasn't the young doctor's fault, and she hated to make a fuss.

"Do you have any questions?"

"Yes. When can I go home?"

"Today, if you really think you feel like it. But you'll have to leave the hospital by 10, or Blue Cross won't pick up the tab. If you stay past 10, you'll be charged for another day."

"Oh, dear, that's only a half an hour from now. I'll have to hurry and call my husband. I really don't want to stay another night."

"Any other questions?" The doctor stood up.

"Well, yes." Because Eloise was always flustered around doctors, she had written down her questions on a slip of paper the night before the operation, when she was expecting a visit from Dr. Russell. The few that had to do with surgery and anesthesia no longer applied. She did ask Dr. Jacobs whether she could lift grocery bags and laundry baskets, how soon she could drive and how soon she could go up and down the steps of her two-story house.

"As soon as you feel like it," he replied, chuckling. "You must have stayed up all night thinking up those questions."

The comment nettled Eloise a little but she let it pass. The doctor tossed a mimeographed sheet of postoperative instructions on her bed on his way out. It said to avoid wine and beer, wipe with wet cotton balls after bowel movements and take several sitz baths a day.

"Wait, doctor, please. Before you go, what's a sitz bath?"

"The nurse will show you," he called over his shoulder as he hurried out. Eloise took advantage of the option the doctor had given of leaving that day.

By the time Eloise had carried her gear up to her own bedroom and unpacked, she was exhausted and hurting. She flopped on the bed fully dressed, and only got up once all morning, to cut the hateful hospital bracelet off her wrist. During the first few days, the least exertion made her tired to the point of weepiness. She could eat only thin soup, crackers and soft drinks without throwing up. The Demerol the doctor had prescribed took the pain away but made her disoriented—and distorted her sense of time.

Going up and down steps seemed to make her bottom more sore, as did walking any distance. It was hard to find a comfortable position to sit or sleep. She had a slight fever and mild pain at night. Although the first bowel movement was painful, it wasn't as bad as she had feared. Within a week, she was back on her regular schedule; within 10 days, she felt better than she had before the operation.

The bill from the hospital came, showing that the insurance company had to pay $600, while the only out-of-pocket charge to the Williamses was $2 for the phone. Harry joked that they had saved money since he had eaten his meals from her hospital tray.

Eloise had 3 postoperative checks over the next 2 months, starting 2 weeks after the surgery. For each appointment, the nurse positioned her on the kneeler, where she waited 5 to 15 minutes for her exam. In no case did any of the doctors look at her face or greet her by name before examining her behind. Each time she was seen by a different doctor—once by Dr. Russell, once by Dr. Jacobs, and once by the third doctor in the group practice. None of them told her when to stop taking sitz baths and pain pills, although all asked how often her bowels moved and told her to drink lots of water.

When Dr. Baxter, Eloise's gynecologist, asked at her annual checkup how the operation had gone, Eloise told him she liked Wardville Hospital.

"The operation went just fine," she smiled.

Eloise dismissed the surgery from her mind as soon as the postoperative discomfort waned. Although she was not taken with the surgeons personally she believed she had had basically good medical care.

"Well, hospitalization and surgery are never pleasant," she told Harry after she recuperated. "But I think they did a good job on me, and what counts is that I feel fine now."

All that you've just read is the *bad* news—what happens when you have a fairly advanced case of hemorrhoids and must face some kind of surgery. The *good* news—that hemorrhoids can be avoided or cleared up without surgery (if caught soon enough)—is considerably shorter and, of course, sweeter. But there is a catch. We've got to deal with a good-sized medical controversy to get to this happy news.

The standard medical opinion these days is that hemorrhoids—like varicose veins elsewhere in the body—are caused by some impairment to normal circulation. There are, however, a body of medical thought and a bunch of medical/legal wrangles that question this opinion. People frequently seek Workmen's Compensation for cases of hemorrhoids, claiming that the hemorrhoids were caused by long hours of sitting at work, by the hard, cold sitting surfaces there, or by the same kind of straining and lifting that many say causes hernias. Their bosses usually counterclaim that the hemorrhoids in question were caused by constipation, something for which the employee—not the employer—is responsible. When such arguments get to court, doctors called to testify say that it's not as simple as either side claims, and that both points of view have some merit. Hard chairs themselves are not the cause of hemorrhoids so much as sitting for long hours on *any* surface. A chair's pressure on the knee and buttocks can dam up the flow of blood between the lower limbs and the heart, and the added push needed to break the dam may result in varicose veins in the rectal canal.

When they get to the other side of the question, constipation, these doctors pretty much repeat themselves. Sporadic bouts of constipation do not cause hemorrhoids, they say, but again it's not that simple. Years of straining to pass hard, small stools may contribute to the condition. The lack of natural bulk or fiber in nearly *everyone's* diet produces the small, hard stools (which *are* a kind of chronic, low-grade constipation), and this condition—if it doesn't actually cause hemorrhoids—certainly aggravates problems that get started in other ways. To a certain extent both these controversies—the argument over the role chairs play in hemorrhoid conditions and the one over constipation's contribution—have been swept under the rug by medical insurers. Most insurance companies are swayed by the diagnosis of impaired circulation and studies which show that hemorrhoids tend to run in families, and they pay off without question, rendering academic most Workmen's Compensation claims.

But we shouldn't let the subject go that easily. There is evidence in the constipation flare-up to suggest that mild hemorrhoids *can* be stopped short without surgery and that cases just beginning can be kept to the first degree with a high-fiber diet.

To Prevent Hemorrhoids, Put More Fiber in Your Diet

Whatever the cause of hemorrhoids, whether it's evolution punishing man for choosing to walk upright without permission, or heredity, or a basic flaw in the muscle structure that allows the anus to function during elimination (all of which are theories recently advanced without proof), one thing is very clear. Hemorrhoids are terribly common among people who eat a highly refined and synthetic (they, of course, would say "sophisticated") diet and next to nonexistent among folks who favor simpler, more natural fare. Pioneer studies of diet and disease done by Denis Burkitt, a British surgeon, have shown that the incidence of hemorrhoids is very high in Western Europe and the United States, where "Ding Dongs" and french fries abound, and very low in most African countries, where whole grains and root vegetables are staples. His studies—first reported in the *British Medical Journal* in June, 1972—have even shown that the number of hemorrhoid cases is greater among urban Africans than among their rural neighbors, and that this increase corresponds to the city folks' tendency to adopt the puny diet of the European colonists who originally built the cities.

The magic ingredient in these "primitive" diets, of course, is fiber. Its presence in food makes for large, soft stools, and they produce less wear and tear—literally—on the anus and rectum. In some ways, then, it doesn't matter what produces hemorrhoids. They usually start out as small problems which are aggravated by things that have nothing to do with their cause. It's the worsening of these aggravating factors and symptoms we must fight. Because the large, soft stools of a bulky diet pass easily through the system, they tend *not* to irritate minor varicose veins in the rectum and anal canal. African women, obviously, are just as prone to circulatory disorders (and hence hemorrhoids) during pregnancy as Western women, but the roughage-filled foods they eat keep the swellings small and allow them to be slowly pulled back into place by the natural elasticity of the canal lining. Western women, with their relatively fiberless diet, tend to enlarge their hemorrhoids each time they have bowel movements. The point is that if—as we have seen—simple, no-trouble, first degree hemorrhoids often become big-trouble third or fourth degree hemorrhoids because of hard, small stools, they can be kept down and surgery can be avoided by adopting a stool-softening, high-fiber diet.

The most convenient way to get more fiber into your diet is to make friends with wheat bran. For the best results, get plain, unprocessed, inexpensive bran, not bran cereals. Begin by eating 1 tablespoon a day mixed into oatmeal, yogurt, soup or even juice. A few days later, raise your intake to 2 tablespoons a day and see if the results are any better. At some point between 1 and 3 tablespoons a day, you should notice the desired effects. Although your stools will be larger, they will be much softer and will pass much more quickly and easily. But remember, in order for bran to do its work, it has to have water to absorb; if you aren't in the habit of drinking much water add a glass or so a day to your routine.

Other than bran, the kind of fiber you need is also found in whole wheat bread (which contains about 4 times more total fiber than white bread), whole grain cereals such as oats and corn, as well as potatoes, beans, peas, carrots and apples. Stay away from prune juice, because it doesn't work by softening the stools; what it does is mildly irritate the bowel, producing a defecation reflex. And don't try to get your fiber from salads, either. Lettuce, cucumbers and tomatoes are nearly all water, and you would have to eat mammoth portions to get results comparable to those a tablespoon or two of bran can produce.

14
Hysterectomy

Take any assemblage of 100 American women. They can be chaperoning their children and grandchildren to a Saturday matinee, "couponing" their way through a crowded aisle of supermarket specials or circling the track at the YWCA. If current surgical trends continue, 62 of them will have had hysterectomies before they have reached age 70.

Topping tonsillectomy, hysterectomy has risen to become our nation's number one major operation. And the figures keep climbing. According to the Hospital Record Study, 702,000 hysterectomies were performed in 1977—a 31 percent increase over 10 years ago.

Clearly, hysterectomy rates in this country are high—too high, say certain consumer research groups who charge that 15 to 40 percent may be done unnecessarily. What they want to know is:

- Why do U.S. surgeons remove twice as many wombs as British or Welsh physicians do?
- Why does our hysterectomy rate continue to soar despite the fact that uterine disease is actually on a downswing?
- Why is it that of all the hysterectomies performed, only about 10 to 20 percent are done to curb cancer or other life-threatening disease?
- And why does the same gynecological complaint result in hysterectomy for one woman, nonsurgical treatment for another and no treatment at all for still another?

It's enough to make you suspicious, at the very least. But, before you become so scalpel-shy as to avoid surgery when it would be in your best interest, there's more to the hysterectomy story than meets the critical consumer eye.

For one thing, if money is a motivating factor in recommending hysterectomy—as some consumer advocates have charged—why is it that the operation rate is higher than average in physicians' families?

In defending the number of hysterectomies performed, physicians point to some obvious problems justifying surgery.

"I think you are going to find that there are unnecessary hysterectomies being performed. No question about it," says John Mikuta, M.D., chief of gynecological oncology at the Hospital of the University of Pennsylvania. "But you have to be careful about what you're calling 'unnecessary.' Sometimes, it's a matter of opinion. . . ."

Stanley J. Birnbaum, M.D., professor of obstetrics and gynecology at Cornell Medical College, explains. "A prolapsed uterus is a perfectly legitimate indication for performing a hysterectomy. Yet, outside of the body, the uterus appears normal. That doesn't mean that the operation was unnecessary. Sometimes the indication for hysterectomy is not a disease in the uterus; it's a mechanical problem with the uterus. And that's difficult to substantiate with just a pathology report."

At least one stumbling block to determining whether hysterectomy is warranted is the definition of "necessary."

Years ago, when hysterectomy was an extremely risk-ridden surgical procedure, it was considered acceptable or "necessary" when the only other alternative was death. In other words, if your life depended on the surgery, you'd have it. And if it didn't, you wouldn't. Simple.

Today, however, since hysterectomy has become a relatively safe surgical procedure (that is, as far as surgery can be called "safe"), it is no longer reserved for life-or-death ordeals. Indeed, the majority of women have hysterectomies to improve the quality—not the length—of their lives.

This is not altogether wrong. A fibroid tumor may not put a woman's life on the line, but it may cause enough pain to drive her off the brink of despair. Likewise, a prolapsed uterus won't kill you. But if surgery can correct the problem and make life more livable, then why not have it? There are many acceptable reasons for hysterectomy, albeit not exactly lifesaving or "necessary" in the previous sense of the word.

The main trouble with this liberalization of hysterectomy indications is that—aside from a few life-threatening conditions including cancer of the lining of the uterus or advanced cervical cancer—there are no absolute criteria for determining when the surgery is warranted. Elective hysterectomies are performed for fallen wombs, fibroid tumors, endometriosis, profuse menstrual bleeding, backaches, headaches and other premenstrual miseries, sterilization and, even cancer prevention—again, all perfectly valid indications for hysterectomy, but none appropriate to all of the women all of the time. Much hinges on the severity of the problem, the degree of discomfort, the age and childbearing status of the woman, the availability of alternative treatment, and the expertise and judgment of the physician.

Sometimes the necessity for surgery is easy to evaluate. For example, a 50-year-old woman suffering from backaches and loss of urinary control as a result of a uterus which has fallen to the bottom of her vaginal canal is a prime candidate for a hysterectomy. But a 33-year-old woman who wants another child and whose uterus is only slightly prolapsed isn't. Now, where does that leave the 40-year-old woman with a partial prolapse? Or, the 35-year-old newlywed with a more severe prolapse problem? There are many gray areas.

Unfortunately, if you don't understand the exact state of your condition or the options available in treating it, you could be misled to believe that surgery is the only way out of a gray zone. A New York woman we spoke with discovered this in the nick of time.

> I had been going to a gynecologist for many years, every 6 months or so. He was a very prominent doctor and a busy man. Every exam, he would ask me if I was losing water and I would say no. This went on for several years. Eventually I did lose a little water—it was just a matter that after urina-

tion, when I stood up, a trickle would go down my leg. It was a very minor problem, and if it bothered me at all, I would never have thought in terms of surgery. But since he had been asking so many times, I wondered if possibly it was important and I told the doctor about it. I thought it might have to do with something he was seeing and not telling me about. When I told him about it, he said probably the muscle was a little slack from having 2 children. He said he could do some plastic work to repair it. He added that when that plastic work was done, he usually would take the uterus, too. Well, that frightened me because I have a very healthy uterus, and I've never had any problems with it whatsoever. I was in my 40s. I didn't plan to have any more children, but I saw no reason for having my uterus removed.

The doctor told me to think about the surgery and he gave me some exercises to do to tighten that muscle. These exercises, by the way, practically eliminated the problem—or else it eliminated itself. I don't know.

The next time I was in, he asked me if I had been thinking about the surgery. I said I had, and he asked if my husband was in the office. I said yes, and he brought my husband into the office and started showing him diagrams of a prolapsed uterus and said this was what I had. Now I had never had any of the symptoms of a prolapsed uterus and the doctor had never, in all of his examinations, mentioned this possibility to me. He asked us if we thought I would have the surgery and we said that if he really thought it was necessary we probably would. He was a busy and respected man. It certainly never occurred to me that he might want to create surgery.

So we took it through my union [source of this woman's health insurance] and I decided to get a second opinion. The second doctor told me that my uterus was in excellent condition for a woman my age. He said there was no prolapsed uterus, that in fact my uterus was in a good position.

Well, that confused me, because here I had this second report conflicting with the recommendation of this doctor I had been going to for years. So I went to a third doctor. He agreed completely with the second doctor and said there was no need for a hysterectomy whatsoever. So of course, I didn't have it. I never told the first doctor. I just never went back to him.

Fortunately, this woman was spared unneeded surgery. But how many more are less fortunate? Probably more than you'd think. Philip Cole, M.D., professor of epidemiology at Harvard School of Public Health, blames the rise in hysterectomies on what he terms "borderline symptomatology." In other words, the woman's symptoms may just hint of an indication for hysterectomy, and the physician will recommend surgery—often "based on the rationale that if a woman is 35 or 40 years old and has an organ that is disease-prone and of little or no further use, it might as well be removed."

Apparently, too, that is a position held by more than a small minority of gynecologists. Several years ago, for example, while one of the authors was waiting her turn to see a very prominent GP, she overheard his words of consolation to a distraught hysterectomy patient.

"Don't look at it *that* way," he admonished her wails over the impending loss. "The uterus is a useless organ anyway—at least once you've had your family. Besides, it's best to get it out now before any *real* trouble starts. Would you rather wait until you got cancer?" he asked as if the disease were inevitable. "Or risk the possibility of another pregnancy? You're at that age now when you have to start thinking about these things."

Then—and the writer remembers this statement quite clearly—he said point-blank with Billy Graham conviction, "In my opinion, every woman should have a hysterectomy by the age of 40."

Another woman we interviewed complained that when she objected to her physician's suggestion that she have her uterus removed, he snapped, "What do you need it for anyway?" "You'd think," she said, "we were discussing the removal of a wart."

There is no comparison—hysterectomy is major surgery, and its complication rate is relatively high. For one thing, it presents all the usual hazards of major surgery—infection, hemorrhage, postoperative blood clots and the risks of anesthesia. In addition, because of the close proximity of the uterus to other pelvic structures, there's always the possibility of incurring damage or operative trauma to pelvic blood vessels, the rectum, the bladder and the ureters (the tubes connecting the kidneys to the bladder). In fact, one of the more common complications of hysterectomy is the accidental severing of a ureter.

Vaginal hysterectomies, moreover, carry with them the additional risk of creating a somewhat shortened or narrowed vagina which could make intercourse painful. And, if the ovaries are removed, the abrupt drop in estrogen level is likely to cause an immediate "surgical menopause" which is more severe than a natural menopause.

There is even some evidence that the uterus itself influences hormone production. According to D. H. Richards, a British physician, 61 percent of the women under age 45 who had a hysterectomy but who had one or both ovaries preserved suffered from hot flashes, urinary symptons, extreme tiredness, headaches, dizziness and insomnia. Most of these symptoms, he says, can be attributed to a hormone imbalance (*Lancet*, October 26, 1974). A follow-up report from the famous Framingham study also indicates that hysterectomy patients are at greater risk of coronary heart disease whether or not their ovaries are removed (*Annals of Internal Medicine*, August, 1978).

But by far the most common reaction to hysterectomy is depression. Women who have had normal or near normal uteruses at the time of hysterectomy had more than twice the rate of psychiatric referral. All the more reason to make sure there's good cause to have surgery before you go through with it.

The important thing here is to weigh the odds. Consider the risks and benefits of surgery in terms of your own health and well-being. Understand your condition fully and be aware of the possibility of alternative treatments. Only with such knowledge can you make an informed decision.

To help you determine why and when hysterectomy may be indicated for you, the following is a discussion of 8 of the most common indications for hysterectomy. Again, keep in mind, that few indications are absolutes. And that one of the most important considerations is in coming to terms with your own feelings—to know when it's right for you.

Fibroid Tumor (Myomas)

Since nearly one-quarter of all women over the age of 30 have fibroids, it's no wonder most abdominal hysterectomies done in this country are performed for this reason. Despite what you may think, it's not true that most fibroids result in hysterectomy. "For the vast majority of women with fibroid tumors, the only treatment is observation," says Dr. Birnbaum.

To understand why and when hysterectomy becomes necessary, then, you've got to understand the nature of the tumor.

Basically, fibroids are noncancerous (and non-life-threatening) lumps that erupt from the uterine walls. They're made up of the same smooth muscle tissue as the uterus, plus some fibrous connective tissue—hence the name "fibroid" tumor. Fibroids grow very slowly. They can be anywhere from the size of a pea to that of a full-term fetus. And when they occur in multiples, they can give a uterus the curious appearance of a lumpy potato.

No one knows exactly why fibroid tumors develop. It's not even known whether heredity is a factor, since they are as common among friends as they are among sisters. One thing is certain, however: their growth depends on a steady diet of the female hormone, estrogen. This is why fibroids are known as the disease of menstruating or estrogen-producing women, why they tend to shrink after menopause and why—according to Dr. Birnbaum—treatment with synthetic estrogen compounds such as the Pill just makes matters worse by accelerating their growth. Don't let anyone tell you otherwise!

In our investigation of fibroid tumors, we discovered some good and bad news. The bad news is that if you're destined to develop fibroids, there's nothing you can do to prevent them. But the good news is that fibroids are seldom cause for serious concern. In fact, the majority of women who have these tumors aren't even aware of them. Others find that they can live with the mild pain and minor inconvenience.

Of course, pain thresholds vary, as do the tumors which cause pain. But it's important to keep a clear perspective—to know *why* you are choosing to have a hysterectomy, if you have made that choice.

"Some women who have a fibroid as big as a pea are going to panic," says Dr. Birnbaum. "Nothing you say can reassure them." One woman's story seems to illustrate this:

> For about a year-and-a-half I was having trouble with my period; I never knew when I was going to get it. When I went to the doctor he found fibroid tumors and recommended a hysterectomy. I could have waited but I was so frightened. It was a Thursday when I found out I needed the surgery and I went into the hospital that Sunday and had it done on Monday morning.

Chances are, this woman would have had the hysterectomy even if she had taken the time to mull over her options. For her, the symptoms were troublesome enough to warrant the surgery. But for others who might not be troubled so much by the symptoms as by the fear of what might happen if they *don't* have the surgery, having it could produce serious consequences.

Just to set the record straight, a fibroid does occasionally develop into a cancer but this is very unusual. "Less than one-tenth of 1 percent undergo degenerative malignant change," according to Dr. Birnbaum. What's more, there is not much chance of this tumor's causing other life-threatening trouble either.

Alan Kaplan, M.D., chief of the division of gynecological oncology at Baylor College of Medicine, Houston, Texas, explains the worst that can happen: "If a fibroid is large enough and in a particular location it could conceivably interfere with urinary or intestinal function, but in my practice I've found this to be extremely rare," he says. "Probably the most common health problem associated with fibroids is anemia caused by an excessive loss of blood. That can be serious. But, again, it's not acutely life-threatening."

The main problem with fibroids—and the primary reason women undergo hysterectomy to have them removed—is not so much that they can shorten life but that they make life miserable. Depending on their size, shape, location and the number of fibroids present, they can cause abnormal bleeding—that is, heavy or prolonged menstrual periods—and excruciating pain. *Severity of symptoms usually dictates treatment.*

What's important is that any abnormal menstrual symptom should be discussed with a qualified physician so that he can rule out serious problems.

Diagnosis is literally in the hands of your physician. By inserting 2 fingers into the vagina and pressing gently on the lower abdomen (just above the pubic bone) with the other hand, a physician is able to feel any unusual bumps on or contours of the uterus. The procedure is known as bimanual palpation and like the Pap smear, it is a routine part of every gynecological exam. Unfortunately, however, it isn't as accurate as the Pap smear. In a heavier woman, it's nearly impossible to feel internal organs. And even in a thin woman, a larger uterine growth which juts out on the outside walls near an ovary may be indistinguishable from an ovarian tumor which poses a much greater threat. Surgery is often the only way to sort them out. And many doctors feel that, at that point, a hysterectomy might as well be performed.

Fibroids can also be diagnosed during a D and C (dilation and curettage), an office or hospital procedure in which the cervix is gently coaxed open using a dilator and then either a spoon-shaped instrument called a curet or a suction device is used to peel off the lining of the uterus. In the process, a physician can usually detect any abnormality in the contours which would indicate fibroids, at the same time analyzing the uterine lining to rule out cancer.

During a D and C, small, "pedunculated" fibroids (mushroom-shaped fibroids propped atop a connective stem, as opposed to rocklike masses resting directly on or in the uterine lining) may be removed with little trouble.

If the tumor or myoma is larger and somewhat embedded in the uterine lining, it may be removed by itself (without taking the uterus) in a surgical procedure known as myomectomy. That procedure is usually reserved for women with 1 or 2 fibroid growths; obviously, it wouldn't be practical to poke holes in a uterus full of fibroids. Also, since the chance of hemorrhage is even greater in a myomectomy than in a hysterectomy, most physicians prefer to use this alternative only for women who are troubled enough by a fibroid tumor to request treatment but who are still young enough to become pregnant.

Otherwise, for the woman plagued by heavy bleeding and pain and who is too far from menopause to grit her teeth and wait for relief, there's always hysterectomy.

Fallen Uterus (Prolapse)

One woman who had a fallen uterus told us:

> I was 34 years old, still a slim 5-foot, 2 inches, 93 pounds, and had my children in the early 60s when episiotomies were done routinely and considered a preventive measure against prolapse problems in the middle years. Besides, I came from a long line of peasant women who were accustomed to bearing large families. . . . So, why me?

Sometimes, the root of a prolapse problem isn't easy to trace. Usually it relates directly to childbirth—the last blow of an extremely long or tough labor. But there are more factors at fault here. In fact, a fallen uterus can just as easily be the result of a clandestine collaboration involving genetics, gravity and the aging process.

A healthy young woman's uterus is propped high atop the vagina. The cervix, or mouth of the uterus, droops into the vaginal canal for about an inch or so. But it doesn't fall further. Connective ligaments pull at it from the top, a tight narrow vagina pushes at it from below, and a very important muscle known as the pubococcygeus (pronounced pu-bo-cocks-uh-*gee*-us) muscle stretches taut from the pubic bone to the tailbone to support all the pelvic organs across the line.

The weakening of any one of these structures can cause a perfectly healthy uterus to slip down and out of its lofty position—much as a telescope collapses.

It could be a set of supportive ligaments drawn progressively lower by gravity and the excess weight of a heavy woman, a vagina that's lost its snap after accommodating a couple of children, a pubococcygal (PC) muscle weakened by recurrent constipation and childbirth so that it resembles a loosely slung hammock, or just a genetic weakness which renders those ligaments vulnerable to stress. Whatever the cause, a simple exercise program can prevent prolapse problems or coax a slightly slack PC muscle back into place.

Begin with some daily yoga postures, such as the shoulder stand—or for more experienced yoga enthusiasts, the head stand—to give your innards a brief respite from the steady downward pull of gravity. Simply lying flat on the bed with your legs elevated by a few pillows will also help.

To strengthen the pubococcygeus muscle, try some Kegels. No, you don't eat them. They are a series of exercises devised by UCLA surgeon, Arnold Kegel, M.D., who discovered that most of the vaginal repairs he performed could have been avoided if women had taken care of their PC muscles.

Basically the exercises call for contracting the PC muscle—simple enough. Initially, however, the most difficult part of the exercises is locating the muscle. Since the PC muscle surrounds the urethra, vagina and rectum, contracting it will produce a tightening sensation across this entire area. Women describe it as "pulling up," or "drawing in." If you're not sure you've got the right muscle in mind, the next time you go to the bathroom, alternate stopping and starting your urine stream until you've emptied your bladder. Stopping urination requires contracting that muscle.

Now that you know where the muscle is located and how it feels when it's contracted, just pull it in as forcefully as you can, hold it for 3 to 5 seconds and then relax for an equal count. Do 8 to 10 repetitions approximately 5 to 10 times each day.

Once you've mastered that exercise, try this one: Imagine

that your pelvic floor is a slow, flat, freight elevator with a heavy load, and it has just closed its doors on the first floor. You slowly start to tighten the muscles and the elevator moves up to the second floor. You tighten a little more and move to the third floor—hold tight for 5 full seconds and then move up to the fourth floor. Now you discover you can't unload yet so you *slowly* start down to the third floor as you relax just slightly. Gradually go to the second and then first floor. Repeat the exercise 5 times and do it slowly at least 10 times a day for a total of 50 times.

It may sound like a lot of work but Kegels are actually simple and convenient exercises. They don't require equipment, a change of clothes or even a special position. You can do them sitting, standing, walking, lying down or standing on your head. So, there's no excuse for *not* working them into your daily routine.

You won't be sorry you stuck to this program either. Regular exercise of the pubococcygeus muscle not only promotes firmer healthier muscle tissue, but also increases the blood flow to the pelvis. With better circulation your reproductive organs will feel better and function better. You may even say goodbye to hemorrhoid problems. And talk about improving your love life!

But—before we leave the impression that exercise is an easy alternative for surgery—we must point out that this program benefits the woman whose uterus is only slightly fallen. More serious prolapse problems usually do not respond to mere exercise alone.

As the uterus slips into the vaginal canal with the cervix leading the way, the cervix becomes an obstruction during intercourse. As it advances even further, the woman may notice a heavy dragging sensation in the pelvis and perhaps an occasional low backache. Stress incontinence (small involuntary loss of urine) can also become bothersome, particularly if the bladder is dropping down along with the uterus.

When the uterus descends so far down that it completely or nearly fills the vaginal canal, hysterectomy becomes a possible solution and probably the most effective one. And in extreme cases there may not be much choice.

> I had my hysterectomy when I was 29—14 months after my last child was born. After 2 hard 36-hour labors my uterus was completely prolapsed. I was in extreme pain. There was no way you could shove that uterus back in place. Anyway, we were planning to limit our family to 2 so there wasn't any question in my mind about whether it was the right thing to do. It was the only thing to do!

For the woman too young or unwilling to give up her child-bearing capacity or the woman too old or too ill to withstand the surgery, however, there are other alternatives.

For one thing, some women can be fit with a pessary. This small plastic ringlike applicance (similar to the diaphragm used for contraception) acts as a support for the slipping uterus and slackened vaginal walls.

Pessaries come in various shapes and sizes to suit all degrees of prolapse. Your physician should be able to tell which type and size would best suit your condition.

But be forewarned; these doughnut-shaped devices have their shortcomings. They must be inserted by a physician, and removed regularly for cleaning, which involves repeated trips to the doctor's office—often, as frequently as every 6 to 8 weeks. Also, because they are a foreign substance and a hard piece of matter, they can cause some vaginal irritation.

But for the elderly woman who might be a poor risk for surgery these small devices are a blessing. For example, a 68-year-old woman we spoke with has been bothered by a prolapsed uterus for many years. For a long while she tried to ignore the problem, but the backaches and frequent time-outs in the john became particularly bothersome on a recent coast-to-coast trip—no doubt aggravated by long hours in the car. On her return, she went to her gynecologist for an exam. It wasn't difficult to diagnose her problem because the uterus was actually visible outside her vagina. Her gynecologist immediately recommended hysterectomy. But she hesitated. About 20 years ago, she had lost a kidney as a result of a serious injury, and she knew that that, plus her age, made her a pretty poor surgical risk. So she consulted a second physician—this time the head of gynecology at a prominent medical college. He didn't even mention hysterectomy. Instead he fitted her with a pessary. She returns to him twice a year to have it checked and cleaned—which to her, is no trouble since she is delighted that she's been spared surgery.

In other women, a type of plastic surgery can sometimes take the place of a hysterectomy. The uterus is pulled back up to its position, the supportive ligaments repaired, and any defects in the underlying muscles of the vagina fixed. In addition, a slack or too-wide vagina can be tightened up to your specifications. And, at the same time, repairs can be made on a sagging bladder (cystocele) or rectum (rectocele).

In cases where the woman is older or feels that she no longer cares to have children, a hysterectomy is combined with whatever vaginal, bladder or rectal repairs have to be made. Since the repair work must be done from the bottom, most hysterectomies performed for prolapse are done vaginally. Otherwise the surgeon must make 2 entrances—once through the abdomen to remove the uterus and again through the vagina to take care of any reconstructive work.

Endometriosis

Endometriosis (pronounced en-doh-me-tree-oh-sis) remains an enigma to the medical profession. They don't know what causes it. They're not sure why it develops. And they're more or less at a loss as to how it's best treated. In fact, in the century or so since this pelvic disease was first diagnosed, the only thing we've managed to learn from doctors is what it is.

In endometriosis, fragments from the endometrium or uterine lining somehow become misplaced during menstruation. Instead of flowing out of the uterus via the vagina, a few leave by way of the Fallopian tubes and spill out into the pelvic cavity. There they become imbedded and grow on the outer wall of the uterus, along the Fallopian tubes, or around practically any other pelvic structure.

Although the condition is noncancerous and again non-life-threatening, it can create a mess of trouble by swaddling the pelvis in a mass of scar tissue. The most common complaint is pain—increasing painful periods after perhaps years of relative comfort, a nagging soreness in the lower abdomen which precedes menstruation by 2 or even 3 weeks and an unbearable shot of pain on deep penile penetration during intercourse.

But what many women find even more distressing is their inability to conceive. If the Fallopian tubes are tied up with endometrial adhesions, there's no way they can swing over to the ovary and scoop up an egg at ovulation. As a result, approximately 40 percent of the women with endometriosis are infertile despite regular periods, normal monthly ovulation and normal Fallopian tubes.

As a matter of fact, endometriosis affects *only* women who menstruate and ovulate regularly—usually young women between the ages of 25 and 45. Apparently, the longer a woman goes without interruption of her normal ovarian function, the greater her chances for developing the disease. And the only known way to curb the progression of the disease is by periodically disrupting the menstrual cycle.

For younger married women who might already have symptoms of early endometriosis—and who might have been postponing parenthood—the best solution might be to get pregnant. With the 9-month leave from ovulation and menstruation, areas of endometriosis often shrink and may even disappear. Of course, regression isn't the rule. But for some lucky women the problem leaves with the pregnancy and never returns.

Older women might do well to just sit tight until menopause. The cessation of menstruation and ovulation often brings a spontaneous improvement of the condition.

For those who are too far from childbearing or change-of-life to use either of them as a "cure," medication or surgery may be the only ray of hope.

But before you select your mode of treatment, make sure your condition is properly diagnosed. Because endometriosis affects the pelvic cavity *outside* the uterus, internal exams won't be of much help. Also, endometrial adhesions are not easily distinguishable from normal tissue using bimanual palpation. The only sure way to make the diagnosis is by laparoscopy—that's one-half of the "band-aid sterilization" procedure.

Granted, this is not the easiest diagnostic procedure. Under either local or general anesthesia, the physician will make a small incision just below your navel. Carbon dioxide will be pumped into the abdomen to lift the outer covering of skin and muscle tissue away from the internal organs. Then using a laparoscope, a kind of slender telescope, the physician can check the pelvic organs for any endometrial adhesions.

Once diagnosed, endometriosis is usually treated by one of 2 ways: medication or surgery.

Until recently, the only medication available was hormones. Doses of estrogen or progesterone much higher than those available in the Pill are administered by mouth or more commonly through injection to bring on a state of pseudopregnancy by temporarily suspending ovulation and menstruation. It works all right. The adhesions melt away and the pain subsides. The only problem is that long-term use of these synthetic hormones brings on a whole host of adverse side effects, and short-term use offers only temporary relief from symptoms but no relief from the progression of the disease.

Recently, a new drug called danazol has come onto the medical market. Unfortunately, danazol is not without potential side effects; namely, it may produce masculinizing reactions such as acne, mild hirsutism (abnormal hair growth), decrease in breast size, slight deepening in the voice, oiliness of the skin or hair. Of course, these side effects don't occur in every woman who tries it. For those women so affected, the distressing problems usually last only as long as the medication is taken, but some symptoms may persist for a few months after treatment stops. And, according to one physician, those effects are "trivial" compared to the potential adverse effects of hormonal agents commonly used for endometriosis. Besides, the benefits may be great.

Although danazol is a newcomer in the treatment of endometriosis, reports of its effectiveness have been very promising. In one small study of women suffering from infertility as a result of endometriosis, half became pregnant after danazol treatment. In another investigation, more than 50 percent of the endometriosis-afflicted women treated with danazol were found to be completely free of any pelvic disease upon laparascopy exam.

An alternative to danazol treatment is conservative surgery in which a lower abdominal incision is made and the endometrial adhesions are removed without removing the uterus. But if fertility is not the main aim of endometriosis therapy, most physicians still favor hysterectomy (usually total abdominal hysterectomy plus the removal of diseased Fallopian tubes and ovaries)—particularly for older women with severe pain.

Profuse or Prolonged Menstrual Bleeding (Dysfunctional Bleeding)

Every once in a while, a physician comes across a case of menorrhagia (extremely heavy or prolonged menstrual bleeding) that defies diagnosis. There's no evidence of fibroids. Pap smears are normal. Even a D and C fails to uncover any concealed malady. Basically, the uterus is in A-1 condition but the woman, obviously, is not.

The patient might be using as many as 14 tampons a day. Or waiting out a menstrual period that lasts for weeks or even months. Her blood count is understandably low as is her stamina; she complains that she doesn't have the energy to go to work or take care of her kids. Does "help" have to be in the form of a hysterectomy?

Well, if the situation cannot be remedied by other methods, hysterectomy is considered acceptable treatment. In fact, some women suffer so greatly that surgery is a welcome relief. Beware of the doctor who talks hysterectomy after you've had only 2 or 3 heavy periods. Occasionally the situation corrects itself. And many times it responds to more conservative treatment.

Unfortunately, what causes this problem is not always easy to assess. When it isn't related to disease (which should be determined by a Pap smear and, if necessary, a D and C), the condition is simply labeled "dysfunctional bleeding," meaning that it's a result of some functional problem in the reproductive organs. Sometimes—and particularly in women nearing menopause—the problem is in the ovaries' failure to produce eggs or ovulate.

To carry off a perfect period, the ovaries must perform several functions. First, they must produce enough estrogen to stimulate the buildup of blood on the uterine lining. Second, they should release an egg midway through the menstrual cycle, which in turn stimulates the production of another female hormone, progesterone. When progesterone production drops, the uterus sheds its lining.

A problem arises, however, when estrogen production keeps stimulating the growth of the uterine lining, but—because the ovaries aren't putting out their monthly egg quota—there's no rise and fall in progesterone to signal the uterus to shed its lining. The blood continues to build, eventually breaking down of its own weight and bringing with it a deluge of blood.

Typically, medical treatment includes a D and C to clean out the excess blood buildup and temporarily stop the bleeding as well as to rule out any malignancy, and hormonal therapy—usually a progesterone pill or an estrogen-progesterone compound—to initiate the periodic shedding.

That combination treatment is often successful in controlling the bleeding, particularly in women who are biding their time till menopause, when dysfunctional bleeding should subside. Yet, hormones are not without their side effects, including the increased risk of uterine and possibly even breast cancer.

For those who'd rather not take the chance, a study published in the *South African Medical Journal* which suggests that moderately high doses of vitamin A can reduce heavy menstrual bleeding may be just what the doctor ordered (February 12, 1977).

Although the effect of a vitamin A deficiency on the reproductive system of women has never been clearly documented, it's known that vitamin A levels in women fluctuate in a cyclic pattern during the menstrual cycle. That fluctuation—in addition to animal studies which showed that a laboratory-induced vitamin A deficiency decreased hormone production and suspended the menstrual cycle—suggests a strong correlation between vitamin A levels and female hormones.

With that information at hand, Drs. D. M. Lithgow and W. M. Politzer of Johannesburg, South Africa, tested the vitamin A levels in 71 women suffering from menorrhagia and found, on the average, only 67 International Units of the vitamin per 100 milliliters of blood. By comparison, a group of healthy controls with normal menstrual periods had about 166 International Units per 100 milliliters—almost two-and-a-half times the amount measured in the first group.

To make sure this wasn't a coincidence, the researchers then decided to treat 52 women with symptoms of dysfunctional bleeding with 60,000 International Units of vitamin A a day for 35 days. Close to 93 percent of the women treated were either cured or helped by the vitamin A. One woman we spoke with reported similar success:

> I had been having heavy bleeding during my periods for at least a year. I've never been able to do much on the first day, but this kept me down 5 days a month. I was hemorrhaging. I had to change every 10 or 15 minutes, and I couldn't do a thing. I went for one-and-a-half years to doctors: first, my family doctor, a gynecologist and a hematologist. The hematologist suggested a hysterectomy. So I went to see the gynecologist again and he was hesitant about operating. He said he hated to do it since internally I appeared to be perfectly normal. However, he wanted to prescribe the Pill. Some choice, hysterectomy or the Pill! About a week later I read about vitamin A for heavy bleeding, so I

> started taking 10,000 units of the vitamin twice a day. I was due for a period in two-and-a-half weeks. When it came, there was no hemorrhaging. There was a heavy flow, but I could carry on normal activities. After that my periods were normal. That was several months ago and I haven't been to a doctor since.

(Vitamin A is one vitamin you can take too much of, but 25,000 International Units a day will not cause adults any problems. Nearly all cases of toxicity involve taking hundreds of thousands of units every day for months or years.)

Sterilization

One out of every 5 hysterectomies is done for sterilization, according to a survey by the U.S. Department of Health, Education and Welfare (HEW). Imagine . . . submitting to major surgery when relatively minor procedures could do the same job.

"It's like cracking a nut with a sledgehammer," says Dr. Stanley Birnbaum.

". . . subjecting a woman to this relatively dangerous operation for sterilization alone is an outrage," says Sidney Wolfe, M.D.

"There's no reason for a woman to submit to major surgery when a relatively simple laparoscopic tubal ligation will do the same job. Better yet, I think that the vasectomy should be given serious consideration by couples desiring sterilization," says Dr. Mikuta.

These assertions are supported by statistics from the Center for Disease Control in Atlanta, Georgia, which show that reproductive-age hysterectomy patients are over 6 times more likely to suffer serious surgical complications and 5 times more likely to die than women who undergo tubal sterilization.

These opinions sent HEW scurrying to reevaluate their policy and withdraw a popular pamphlet they had distributed entitled "Your Sterilization Operation: Hysterectomy." The new regulations state that hysterectomy may *not* be performed solely for the purpose of sterilization.

Still, there are physicians who, for whatever reason, are pushing hysterectomies as casually as they dispense Valium. One woman explains:

> When I was 34 years old and had just given birth to my fifth child, my doctor and I discussed the possibility of having my tubes cut and tied. I told him I'd rather wait a few months to be absolutely sure. He said, "Well, when you come back we might as well do a hysterectomy" (although he assured me that there was absolutely nothing medically wrong). I was so flabbergasted that I left the office and never went back.

There are a couple of exceptions, however, when gynecologists agree that a sterilization hysterectomy is OK or even preferred. That is, when other gynecological problems may require a hysterectomy in the immediate or not-too-distant future. Or when there exists a pelvic condition such as prolapse or fibroids which will probably grow worse.

"We see over and over again, women with minor to moderate gynecological problems who had tubal ligations come back requiring a hysterectomy within the same year," says Baylor's Dr. Kaplan. "This can require 2 surgical procedures and 2 anesthetics, thereby doubling the risk."

Just be sure that the "other" reason for the surgery is valid. And beware of the surgeon who might shield the actual reason for the surgery under an umbrella of invented or grossly exaggerated symptoms. According to Jane Hodgson, M.D., professor of surgery at the University of Minnesota School of Medicine, many gynecologists—including those at Catholic hospitals—"cover" sterilization hysterectomies by saying that the reason for the operation is heavy menstrual bleeding, prolapse of the uterus, dysfunctional uterine bleeding or an abnormal (but not cancerous) Pap test. None of these problems, she states, is justification for subjecting women to the risk of hysterectomy.

One woman we spoke with implied that she may have been so coerced:

> I was thinking of having a tubal ligation but when I brought it up with my gynecologist he changed the subject to hysterectomy. . . . Said I had a slightly prolapsed uterus that would just get worse and I'd eventually need to have a hysterectomy anyway. So why not get it all taken care of at once? The funny thing was, I'd been going to this doctor for several years and he had never before mentioned that I had a prolapsed uterus. Besides that, I wasn't having any discomfort. . . . But he's a well-respected physician in my community and I figured he knew what he was doing so I went through with the operation.

An informed health care consumer can immediately spot some flaws in her rationale. For one thing, if she found the prolapse excuse hard to swallow, she shouldn't have bought it so readily. And second, just because her doctor's office sports an impressive sheepskin and a slew of idolizing patients, she shouldn't have assumed him God. *Maybe he was right.* But a second opinion would have certainly cleared up any doubts in her mind, and it might have even prevented her surgery.

Cancer of the Cervix

Each year, invasive cervical cancer singles out 16,000 women—most of them relatively young women between the ages of 35 and 55—and kills 7,400 of them. Does that sound bleak? Actually when you consider that 50,000 people die each year in traffic accidents and 300,000 of heart attacks, cervical cancer is mildly destructive by comparison.

The thing is, though, that *no one* should die from it. Through the Pap smear, nearly 90 percent of all potential cervical cancers can be detected early enough to insure 100 percent cure—a cure in which, by the way, hysterectomy is rarely crucial.

The cervix is the lower section of the uterus. If you envision the uterus as an upside-down pear, the cervix would be its neck projecting an inch or so into the vagina.

Actually, the location of the cervix—somewhere between the outside world and the inner sanctum of the womb—probably makes it more vulnerable to disease. Bacterial, viral and fungal organisms attack it, causing infections. And a penile battering ram periodically pounds it.

Of course, it's not known for sure what causes cancer of the cervix. But since promiscuous women or women who've begun sexual activity early and had their first baby while still in their teens face the highest risk, while nuns are virtually immune, sexual intercourse seems to be the common denominator in its development. Several factors, including herpes (a sexually transmitted virus), poor hygiene and even the protein makeup of sperm, have been suggested as possible causes.

Presumably, then, prevention of cervical cancer could be achieved by living the life of a celibate. But, for those of us not willing to sacrifice sex, the next best solution may be switching contraceptives. According to a group of Oxford University researchers, diaphragm users had only one-quarter the incidence of cervical abnormalities including dysplasia (possibly an early stage in cancer development) and invasive cancer that users of the Pill or I.U.D. had. Why that is, no one knows for certain. But, these researchers suggest that it could have something to do with the fact that the diaphragm, like the condom, protects the cervix from direct contact with sperm (*British Journal of Cancer*, vol. 38, 1977).

Evidence that the hormones in the Pill may be contributing to cervical cancer comes to us from the University of California. There researchers have discovered a close correlation between use of the Pill and the conversion of cervical abnormalities called "dysplasia" to cancer. Apparently, cervical dysplasias can go either way: they can shrink to the point where they actually disappear or they can grow into a cancer. Based on this study, women who continue taking the Pill after a dysplasia has been diagnosed stand a greater chance of falling victim to cancer (*Science*, June 24, 1977).

But no matter what the case against contraceptives, your best safeguard against advanced disease is a regular Pap smear.

This test, developed in the 1920s by Dr. George Papanicolaou, is still one of the best known methods of early cancer detection. It's fast, simple, painless, and, unlike other diagnostic procedures, it involves no risk for the patient.

Theoretically it makes a lot of sense, too. Based on the little we know of cervical cancer, it looks like the Pap smear may be able to detect abnormal cell changes in the cervix 10 to 15 years before a full-fledged cancer develops. With prompt treatment, then, advanced life-threatening cancers can be prevented.

There is some question, however, concerning how often Pap smear screening should be done. Until very recently, it was generally recommended as an annual health measure. That recommendation was based in part on the realization that although the Pap test isn't 100 percent accurate, repeating it at yearly intervals reduces the margin of error. Yearly tests would also increase the likelihood that any new lesions would be detected.

Today, some authorities including New York University health researcher, Anne-Marie Foltz, suggest that every 3 to 5 years is adequate—at least for educated middle-class women who are at low risk of developing the disease anyway.

Margaret Sloan, M.D., of the National Cancer Institute (NCI), explains that although the NCI still favors the yearly Pap test, new guidelines may soon be adopted. Basically, they will state that a low-risk woman should be tested for 3 consecutive years beginning with the year of her first sexual intercourse, or at age 20, whichever comes first. Then she should have a Pap test every 3 years thereafter. Women who became pregnant in their teens, who have multiple sex partners, or who suffer from genital herpes might be best advised to undergo a Pap test every year.

The Pap smear shouldn't be unfamiliar to female readers. A recent Gallup poll tells us that nearly 80 percent of American women over the age of 20 have had at least one in their lives. Yet, there is a certain mystique associated with a procedure which takes place under the cover of a white sheet.

Actually, what occurs in those few minutes takes longer to explain then it does to experience. First, the physician inserts a metal instrument called a speculum into the vagina. Once in place, the 2 shoehornlike wings are spread apart to permit a clear view of the cervix. Then, with the blunt tip of a depression stick or a cotton swab, the doctor takes 2 or 3 sample scrapings: 1 from the outer cuff of the cervix; 1 from the area just inside the cervical canal; and possibly 1 from the vaginal wall.

Aside from the pressure of the speculum, you shouldn't feel any discomfort. For one thing, the cervix has no nerve endings. And, since the cervix is shedding cells all the time, it is only this loosened cellular debris that is scraped away to be smeared onto slides for microscopic analysis. Indeed, some women remark that the most painful part of the procedure is waiting to hear the results.

And, says NCI's Dr. Robert Bowser, even that nervousness is uncalled for. The vast majority of Pap smears are normal. And even if a woman is called back for a follow-up test, it doesn't mean she should panic. She could be asked to come back for another test for any of a dozen reasons. Maybe the slide wasn't prepared properly. Or she might have trichomoniasis (a type of parasitic yeast infection). Or maybe it's some slight abnormality labeled "precancerous" but which might disappear on its own. Whatever it is, if she's been having Pap tests regularly, chances are *extremely remote that the first hint of trouble is going to signal a serious invading cancer.*

Unfortunately and understandably, more than one woman has been confused by Pap smear terminology. After all, what health-minded person can comprehend that a "negative" test result could bring anything but bad news? But it's actually good news. "Negative" to the physician means negative for disease. It means that the cells of your cervix are normal; there's no sign of cancer.

"Positive," on the other hand, implies the presence of cancer. But, again, don't panic. Early cervical cancer is very treatable. It may not even require hysterectomy. In fact, thinking in terms of cancer or surgery at this point is jumping the gun. No competent doctor would base a diagnosis solely on the findings of a single Pap smear. And neither should you. A recently published study disclosed that of a group of 53 women with "positive" cervical smears who refused follow-up diagnosis of treatment, 19 returned 2 or more years later with "negative" Pap results. Either the original test reports were mistaken or the cancers had completely regressed (*Lancet*, August 26, 1978).

Actually, sorting out the good slides from the bad ones is not as easy as distinguishing between black and white. There's "positive" and there's "negative" and then there's the suspicious group. And deciding which classification a specimen falls into is not an easy task.

"It's like how do you recognize your grandmother. . . . Well, she has gray hair, a long nose and wears glasses," explains John Seybolt, M.D., chief of the Cytology Laboratory at the New York Hospital-Cornell Medical Center. "Now you look at someone and say 'Well, she has gray hair only.' That's not enough to call her your grandmother. You need more criteria. The same holds true for classifying Pap smears. A slide may have 2 or 3 criteria for a 'positive' classification but if it doesn't have enough of them, it doesn't qualify." For that reason Pap smears are graded according to degree of cellular change (see box).

If a report of suspicious cells calls you back to the examination table and stirrups, here's what to expect from further diagnostic tests:

- *Colposcopy*. That may sound frighteningly invasive, but it's no more of a hassle than a Pap smear. After a speculum is inserted and the vaginal walls swabbed with a vinegarlike solution to remove mucus, the exposed cervix is viewed through a binocular instrument called a colposcope, which magnifies the surface features. The instrument is held outside the body, so don't freeze up in anticipation of pain. It won't hurt and, in fact, it may save you additional and perhaps unnecessary follow-up.
- *Biopsy* and preferably a colposcope-directed biopsy. Once

PAP SMEAR CLASSIFICATIONS

Current Guidelines*

Class I— Negative (Normal)
Class II— Inconclusive (Abnormal changes in cell formation, which could be anything from a trichomoniasis infection to an early precancerous problem)
Class III— Suspicious (Abnormal cellular changes which are insufficient for a definitive diagnosis)
Class IV— Highly Suspicious (Markedly abnormal cellular changes which, however, cannot be definitely called positive)
Class V— Positive for Cancer

New Guidelines Proposed by the National Cancer Institute

Unsatisfactory Cellular Specimen (Slide quality too poor to obtain an accurate reading)
Normal Cellular Pattern
Benign Cellular Changes (This category includes any abnormal changes caused by infection or injury, none of which are precancerous)
Dysplasia: Mild, Moderate or Severe (Abnormal cellular changes thought to be precancerous; rated according to the proportion of abnormal to normal cells present on the slide sample as well as degree of change in size and shape of abnormal cells)
Carcinoma in situ (A localized cancer condition)
Invasive Carcinoma (A cancer which has invaded the underlying tissues of the cervix)

---

*This is an example of the type of classification system used in some Pap smear screening laboratories. There are slight variations, however, from one hospital to the next.

the problem is located, and evaluated through colposcopy, the physician can take a tissue sample from the suspicious area. That can be done in the office. At most you might feel a little pinch, but it isn't enough to require anesthesia or hospitalization. *Certainly no treatment—least of all, hysterectomy—should be undertaken without a biopsy.*

- *Conization.* If, on colposcopic examination, the physician discovers that the suspicious area reaches into the cervical canal, or if the biopsy results return from the lab labeled moderate to severe dysplasia, it may be necessary to evaluate the extent of disease further by cutting a cone-shaped wedge out of the cervix. Since half of the volume of the cervix is actually removed during this procedure, hospitalization and anesthesia are required. Possible immediate complications include hemorrhaging, and long-term complications such as infertility can result. Obviously, this is not your basic biopsy. Yet, it remains an invaluable diagnostic tool which could save you from a hysterectomy. And, by comparison, the risks are minimal.

Treatment of cervical cancer is tailored according to the extent of the trouble and the stage of cancer development. As mentioned earlier, it usually takes many years for a full-fledged cervical cancer to take hold, 10 to 15 years by many accounts. And it isn't even known for a fact whether every problem labeled "precancerous" will develop into a cancer. But most are removed as a precautionary measure. Other minuscule lesions diagnosed as "mild dysplasia" may disappear on their own, perhaps due to some kind of body defense mechanism. But generally speaking, the earlier the diagnosis, the less drastic the treatment and the more effective the cure. It's rare that any dysplasia diagnosed "mild" to "moderate" or lesion diagnosed "suspicious" (Class III) requires hysterectomy.

Sometimes, the method of diagnosis doubles as treatment. In a small lesion, for example, a biopsy might whisk away every last trace of trouble. Similarly, conization can clear up certain larger but still localized dysplasias with no need for further surgery, depending on their location. In fact, there is a growing number of American physicians who consider conization adequate treatment for cancer *in situ* (a definite cancerous condition which has not yet spread to underlying tissues) particularly in younger women. They believe that success of conization can be determined by examining the wedge and taking a Pap smear. Myron Melamed, M.D., chief pathologist at Memorial Sloan-Kettering Hospital, is among those physicians. And Dr. Mikuta points out that this may be one reason for the high hysterectomy rates in the U.S. relative to other foreign countries, where conization rather than hysterectomy is considered routine for cancer *in situ.*

With smaller, less advanced abnormalities, hysterectomy is never an acceptable option. If they cannot be removed entirely at the time of biopsy, and the results of the biopsy show no further invasion, they can be quickly eradicated in another office visit.

Cauterization, which uses a heated wire to burn away abnormal tissue, is the long-standing treatment of choice for minor abnormalities. Years ago, it was customary to cauterize women after childbirth, to clean up any coating left behind by the pregnancy and give the uterine cervix a nice shiny covering. Today, you'd be hard pressed to find an obstetrician who still practices cauterization routinely, but according to Dr. Mikuta, there are some papers suggesting that women who have had routine cauterization after delivery have a lower incidence of cancer of the cervix. Whatever the case, it does seem to destroy diseased tissue and promote new growth of healthy cells.

Another procedure making its way into the gynecology suite is cryosurgery. That procedure, which destroys the abnormal cells by freezing rather than burning them, is preferred by some physicians because it is easier and less painful than cauterization. However, one physician we spoke with regarded it as still an experimental procedure.

Both cauterization and cryosurgery can be performed in the doctor's office without anesthetic. Possible side effects include bleeding and discharge—nothing that a vinegar and water douche can't clear up.

A biopsy that verifies a more serious dysplasia or cancer *in situ* is more likely to lead to hysterectomy than to conization in this country. Again, much hinges on the age and emotional maturity of the woman. But, at this stage, surgery is still relatively limited. For noninvasive cervical cancers, only the uterus, including the cervix, is removed. The ovaries and the Fallopian tubes may be left intact. Once the cancer has invaded the underlying cervical tissues, much more extensive surgery may be necessary. Dr. Mikuta explains; "You can't solve this problem with just a simple removal of the uterus and the cervix. This requires taking out the uterus and cervix plus 3 additional things: the tissues at the side of the uterus all the way over to the pelvic wall; the pelvic lymph nodes; and the upper third of the vagina. Along with this, we usually remove both tubes and ovaries. This is called a radical hysterectomy. You can treat cancer of the cervix by radiation just as well in terms of survival. But I feel that you get a better result with surgery, particularly in younger women where you might be able to preserve an ovary or two. Radiation wipes everything out. Plus you have to deal with possible damage to the bowel, bladder or to the vaginal tract itself. There can be some fairly significant shrinkage to the vaginal tissues with the radiation therapy."

That kind of surgery requires the skill of a gynecology specialist known as a gynecological oncologist. It is an extremely complicated and risky procedure which should be performed only by surgeons with adequate training, with fully certified anesthesiologists, in hospitals which can supply good backup facilities. Don't expect your GP or even your obstetrician to take care of this problem in a small-town community hospital. Invasive cervical cancer is definitely a case for the "big boys."

Cancer of the Lining or Body of the Uterus (Endometrial Cancer)

It's still cancer, but cancer of the lining or body of the uterus (we'll refer to it simply as uterine cancer from here on in) just doesn't compare to cervical cancer. First of all, it strikes older women—mostly postmenopausal women in their late 40s and 50s. Second it is somewhat less treacherous—its presence is usually signaled by symptomatic bleeding early enough to permit effective treatment—and it is less likely than cervical cancer to spread beyond the pelvic reproductive organs. Third, because of its hard-to-isolate location in the uterine lining and the age of women who develop it, uterine cancer practically always results in hysterectomy, even when discovered in its very early stage.

The risk factors for uterine cancer are different as well. Unlike cervical cancer, sexual activity or social class isn't considered a common denominator. Instead, statistics show that women who tend to be overweight, diabetic or have high blood pressure are more likely to develop uterine cancer. Presumably, then, diet may be the underlying culprit with the typical American smorgasbord of fatty meats, salty seasonings and sugary desserts paving the way for many more problems than bargained for. (Still waiting to slim down?)

Of course, that doesn't explain why one of the thinnest women this writer ever knew—a woman who had neither diabetes nor high blood pressure—died at age 57 of uterine cancer. One reason could be that this curious cancer may be caused in part by some basic genetic or metabolic disturbance. According to Lucienne Lanson, M.D., a San Francisco gynecologist, women who have been plagued with irregular periods, have not ovulated regularly, have had trouble becoming pregnant, and gone through a bloody menopause (a change of life characterized by heavy and prolonged menstrual bleeding) seem more susceptible to its development.

A growing body of evidence suggests that the lining of the uterus in some women may be supersensitive to estrogen. And with so many women taking the Pill for contraception and estrogen for menopausal hot flashes, well, is it any wonder that the incidence of uterine cancer rose sharply in the 70s?

Whatever the cause, our main concern is with cure. As in any type of cancer, early detection is the key to effective treatment. Unfortunately, the trusty Pap smear becomes somewhat undependable when it comes to detecting uterine cancer. In fact, less than half of the women who have uterine cancer will discover it through an annual Pap test. Of those remaining, most will be unaware of any problem until a bloody pool sends them panic-stricken to a physician. Bleeding between periods is one sign that something may be amiss, as is any bleeding in postmenopausal women. Of course, this bleeding can be indicative of other problems as well but it's best to get to a gynecologist and let him or her make the diagnosis. If uterine cancers are detected at the onset of symptomatic bleeding, it is usually early enough to promise effective treatment.

Of course, nabbing a cancerous condition before any symptoms erupt is even better. How? Well, there is a diagnostic test called endometrium aspiration which should be done along with the Pap smear on women who fall in the high-risk category—that is, postmenopausal women who are overweight, diabetic, have high blood pressure or are swallowing synthetic estrogen. Dr. Mikuta recommends this test for every woman over the age of 40. After the physician finishes taking the Pap smear samples, he expels the air from a small bulbous syringe, inserts the tip through the cervical canal and into the uterus where he releases the pressure so that mucus and cellular debris from the uterine walls is sucked into the vacuum. The contents are then emptied onto a slide for examination. Because the cervical canal is somewhat sensitive to invaders, the passage of the syringe might cause cramps. But since the test only takes a few seconds, the discomfort will shortly subside.

Should the cancer weasel by the Pap smear and aspiration without detection, and abnormal bleeding begins, a diagnostic D and C is performed. Again as we mentioned in the discussion on fibroids, this will be able to differentiate between bleeding caused by fibroids, dysfunctional bleeding and cancer.

And should the D and C confirm cancer, a hysterectomy is your safest and best existing method of treatment. In fact, uterine cancer is considered one of the few absolute indications for hysterectomy. And, since most women with uterine cancer are already past menopause, and since uterine cancer can spread to the ovaries, this is one time when a hysterectomy is almost sure to include removal of the ovaries and Fallopian tubes.

Cancer Prevention

Take a patient who is in a low socio-economic and high-risk bracket for cervical cancer. She had her first baby at age 15, maybe 5 kids by the time she is 22. She is unmarried and has a number of different sex partners. Now let's suppose she shows up at a hospital clinic after having a slightly abnormal (but not cancerous) Pap smear or just walks in off the street and requests a sterilization. There's a good chance that she'll be leaving without her uterus.

They call it "prevention." And, say some physicians, with 2 strikes against her, this particular woman stands to benefit from the surgery. Number 1: her background puts her at high risk of cervical cancer. Number 2: if she is sterilized by other means, she probably won't be coming back to the obstetrical service to be screened for cancer.

Removing a perfectly healthy uterus is sometimes justified for persons suffering from cancer phobia (fear of cancer). In fact, often such a patient requests surgery and, says Dr. Mikuta, there may be serious consequences when the physician refuses to comply. Dr. Mikuta tells of a 35-year-old woman who was in good health but who was convinced that because both her mother and sister had died of cervical cancer, it was just a matter of time before it got her. She wanted a hysterectomy. But her physician turned her down; told her not to worry, she was fine. About 15 minutes later, the doctor who gave her this advice turned around and saw a body falling down past his window. The patient had gone up on the roof and jumped off, all because of her tremendous fear of cancer.

Of course, that is an extreme case. But it does illustrate the fact that indications for hysterectomy are rarely clear-cut. Generally speaking, a hysterectomy performed in the absence of disease could hardly be called acutely life-saving. In this case, it might have been.

Also, physicians maintain that having surgery for sheer prevention is the patient's right. "It's just as valid as having plastic surgery," says Dr. Kaplan. "Of course, I would never push a woman into surgery for this reason. But if a patient says, 'Look, my family history is clouded with case after case of uterine cancer and I'd rather have a hysterectomy now than worry the rest of my life about getting cancer,' she is a valid candidate for hysterectomy. As long as she's completely aware of all the risks involved, then the decision should be hers."

Nonetheless, some physicians and consumer research groups balk. Somehow the idea of thwarting the possibility of disease at the cost of serious complications—including depression and even death—not to mention hundreds of dollars just doesn't seem worthwhile. Sure, a woman without a uterus is an unlikely target for uterine cancer. But, by the same token, a castrated male is an unlikely candidate for testicular cancer. And you can bet your bottom dollar few men would be willing to put their money and masculinity on the line based on such a flimsy piece of reasoning.

If a woman is fearful of cancer, she should be offered *reassurance*, not surgery, say the consumer advocates. Her doctor should take the time to explain what cancer is, how it develops, her odds of developing it, risk factors she may be able to avoid and how regular screening and early treatment can catch it before it kills—often with less mutilation than a hysterectomy. Should this information and education fail to convince her, perhaps she will benefit more from a psychiatrist's couch than a surgeon's table. At least, it's worth a try.

Aside from the ethical issue, there's also a problem justifying the bottom-line benefits. What exactly is to be gained—in terms of life years—by having the surgery before the disease actually occurs? Obviously, those who would otherwise have died from uterine or cervical cancer stand to gain the most and those who wouldn't have gotten the disease in the first place, the least. But we don't know who's who. So, public health authorities and statisticians work with averages. The interpretations of those figures vary with the sources.

Those in favor of "preventive" hysterectomy say that women undergoing surgery by the age of 35 have a slightly longer life expectancy than those who do not have the operation. Those against, including Harvard's Dr. Cole, point out that this increase in life expectancy amounts to an average of only 0.2 years per woman, or roughly 2 to 2½ months. Ironically, this is the time it takes most women to have a hysterectomy and recuperate from the surgery.

Furthermore, in the book *Costs, Risks and Benefits of Surgery* (Oxford University Press, 1977), John P. Bunker, M.D., Benjamin A. Barnes, M.D., and Frederick Mosteller, Ph.D., add an important qualifying remark. According to these men, the increased life expectancy described above relates only to healthy premenopausal women. For the patient who is less healthy or older—for example, a 50-year old woman with moderately high blood pressure—life expectancy is *shortened* by elective hysterectomy because of the tremendous surgical risks.

Discussion shouldn't wind down once the decision to operate has been made. There's much more you should know and there are even a few more decisions you may be involved in.

Ask for Details about Your Hysterectomy

For starters, find out exactly what your surgeon intends to remove. It may sound silly, but despite the popularity of this procedure, many women are not clear on what a hysterectomy entails. The term hysterectomy refers to the removal of the uterus. Period. Whether your physician chooses to call it a simple, a complete, a total, or a pan-hysterectomy, technically they all mean the same thing—the removal of the body of the uterus plus its cervix. Two less common procedures include the subtotal hysterectomy, which implies the removal of the body of the uterus but not the cervix and the partial hysterectomy in which only a portion of the body of the uterus is removed. The radical hysterectomy, as we mentioned earlier, is a more extensive procedure in which the uterus plus adjacent lymph nodes and possibly part of the vagina are removed, usually to stop the spread of cancer.

Whatever the case, you'll notice that none of these procedures includes the removal of the ovaries or Fallopian tubes. Although about half of all hysterectomies are performed in conjunction with the removal of these adjacent structures, the procedure is referred to separately by a very long, fancy term: bilaterial salpingo-oophorectomy. "Salpingo-" refers to the Fallopian tubes; "oophor" to the ovaries; "-ectomy," to the removal of; bilaterial simply means both sides. Therefore, a bilaterial salpingo-oophorectomy means removal of both tubes and ovaries.

Unfortunately, even physicians become casual in their use of terminology and may at times use words like "total hysterectomy" or "complete clean-out" to mean the removal of the uterus plus ovaries. Your best bet is to check with your surgeon and have him or her spell out exactly what you can expect.

If the procedure planned for you includes a bilaterial salpingo-oophorectomy, that's definitely something you should know about beforehand. And, depending on the circumstances, it may be one decision in which you'll have a voice.

Every physician we consulted agreed that the patient has the right to decide whether or not she shall retain one or both ovaries. (Remember, retaining one ovary or even a part of an ovary should preserve hormone production.) This, of course, is contingent upon the health of the ovaries and the extent of uterine disease—something which cannot always be determined prior to surgery. But, the variables should be discussed fully and the patient's wishes clearly made known to the surgeon before any consent forms are signed.

Generally speaking, physicians favor the let-be policy for healthy ovaries in any woman under 40 years of age. This woman has not yet reached menopause, so the removal of her ovaries would abruptly cut off her estrogen supply and throw her into a sudden change of life. And since surgical menopause is notoriously more severe than natural menopause with its gradual tapering off of estrogen, most physicians would just as soon let the ovaries be if at all possible.

For women over 45 or past menopause many surgeons believe that there's no further need for the ovaries; they've already slowed down their estrogen production. And since cancer of the ovary, an extremely virulent and elusive disease, becomes a potential threat in postmenopausal women, physicians often suggest oophorectomy as a preventive measure. In fact, a few go so far as to insist that leaving the ovaries in the postmenopausal patient borders on criminal negligence.

That may be a bit extreme. The mortality rate for ovarian cancer is about 10 per 100,000—less than the number of women who die each year from complications directly attributable to either pregnancy or delivery. Also, the ovaries do continue to release a trickle of estrogen after menopause—even up to age 60 in some women.

It is true that the ovaries are susceptible to a whole host of ills. And occasionally, the woman who declines to have them removed at the time of hysterectomy may find herself submitting to a second surgical procedure later to rid herself of a painful or even life-threatening ovarian situation.

On the other hand, the woman who has her ovaries removed and then makes up for the lost hormone by taking replacement estrogen, may be incurring a whole new set of risks. Of course, as a hysterectomy patient, she won't have to fear the development of uterine cancer, the major risk related to snythetic estrogen. But other studies have shown that she may have a greater than average chance of developing benign breast cysts and possibly breast cancer (*Journal of the American Medical Association*, October 13, 1978).

Another question to be resolved before surgery is whether your physician proposes to do the surgery through an abdominal incision or through the vagina. There are advantages and disadvantages to both. For example, those who favor the vaginal hysterectomy point out that postoperative pain, hospitalization and recuperation time are reduced simply because there is no incision. Also, for some women concerned with scars, this approach has definite psychological benefits. On the other hand, those who prefer to perform abdominal hysterectomies point to the high rate of infections and possible foreshortening of the vagina incurred during vaginal hysterectomies. They also argue that blatant pelvic disease might be missed by operating blindly from below. To get the full picture of pelvic condition, they say, you've got to go in through the abdomen.

Actually, you probably won't have to wrestle with this decision. It's more than likely that the nature of your problem will dictate the appropriate hysterectomy approach. For example, if you're undergoing surgery for a prolapse problem, the uterus is already on its way out via the vagina; the surgeon has only to complete the job. On the other hand, if the uterus is being removed because of a large fibroid, chances are the physician wouldn't be able to deliver it through the vagina, anyway. The abdominal hysterectomy is its only way out.

Many times too, the approach is determined by your physician's area of expertise. Robert Henry Barter, M.D., professor of gynecology at George Washington University and member of the Society of Vaginal Surgeons, believes that although 70 percent of all hysterectomies could be handled successfully through the vagina, most physicians prefer not to do them that way because they just don't know how. "It's a much more demanding type of surgery," he told us. "You need special equipment, special lighting and so forth. Besides which, you must have special training. There are very few people in this country capable of performing them properly."

Obviously, then, it would do you little good, and possibly some harm to insist that your physician perform a vaginal hysterectomy when he's skilled in doing abdominal procedures. If you are determined to have a vaginal hysterectomy, you might be better off finding a surgeon who performs them frequently.

Or, if its just a matter of placating your vanity, talk to your physician about the placement of the incision. According to Dr. Birnbaum, the strongest and least noticeable scar is one which runs horizontally across the hair line. The stress of the muscles pulls the incision closed so it heals very nicely. Also, once your hair has grown back, the scar will be neatly hidden. Who said your two-piece bathing suit was destined for the Salvation Army?

Fear of a flabby belly following abdominal hysterectomy is also unfounded, says Dr. Birnbaum. Of course, a lot hinges on what you've got to start with. But if you're toned up before surgery, there's no reason why you can't be as firm and flat afterward, because, with rare exception, the muscles are not cut. They're just pulled back, so that the surgeon can get to the organs underneath. That little bit of stretch—nothing compared to pregnancy—can be shaped up with some sit-ups or leg-lifts once the incision is completely healed.

By the time you sign in at the hospital you should be perfectly clear on all the major issues—why you're having the surgery, what's going to be done and how the surgeon is going to do it. If you're not—if you've got any questions or reservations—don't expect them to be resolved on the eve of surgery. You'll have enough to keep you occupied.

Usually, the night before surgery is fraught with routine procedures: blood tests, x-rays, gynecological exams. In preparation for the surgery, you will also be given an enema and douche, and your pubic hair will be shaved. The rest of the preparation reads like it does for any other surgical procedure: no eating or drinking after midnight, a tranquilizing shot or two in the morning, and then off to the OR.

A hysterectomy may be performed at any time of the month—even during your period. But there may be some advantage to scheduling the surgery sometime during the second half of the menstrual cycle. According to a group of British physicians, bacteria were found in the vagina and postoperative infection occurred more often in the first week of the cycle (*Lancet*, December 8, 1973).

A hysterectomy is practically always done under general anesthesia. And chances are you'll be under the influence of these stupefying drugs for about 3 hours, or the time it takes to complete the surgery.

Afterward, you'll be wheeled to a recovery room until you awaken and then back to your room for further recuperation. As in all other surgical procedures you'll still have the IV bottle hanging over your head. And because hysterectomy is an abdominal procedure, you might have some swelling of the bladder, requiring a catheter for a few days. That is all routine.

What You Can Expect after a Hysterectomy

Probably the most painful postsurgical problem—at least so far as abdominal hysterectomy is concerned—is not the incision (though that will be extremely tender for a week or so) but gas. In fact, it's liable to be the most bloated feeling you'll ever have. It will subside in a few days. And by the time you're homeward-bound—usually in as short as 5 days for a "vag hyst" and 7 to 14 days for abdominal—all bowel and bladder function should be back to normal.

Just because you're home doesn't mean you're home free. It takes a long while to get over the trauma of hysterectomy. You'll feel weak, tired and maybe even a little weepy for several weeks after the surgery. And although physicians insist categorically that recuperation should not take longer than a month or two, sometimes it does. And there's nothing abnormal about it.

One woman we spoke with told us that it took her a year to recover completely from the "wiped-out" feeling. She even felt guilty because her physician acted as if she were dragging out recuperation in order to elicit attention and sympathy. Another woman explained that she had been programmed before the surgery to think that recuperation was going to be a breeze. When the pain, depression and weakness was with her 4 months later, she sought another physician. The second physician just reiterated the opinion of the first—recuperation from surgery shouldn't take longer than 2 months. "I know," he said, "I had a hernia operation a couple of years ago."

Unfortunately, some physicians treat hysterectomy as "just another operation." Anyone who's gone through it will tell you that it's just not so. The deep cutting into the abdomen and the removal and rearranging of internal organs take time to heal. In addition, hysterectomy is commonly followed by several distressing symptoms not related to other operations. According to D. H. Richards, 70 percent of his hysterectomy patients had postoperative depression and an almost equal number had hot flashes, urinary symptoms and extensive tiredness. About half suffered headaches, dizziness or insomnia postoperatively (*Lancet*, October 26, 1974).

For those reasons, convalescence cannot be rushed. Dr. Mikuta warns his patients to stay away from work for 6 weeks. And that includes housework! No heavy lifting (more than 5 to 10 pounds). No pushing a vacuum cleaner. Also, sexual intercourse should be postponed until your first postoperative check.

Aside from the vast amount of physical mending that's required after this major surgical procedure, there are also psychological wounds to heal. The uterus is a very intimate and personal organ, closely tied up to a woman's image of femininity and self so that feelings of self-doubt, loss of femininity, sexual inadequacy, barrenness and depression frequently follow its removal. And while many women are reluctant to discuss these problems with their physicians, about half suffer some psychological effects within the years following surgery.

"Women need reassurance that the loss of their uterus is not going to alter their functioning as a woman," says Evalyn Gendel, M.D., director of the Human Sexuality Program at the University of California School of Medicine, San Francisco. "It won't make her any less of a woman sexually."

Dennis Smith, M.D., a gynecologist and psychiatrist at Case Western Medical School in Cleveland, goes on to suggest that the psychological trauma of hysterectomy may be prevented or at least lessened with presurgical counseling.

"First of all, a woman has the right to know exactly what she can and cannot expect from the surgery. That way she is emotionally prepared for any consequences," he explains. "For example, women are repeatedly told that the hysterectomy will have *no* effect on their sexual relations. Yet one of the most common problems women report is that the sensation of intercourse is different. They may still enjoy sex and still have orgasm but something has changed. For some women the difference may be the absence of the cervix; perhaps they had gotten some pleasure from cervical contact. For others it may be that the uterus isn't there anymore so they miss the sensation of uterine contractions during orgasm. Actually, it's not too much to deal with—unless, of course, it completely takes her by surprise."

Second, says Dr. Smith, a woman should plunge into her psyche *before* plunging into surgery. It's important that she evaluate her own feelings of femininity and self prior to the surgery. "I can think of a woman right now who has severe pain caused by endometriosis and who would greatly benefit from a hysterectomy," Dr. Smith explains. "She came to me in anticipation of the surgery to discuss a psychological hang-up. Apparently she didn't want any more children but she was having trouble coping with the anticipated loss of her ability to give birth. We discussed the issue openly. And her eventual decision was to put up with the pain rather than go through with the surgery. I respect that decision. She must come to peace with herself. And this must be done *before* the act is committed.

"Probably the most important consideration is in understanding why the surgery is being performed," Dr. Smith adds. "Pump your physician for information. If you still don't understand, get a second opinion from someone who is willing to sit down and discuss your situation. Don't stop until you can go to yourself and answer without hesitation why the surgery is needed. Women who understand the reason for the loss—even though they may still feel it—are better able to come to terms with any problems which may occur afterward."

15
Breast Problems

From the time a young woman slips out of cotton T-shirts and into her first training bra, her awareness of breasts probably drifts in and out of focus. Even if she accepts them casually, magazines and movies don't. Bare-bosomed ladies on the covers of *Cosmo* and *People* stare at her as she stands in the supermarket checkout line, and newspaper headlines cite new achievements in treatment of breast maladies.

All species of mammals except humans take female breasts quite for granted. Mammary glands feed the young, and that's that.

To carry out that life-sustaining function, the human breast contains 15 to 25 separate milk-producing glands, each equipped with its own duct leading to a separate opening in the nipple. The ducts and nipple are surrounded by some small muscles, but the bulk of the breast itself is composed of plentiful fat in which all those glands and ducts are softly embedded which explains why excess dieting trims some women of curves they would rather keep. The breast, like other body structures, is fed by nerves, blood vessels and a system of lymph glands which lie underneath, above and beside it on the chest. All in all, a wonderfully efficient package.

From prenatal life through maturity, the growth and development of the female breasts depend on their response to levels of hormones circulating in the blood. When an error occurs in those normal processes of growth and development, disease results. The cause could be too little or too much of a hormone in the blood or too little or too much response by the breast. The abnormality can be harmless but annoying (benign, noncancerous), acute and life-threatening (malignant, cancerous) or somewhere in between. And at some point in its development, the disease announces its presence by one or more physical signs.

The breast, for all its functional and ornamental attributes, is vulnerable to some very uncomfortable and worrisome ailments, the most alarming of which is cancer. Confusion over risk factors and mass screening for breast cancer, combined with blazing headlines that 1 out of every 13 women faces breast cancer each year, can prompt you to react in either of 2 ways: you nervously devour all the facts and theories and pray that you never have trouble, or else you throw up your hands in utter hopelessness.

Those same hands of yours, however, can easily be educated to examine your own breasts for abnormalities, and thereby help to minimize your chances of becoming a cancer statistic. Early detection can not only save your life, but can increase the feasibility of cosmetically pleasing reconstruction of the breast should surgery be necessary.

Self-Examination of the Breast

The symptom that most often prompts breast cancer victims to see their doctors is a lump (usually painless) in a breast. Sometimes a lump is found during a routine medical checkup, but 95 percent of breast lumps are found by women themselves, either during habitual self-examination or incidentally, while showering or undressing.

Because smaller cancers can be more successfully treated than larger ones, breast self-examination and regular medical screening are a must. Early detection is the surest hedge against trouble, and to rely on the accidental discovery of a lump is to have no hedge at all.

Frequent examinations — monthly self-exams plus yearly physician exams — are more likely to result in diagnosis of cancer in its earlier states, and to check the spread to the lymph glands under the arm. In a National Cancer Institute-supported study of the self-exam habits of 246 newly diagnosed breast cancer patients, over one-third of the patients who never practiced breast self-examination had advanced stages of cancer, compared to only 5 percent of those who had routinely done self-exam. Furthermore, patients who never practiced self-examination showed up with significantly larger tumors than those who practiced it at least monthly (*New England Journal of Medicine,* August 10, 1978). And the larger the tumors, the more lymph nodes that were cancerous.

Only one-fourth of American women practice self-examination. If all women took the time for regular, thorough home and office exams, early detection would result in a more favorable picture for cure. Breast cancer cannot yet be prevented, but the woman who does her homework greatly improves her chances of catching it in its most treatable stages. According to Roger S. Foster Jr., M.D., and his co-researchers in the above study, each woman "destined to develop breast cancer has in her own hands the possibility of increasing her chance of survival through performance of breast self-examination."

Many women do not examine their breasts because of fear of what they might find, when actually what they might find may save their lives. Others are not confident enough or just don't bother.

Not only must self-examination be done regularly, it must be done properly. It's simple and only takes a few minutes. A woman should ideally begin routine exams in the late teens or early 20s — not because of the possibility of cancer but because the unlikelihood of cancer at that time helps her to learn the unique consistency of her own breasts without anxiety over cancer. Self-examination should be continued throughout life, even during pregnancy. Once you get into the habit, you will become familiar with the natural thickenings, bumps and irregularities that occur in the normal, healthy breast, and your hands and eyes will become trained to detect any abnormalities that may develop. That is one reason that self-exam should be performed between your doctor's exams. Another is that it can be done frequently, at no expense or time spent in a waiting room. There are certainly no adverse side effects or risks, and it is only slightly uncomfortable.

It is best to choose a specific time of the month, preferably right after your period if you are still menstruating. That allows for cyclical changes in the breast which normally occur between periods. If you are past menopause, the first day of each calendar month is a good reminder.

Breasts may vary in many ways even when disease-free. On the same woman, one breast may be somewhat larger, shaped differently or more sensitive than the other. Both may be very tender all over or only in certain areas, or tender only at certain times of the month or year. They may be lumpy, or free of any nodules at all. They may be firm, full, small, a little saggy or very saggy. They may change slightly from one year to the next. The nipples may be flat, erect, inverted, large or small, and the surrounding areola may be dark brown or pale pink. The purpose of regular self-examination is to keep in touch with any *changes* that may suddenly occur. That requires both looking and feeling.

How to examine your breasts. Disrobe to the waist and stand or sit before a mirror in a well-lit room, with arms down at your sides. Look for changes from one exam to the next, such as dimpling of the skin or pulling in of an otherwise turned-out nipple. Observe any crustiness or scaling of the nipple. Watery, yellow, pink or blood discharge from the nipple should also be noted at any time. (Milky discharges are not uncommon, and are caused by benign changes in the breast.)

Still sitting or standing, lean forward slightly, watching for those same changes.

Raise your arms slowly and evenly overhead and press your hands together behind your head, observing any changes in contour of one breast, puckering or dimpling of the skin, or "pulling" in the skin (that is, tendency of the breast tissues to fail to slip easily over the underlying muscles). Raising the arms in this way may accentuate changes that might not otherwise be obvious.

Next, place your hands on your hips and tighten your chest and arm muscles by pressing firmly inward. Again, observe the breasts for changes.

To feel (palpate) the breasts themselves, lie flat on your back with a small pillow or folded towel under your left shoulder. Raise the left arm itself overhead. With the right hand slightly cupped and the fingers together, feel for any unusual lumps or change in the texture of the breast skin. Use the flat of the fingers, not the tips. Lumps are palpable at about the size of a pea or larger. Avoid compressing the breast tissue between the thumb and fingers, as that may give the impression of a lump that is not actually present.

Begin either at the nipple, proceeding in a rotary direction toward the outer regions of the breast, or palpate each half of the breast at a time. If you prefer the latter method, start with the inner half of the left breast, examining the areas from the collarbone to the underportion and from the nipple to the breastbone (sternum) in the center of your chest. Then feel the outer half from bottom to top and from the nipple to the underarm. (A ridge of firm tissue in the lower curve of each breast is normal.)

Transfer the towel or pillow to the right shoulder and repeat, using the left hand to feel the right breast.

It may be easier to feel for lumps with the skin of the hands and breasts wet and soapy. The soap allows the hands to glide very lightly over the skin surface, as you would stroke a length of fabric to determine the nap or grain. That will help you to detect any small changes underneath the breast surface. You may find it convenient to practice this in the shower, either before or after the rest of the exam.

Other signs to be alert to are breast pain, itching of the nipple, noticeable enlargement or shrinking of both breasts and generalized hardness or redness. Very rarely, a lump in the armpit, arm swelling for no apparent reason, or bone pain may prompt you to call for a doctor's appointment.

The Physician's Exam

Self-examination is very similar to but not a substitute for an annual exam. You will be asked to lie on an exam table. In some clinics, a nurse or other specially trained professional may perform the exam. For one thing, it is possible for you yourself to miss lumps, even when you have been very thorough. In the examining room, insist on a complete exam — it should take more than just a minute or two — and have the physician or nurse review the self-exam with you to be sure that you are performing it correctly and to point out the normal ridges, muscles and bumps in the breasts.

Like the story of the princess and the pea, it takes a sensitive hand to feel a lump buried under layers of fatty tissue, and it takes professionally trained hands to detect more elusive, hard-to-feel lumps. That is particularly true if you are older or have large breasts. In a small breast, even a very small lump can be felt. As the breasts become larger, fattier or more pendulous after menopause, childbirth or weight gain, even a large growth may be difficult to detect. Tumors developing in the milk ducts are often not readily felt. You may feel more confident having the exam done in an obstetrician-gynecologist's office rather than by a GP because of the gynecologist's expertise gained from examining many, many women.

The physician may record the location, size and consistency of any lumps or thickenings on a sketch of the breasts, for future reference. At that time, he or she should also record or update your complete medical history, including previous benign breast problems, childbearing and menstrual history, and any breast cancer in your mother or a sister.

Physicians estimate that breast cancer mortality might be reduced by nearly 20 percent through widespread self-examination and up to 48 percent when combined with yearly physician's exams (*New England Journal of Medicine,* August 10, 1978). Of course, any time you find a lump or notice an abnormality in the breast, it is wiser to check with your doctor rather than wait for an appointment scheduled way off in the future.

Mammography. Depending on your age, your physician may order a yearly mammography — a special x-ray which shows considerable detail of the breast — to screen for unpalpable masses. A mammogram may also be ordered if your breasts are rather large and fatty, making manual detection of lumps difficult and unreliable. Ninety to 95 percent of breast cancers can be detected by mammography alone, while only 60 percent are felt during physical examination. Recent studies show that combining mammography with physical examination reduces death from breast cancer by one-third over chance finding of lumps, because mammography can detect localized tumors before they spread to the armpit glands or beyond (*Mayo Clinic Proceedings,* March, 1977).

Mammography is the most reliable way to detect whether or not unpalpable masses are present. It also helps to determine whether they are benign or malignant. So it is used both to screen women who have no symptoms and to help diagnose a suspicious sign.

You will be asked to disrobe to the waist and be given a dressing gown to wear into the closed-off examination room. You will either stand or sit against the mammography equipment, depending on the type of machine used. One breast at a time is exposed, and the chest itself is not involved. (A chest x-ray is a low radiation shot of the whole chest and should not be confused with a mammogram.) The rest of your body, including the ovaries, is not exposed to the radiation and need not be shielded.

Each breast is slightly compressed between a small shelf projecting from the machine and a cone lowered from above. Two exposures are made of each breast, to view the breast from the side and the front. Mammographic equipment is calibrated to indicate exact exposure time and consequently the amount of radiation delivered to the breast. That is measured in rads (radiation absorbed dose) and will be about one rad or less to the midpoint of each breast. The amount will depend on the size of the breast. Larger breasts require slightly more exposure time. Ask the x-ray technician or radiologist (a physician specializing in use of x-rays) how many rads will be absorbed. If your radiologist doesn't know or if it seems high, ask your doctor to suggest an alternative exam site.

Mammography itself only takes 5 or 6 minutes altogether. The result will be images of the interior of your breasts, recorded on film. These images are studied by the radiologist and interpreted to your physician.

As a screening tool, mammography is combined with complete medical history and physical examination of the breasts in women age 50 and over because of the increased likelihood of cancer showing up at that age. It may also be indicated in younger women who show other known risk factors or who have an inordinate fear of cancer and need reassurance.

Mammography is a valuable tool for diagnosing suspicious signs or screening high-risk women, but is not without risks. There is great controversy over the use of routine mammography to screen symptom-free women because of the theoretical possibility that repeated mammography, by exposing the breasts to radiation, may in itself cause cancer, especially in those already at high risk. (That is, precisely those who are recommended for screening.) On the other hand, these hazards are offset by the potential value of mammography in detecting unpalpable masses before cancer has spread to the lymph nodes under the arms or to vital organs, thus making earlier treatment possible and survival more likely. If caught while small and confined to just the breast, there is an 85 to 95 percent chance for survival, compared to only 50 percent if the cancer has invaded the nodes or beyond.

Estimates state that approximately 120 malignancies will be produced for every million women exposed to one rad to each breast in 1 year, and that is after a latent period of anywhere from 10 to 20 years. That's compare to nearly 10,000 early cancers that would be missed if mammography was not done at all (*Journal of the American Medical Association,* August 22, 1977). So its advocates consider it a very important leg of the three-legged stool on which early breast cancer detection stands: self-exam, physician's exam and mammogram.

There is also the possibility of unjustified reassurance from the 10 percent chance of false-negative mammograms. (Negative means "no cancer seen"; false-negative means there really is cancer but it doesn't show up.) On the other hand, repeating the exam yearly offers some protection against false-negatives.

Obviously, there is no question about the use of mammography in women who show any of the suspicious signs of breast cancer. But when expert opinions on use of mammography for regular screening of symptom-free women range from the view that it will save many lives to the belief that the practice will produce potentially fatal illness in those same women, where does that leave you?

The following guidelines, offered jointly by the American Cancer Society and the National Cancer Institute and used in their many Breast Cancer Detection Demonstration Projects throughout the country, should help:

- At any age, mammography can be valuable in determining the nature of suspicious masses in the breast, even if they are recurring symptoms of benign breast disease.
- If you are under 35 and symptom-free, mammography will not be used for regular periodic examination.
- If you are between 35 and 39 and symptom-free, mammography should only be considered if you have already had cancer in one breast.
- If you are between 40 and 49, periodic mammography may be part of your routine checkup if you are at high risk because of previous breast cancer or cancer in your mother or a sister.
- At age 50 or older, the benefits of catching unpalpable masses are greatest in relation to the risk. That is due both to the increased likelihood of cancer showing up at that age and the reduced number of mammograms exposing the breasts to radiation by beginning at that time. Also, the breasts in women over 50 are less glandular and dense than those of younger women, making mammography more accurate. Arthur Holleb, M.D., senior vice-president of medical affairs for the American Cancer Society, feels that childlessness, first childbirth after age 30 or early onset of menstruation may suggest the need for regular mammography in some women under 50.

Ask your physician to review the reasons for any earlier or more-than-yearly use of mammography for you. For some women, the annual clean bill of health is worth repeated exposures. For others, symptom-free breasts and a low-risk medical history suggest they need undergo only the minimum — or none at all.

Mammography for diagnosis of a suspicious sign is covered by major insurance plans and Medicare: breast x-rays as part of a *routine* exam are not.

Newer, higher quality x-ray films are now being used which permit faster mammography and consequently less exposure to radiation than was possible a few years ago. An alternative method is Xeromammography (also called Xeroradiography) in which the images of the breasts are projected onto a Xerox plate. From that, the images are transferred to special paper, much like the photocopier system you may use in your office. Xeromammography yields better quality images, but the dosage is not quite as low as fast-film mammography.

Thermography. Under evaluation is another technique, thermography, which uses no radiation at all, but rather measures the heat radiated by various masses in the breast. Approximately 45 to 70 percent of breast cancers cause an abnormal heat pattern on the skin surface. But so do some noncancerous masses. Although it is safe, the high false-positive rate (indicating cancer when there is none) makes thermography valuable only when combined with physical examination, in order to determine if a woman should have a mammography, or to help clear up a questionable abnormality on a mammogram.

If you or your doctor should discover a lump or other symptoms, that does not automatically mean you have cancer. If your exam falls just before your period, the harmless nodes (lumps) that develop premenstrually may either incorrectly suggest a malignant tumor or obscure an underlying lump. Your doctor may ask you to return to his office after your period to double-check the problem.

Regardless of the controversy, if a lump is present, your doctor may order a mammogram not only to help determine whether it may be cancerous but to discover any other unpalpable masses and their location — in either breast. Even if a mass is palpable, the geography of the breast changes when a woman moves from lying down for a physical exam to sitting for a mammogram. You have probably noticed that difference when you shift position for sunbathing at the beach.

Office biopsy. Once mammography has told your physician exactly where any problems are located, he may remove some of the suspicious tissue for further study. That is usually done in the office by fine-needle aspiration and/or needle core biopsy. Either procedure is simple and takes about 15 minutes.

For fine-needle aspiration, the physician will insert a long, thin, hollow needle through the fatty breast tissue into the growth and drain it of any fluid. Lumps are often just pockets of innocuous fluid, called cysts. If the fluid is clear, it generally means the cyst is noncancerous; the fluid is discarded. If the fluid is bloody, or aspiration doesn't completely eradicate the cyst, the fluid may be sent to the lab for study.

If the mass does not completely disappear, recurs or turns out to be solid rather than fluid filled, some physicians may proceed with a needle core biopsy. First the breast will be numbed with a local anesthetic, like the "local" you get for tooth extraction. By inserting a slightly larger needle through a tiny incision on the breast surface, a core sample of the problem tissue will be pulled out. That leaves a small scar.

The smear of suspicious aspirated fluid or biopsied material is sent to a pathologist for examination under a laboratory microscope. Although truly benign cells do not become malignant, they often mimic the cancerous kind — and can co-exist in the same breast. Therefore, sampled cells are always examined by a pathologist. Based on the size, formation and other characteristics of the cells, the pathologist will tell your doctor if the disease appears to be benign, malignant or questionable. Benign means the abnormal cells have neither gone berserk nor invaded healthy tissue. Besides cysts, benign lumps may be merely masses of scar-like tissue among the fat. Malignant cells are a threat to life because, after first invading the ducts and fatty tissues of the breast, they eventually penetrate the lymph glands and blood vessels, to travel to bones and vital organs, especially the liver and lungs.

The lab test itself takes just a few minutes to process, and your physician will have the results in a few days at the longest.

Benign Breast Disease

Eighty percent of all lumps confirmed by doctors are benign. That is, they are not cancerous. But only your physician can diagnose the difference. Although there is no need to panic, it is just as unwise to "wait and see," hoping the lump will disappear.

Another very common breast complaint is pain and tenderness (with or without a lump), which may send you to your doctor not so much out of fear of cancer but sheer discomfort. Even if disease-free, breasts may become enlarged, painful and tender to the touch due to water buildup in the fatty tissues just before or during your period. That may be caused by an excess of sodium in the body. In some women, fluid buildup is a habitual response to the natural rise in the hormone estrogen which occurs just before menstruation. The waterlogged tissues swell, nudge the nerves, and you feel pain.

Should you suffer unbearable discomfort, your physician may prescribe a thiazide diurectic, a drug which flushes this excess water out of the fatty tissues and out of the body. Diuretics are used in this case for only the few days prior to or during your period, so they don't cause the large losses of vital minerals — mainly potassium — that are common in continuous, unsupplemented diuretic therapy.

Diuretics are drugs, capable of causing toxic reactions such as dizziness, headache, ringing in the ears or nausea. If you should suffer such side effects, your doctor can change your prescription to find a drug you can tolerate.

Another approach to relief from fluid retention is use of small doses of another hormone, progesterone, to counteract the estrogen's effect.

But before resorting to drugs or hormones, try enlisting the support of your bra for relief. For many women, wearing a bra to bed during the problem period is the answer. The elastic support of the bra acts as a second skin, counteracting the pressure within the breast tissues.

Even for daytime wear, and especially if your bosom is a somewhat generous 36C or larger, an inadequate brassiere can aggravate either premenstrual pain or pain due to benign disease. Just choosing a pretty bra from among the underwire push-ups and lacy strapless styles on the rack does not insure that you've chosen the right bra for you.

Determining your proper bra size and style requires some homework. First, measure your rib cage under your breasts with a tape measure. Add 5 inches to that number. The total is your bra size. If it is an odd number, say 37, round it off to the next highest number, 38.

To determine the letter size of your bra cup, measure the largest circumference around your body at bust level (that is, around your back and horizontally across both nipples). If that measurement is 1 inch more than your bra number size, your cup is an A. Two inches more, you are a B cup. Three inches more, a C, and 4 inches more, a D.

Bulges over the bra top mean either the cup is too small or you have the back and shoulder straps adjusted too tightly. The bra style you choose should distribute support or most of the weight of your breasts across your back. If the shoulder straps are forced to carry the burden, they will dig into your shoulders.

Should finding a comfortable bra be difficult for you, ask one of the trained salespeople in women's specialty shops or lingerie departments in major stores to help fit you.

Cutting down on dietary salt intake is very likely to reduce the water retention itself and pain. The drastic change in seasoning may make your food taste bland, but other herbs and spices such as celery seed, parsley, or chives can compensate for the salt.

Physicians ranging from a country doctor in Indiana to a Park Avenue gynecologist in New York report that supplemental doses of vitamin B_6 soothe tender breasts. Backed up with lesser amounts of other B complex vitamins, B_6 has a natural diuretic effect on water buildup. Vitamin B_6 also seems to regulate out-of-proportion hormone levels in some women. Kenneth I. Sheek, M.D., a practitioner in Greenwood, Indiana, sees excellent results in women who take just 40 milligrams of pyridoxine (B_6) a day in B complex tablets. Other women need much more. A New Jersey gynecologist gives his patients up to 600 milligrams a day, beginning at ovulation (about midpoint in the menstrual cycle). Sore breasts are usually only a memory by the second month of supplementation. While your needs for B_6 will not be exactly the same as your neighbor's, a baseline dose is a daily total of around 100 milligrams, according the Gideon G. Panter, M.D., obstetrician-gynecologist in New York City.

If pain lasts for more than a few days of your menstrual cycle, forces you to wear a bra round the clock, wakens you at night, or makes household chores, sports or office work unbearable, you need medical attention. And you probably won't need a pep talk to get you there!

Abnormal but benign growths cause symptoms of redness, nipple puckering or discharge and skin dimpling as well as lumps and pain which mimic cancer but can also characterize a variety of noncancerous breast diseases.

The most common cause of breast lumps is fibrocystic disease, also called chronic cystic mastitis or mammary dysplasia. There is no one distinct fibrocystic disease. Rather, that term covers a range of abnormal conditions that develop in the breast, sometimes simultaneously. It is benign, and it is the most common type of breast disease, usually showing up between the ages of 18 and 50, while the ovaries are still functioning. It then subsides after menopause. Half of the women in the U.S. will be diagnosed as having fibrocystic disease sometime in their lives.

"Fibrocystic" is a tag which explains what has happened to a previously healthy breast, possibly due to the slight rise in estrogen that is normally secreted by the ovaries about midpoint in the menstrual cycle. A deviation from the normal process of manufacturing new cells in glands, ducts and connective tissues may result in 2 types of symptoms. Either long, threadlike fibers aberrantly grow to form a solid, scarlike mass, or a small pocket among the tissues fills with fluid or semisolid material to form a cyst. Both result in unwelcome lumps the size of a grape or larger that cling to healthy breast tissue. And they hurt!

Immediate relief is gained by minor surgery — either in the doctor's office by needle aspiration or in a hospital on an outpatient basis for surgical removal of a lump. Either way, you feel better. However, the disease tends to be chronic. After a few months, the system goes out of kilter again, and you may find yourself returning for repeated removal of lumps or fluid. Repeated aspirations call for removal of the cyst itself. Like lump removal, that too is done as an outpatient procedure under local anesthesia. Recurring discomfort may be somewhat relieved by a supporting bra.

But recurrence may be preventable. Vitamin E (alpha tocopherol) can often reduce not only the discomfort but also the size and number of breast cysts. Alpha tocopherol seems to work by reversing the abnormal ratio of estrogen and progesterone circulating in the body during the menstrual cycle. That change in hormone levels is an antidote to estrogen's disturbing effect of cyst formation in the breast.

Success with alpha tocopherol for fibrocystic disease is very real. Robert London, M.D., director of the Obstetric and Gynecologic Endocrinology Research Lab at Sinai Hospital in Baltimore has seen promising results from daily oral doses of 600 International Units of alpha tocopherol in 80 percent of one group of women studied.

"Some women respond better than others," Dr. London reports. "But relief usually follows within two months at most. That's very encouraging, because there is so little attention paid to the effective treatment of fibrocystic disease other than surgical removal of the cysts."

Benign breast lumps may also regress after a change in dietary habits. John P. Minton, M.D., Ph.D., of the department of surgery at Ohio State University College of Medicine, has seen benign lumps completely disappear within 2 to 6 months in 13 out of 20 women who completely eliminated coffee, tea, chocolate and cola from their diets. And relief eventually came to 3 others within 18 months after the change. Those substances contain chemical stimulants called methylxanthines, which hinder the work of enzymes in cells (*Journal of the American Medical Association,* March 23, 1979).

The next time you shop, bring home one or two of the herbal teas sold in health food stores and supermarkets. They are free of stimulants and refreshing stand-ins for breakfast or coffee breaks.

Another lumpy pest goes by the name of fibroadenoma. These firm, round, nontender lumps range from about the size of a large pea to that of a golf ball, and are somewhat mobile. They usually occur singly, make their appearance within 20 years after puberty and are removed surgically.

The most frequent cause of clear or bloody nipple discharge is small, warty, usually unpalpable growths blocking the ducts underneath the nipple and areola. Your doctor may decide to have the discharge smeared onto a glass slide and examined at a lab, but that test is not totally reliable. More than likely, the growth — papilloma — or the duct itself will be cut out and studied to determine if it is cancerous or benign.

Pain, tenderness and redness are sometimes caused by an inflammation of the milk ducts (mammary duct ectasia). About half the victims of this disease will suffer inverted or cracked nipples, or have difficulty nursing. It may also produce a lump, sometimes with pulling in of skin or the nipple. Suspicions can be overruled only by biopsy of the tissue.

An occasional incident of drawing in of a nipple or dimpling of skin may be due to death of a small area of fatty tissue below the surface. Such fat necrosis sometimes follows a slight injury, perhaps from a fall or a blow to the breast.

Open Biopsy: Is It Cancer . . . Or Isn't It?

If the pathologist and your doctor are certain that your symptoms are due to one of those benign conditions, the growth will be removed on an outpatient basis and that's that.

However, some abnormal cells are neither clearly benign nor are they clearly malignant. Some growths are too small to yield enough tissue for an accurate office biopsy. Fine-needle aspirations are only 92 percent accurate for diagnosis, and a benign reading is not to be trusted in a woman 50 years of age or older, who is more likely to have cancer. A cyst may refuse to disappear, even when repeatedly aspirated. In any of these cases, your doctor may very likely want to take a closer look at the tissue by means of an open biopsy.

That is now widely performed as an outpatient procedure, in an operating room, under general anesthesia. Using a mammogram of the breast as a guide to the location of the mass, a small incision is made in the breast. If the incision is made parallel to the natural skin contours that surround the areola, scars tend eventually to fade, minimizing unsightly marks. That should be a consideration especially in a woman who undergoes repeated surgical biopsies.

Removing only what is necessary, the doctor cuts out a chunk of tissue containing the suspicious cells for immediate study by a pathologist. Then the wound is sewn up. A section of the soft tissue is quickly frozen and stained so that it can be examined under a microscope. The test itself takes about 5 minutes and the surgeon can have the results in 20 minutes.

Eighty-five to 90 percent of breast cancers can be readily diagnosed by frozen section. The remaining 10 to 15 percent are minimal cancers — not yet invasive, but not truly benign — and the pathologist may need more details of the cells to make his decision. In that case, he will make a permanent section from the same soft tissue. He may even request more and better samples of tissue. Instead of freezing the section to make it rigid, the pathologist fixes it with formaldehyde; it is dehydrated, set in paraffin, stained and then read. That whole process takes from 12 to 24 hours, so your surgeon won't have the results until at least the next day.

Half of those minimal cancers can be easily diagnosed based on reexamination by permanent section; the remaining half (or 1 in 25 of all open biopsies) may require the consulting opinion of a second pathologist.

The decision on choice of treatment, including major surgery, is made by the surgeon based on what is seen on either the quick-frozen section or the longer permanent section lab test. Cancers vary from very sluggish growths to those more likely to spread widely (metastasize), with some in a gray area where they are neither. Some are so sluggish they border on benign and may never become malignant. While it is logical to assume that all large cancer tumors were once small, there is no evidence that all small, sluggish growths become large. Those noninvasive cancers smaller than the size of a large pea or confined to a local spot are tricky to diagnose and not very well understood. Not unexpectedly, some surgeons feel that a breast containing clusters of such minimal cancer cells should be removed for fear they may later start growing into a true cancer. Delay in treatment after open biopsy does not affect the course of the disease one way or the other. Because breast cancer is a relatively slow developing disease compared to other cancers, a few more days is not going to make any difference in the success of treatment.

Since only about 1 in every 15 or 20 women who require open biopsy for cancer diagnosis actually has malignant cancer confirmed, that step-by-step approach should eliminate the fear of waking up without a breast. It also avoids unnecessary hospitalization and expensive preoperative tests not needed in those remaining women who do not require further surgery.

There are personal considerations, too, as pointed out by Morton Comess, M.D., a surgeon in Phoenix, Arizona. "If you are a working woman, the boss will want to know if you'll be out for a day or a month. If you have children, you have to arrange for babysitters. (On the other hand, those are not likely to be problems for the woman in her 60s or 70s.) So scheduling the major surgery apart from the outpatient biopsy makes sense that way, too." Discuss the possibility of minimal cancer, should it be found, with your surgeon before open biopsy. He can still remove the breast later, if he feels that the presence of unseen microscopic cancer cells is likely elsewhere in the breast. Amputation of a breast — or anything else — is serious enough business to warrant close observation of those worrisome cells rather than automatic removal.

Mastectomy (breast removal) is an extreme measure for a cancer which affords a 70 percent chance of 30 years of disease-free survival without any treatment at all, according to Gerson Lesnick, M.D., surgeon at Mt. Sinai Hospital in New York. He suggests close observation of minimal cancers, followed by prompt treatment if the cancer should become invasive (*New York State Journal of Medicine,* February, 1979).

But suppose your physician forgoes the step-by-step approach? An alternate scenario can go like this:

Your physician may skip the fine-needle aspiration and you are admitted to the hospital for open biopsy. The surgeon asks you to sign a paper giving permission to go ahead with any treatment deemed appropriate based on the pathology test done while you are on the operating table, unconscious. What that means is that the surgeon goes into the open biopsy all suited up to do a mastectomy based on results of the frozen section. The pathologist announces that the verdict is "malignant," and you wake up without a breast.

One woman whose surgeon separated biopsy from mastectomy described her experience:

> My doctor was quite confident that the lump was benign and reassured me that it would not be a problem. So when a young intern came to my hospital room the night before surgery and said, "You know, Mrs. Smith, you have to sign this paper giving permission to remove your breast if we find cancer," I was really quite stunned. But I was naive and thought you had to sign certain forms before any kind of surgery, so I signed.
>
> It turned out to be questionable, and the doctor let me wake up with my breast. When he came in to see me, I assumed everything was OK, but he said, "Not exactly. . . . " He explained that there were 2 lumps. One was benign, and 1 was questionable according to the frozen section. So the lab started a more extensive, permanent section exam and they let me wake up.
>
> If that exam had been all right, I would have been

> home free. The cancer was very minute, almost infinitesimal, but it wasn't benign and the doctor really felt he should do a mastectomy. Or we could wait and see. We also discussed the possibility of reconstruction of the breast later.
>
> I was very tired and emotional. My husband said it was up to me. I thought about it for about an hour or so. I decided I didn't want reconstruction, and the surgeon did a simple mastectomy 3 days later.
>
> It was very traumatic, but I feel I was lucky not to have to experience the shock of waking up without a breast.

Some women are so overwhelmed by the fear of cancer that immediate removal of a breast is worth some reassurance that they have been cured. For others, the thought of later reentering the hospital in anticipation of definite loss of a breast is more agonizing than the uncertainty of allowing the surgeon the option of performing a mastectomy while they are already on the table. Combining open biopsy with mastectomy also eliminates the risks of a second general anesthesia later.

Much will depend on your surgeon's judgment of what he sees of the cancer at the point of biopsy. Cancer (carcinoma, medically speaking) is not one disease — there are about 15 varieties. Cancer is very sneaky, starting out microscopically, growing gradually and not revealing itself until it is well-established. First it invades normal local tissues and often takes a free ride in the lymphatic system or bloodstream to reestablish itself on vital organs. If open biopsy shows that there is in fact cancer, its location, size, stage of development and type will help your doctor to decide on what treatment is best for you and what your chances for cure are.

At that time, the cancer cells should also be tested for estrogen receptor sites. That information will indicate whether hormone therapy will be useful. Bone and liver scans will indicate whether or not it has spread to those organs.

Breast cancer, like other cancers, is classed according to stages and type. The stage indicates how far it has spread, and the type denotes how aggressively it behaves or is likely to behave.

Stage is determined by size of the tumor (T), involvement of the lymph nodes (N) and metastases (M). Briefly, that TNM system places the cancer at one of 4 stages of development:

Stage I The malignant growth is confined to the breast. There are no signs that it has spread to the armpit or beyond.

Stage II The primary (largest and first discovered) tumor is only at Stage I, but there are suspicious lumps in the armpit.

Stage III The primary tumor has invaded the skin, chest wall and chest muscles. Lumps can be felt in the armpit, and unpalpable masses may also be present. (The presence of those cannot be determined without further surgery. Manual palpation is very unreliable here.)

Stage IV The cancer has spread beyond the breast and armpit region, usually to bone marrow, liver or lungs.

How aggressively the tumor itself grows also determines treatment. Based on examination of biopsied cells, cancer is classified according to the likelihood of its spreading to distant organs (metastasizing) and its potential for destroying healthy tissue surrounding it (invasiveness).

Type I Rarely metastasizes, not invasive. The cells multiply within but not beyond a local tumor or tumors, which makes them easy to remove surgically.

Type II Rarely metastasizes, always invasive. The cells may spread to ducts and other breast tissues, requiring radiation or breast removal.

Type III Moderately metastasizes, always invasive. Most of those cancers originate in the ducts themselves and are called invasive ductal carcinoma; the others originate in glands and are called adenocarcinoma. Both are very likely to spread to lymph nodes and possibly the bloodstream, making local control unlikely.

Type IV Highly metastasizes, always invasive. Those cells spread directly from the original tumor into the bloodstream. Immediate and sustained drug therapy has made them less lethal than previously.

Adapted from *Current Medical Diagnosis and Treatment* (Lange Medical Publications, 1978) p. 421.

Surgical Answers to Breast Cancer

Based on those criteria, your surgeon will decide on treatment. For Stages I, II and sometimes III, long-term survival is a realistic goal. That's why early detection is stressed again and again. Ninety percent of breast cancers fall into the operable categories.

The first item on the agenda is removing the troublesome cells. That means surgery to some extent, possibly followed by radiation therapy. After the open biopsy, you may wait in the hospital for surgery or reenter at a later date.

For the remaining 10 percent which have progressed to Stage IV (or some in Stage III), cancer cannot successfully be treated by surgery. Attempts will be made to weaken the cancer, counteract its physical effects or delay its recurrence. The arsenal for that war includes irradiation, hormones or very powerful drugs (chemotherapy). Those tools hold out hope for improving the overall survival of advanced breast cancer patients.

Obviously, surgery is going to produce disfigurement — some operations result in more disfigurement than others. While cosmetic effects are not to be coldly ignored, your surgeon will choose the method he feels offers you the greatest chance of a cancer-free life with as little deformity as possible. That decision is primarily influenced by his observation of the cancer's behavior at biopsy. During your first visit with the surgeon, ask him about the possibility of reconstruction of the breast after you recover from mastectomy. If the tumor is not located near the nipple, it may be possible to save the nipple and later attach it to a rebuilt breast. (If that's the case, the nipple will temporarily be sewn to an inconspicuous spot on your body, such as the groin or inner thigh.)

The possibility of future reconstruction of the breast may also influence the direction of the surgeon's incision. With the increasing acceptance (and affordability) of breast reconstruction after mastectomy, horizontal incisions are favored. That results in a scar which falls into the skin's natural tension lines, improves the cosmetic effect of reconstruction and doesn't interfere with the blood supply to the reconstructed breast. (A discussion of breast reconstruction surgery appears later in this chapter.)

Artificial breasts (prostheses) that slip into the bra make it possible for a woman who has had a mastectomy without further reconstruction to continue to wear attractive and even slightly revealing clothes; her personal taste in neckline styles may warrant discussing the direction of the incision with her surgeon. A horizontal or slightly diagonal incision can be covered by a prosthesis-filled brassiere, evening dress or even a bikini. Until recently, most surgeons routinely made a vertical incision, which allowed for plunging necklines.

Any surgeon who is board-certified is qualified to do a mastectomy. Survival and recurrence rates depend on the state of the cancer rather than the surgeon's technique, so you need not worry about locating a breast surgery specialist if you do not live near a big city hospital. However, some surgeons may not have enough experience with breast surgery to take great pains about the direction of the incision. While cure is more important than contour, your plans for possible reconstruction should be taken into consideration.

Quality of life after mastectomy is just as important as length of life. Don't hesitate to ask your surgeon any questions about either the operation itself, healing time or side effects. He should explain in detail what is to be removed during the operation and why. How much tissue is going to be removed, particularly in the underarm and chest area, influences healing time and arm motion at the shoulder. At that time, he can also answer your questions about pain and postsurgery depression or anxiety.

After the breast is removed, the edges of the cut area will be pulled together snugly over the ribs and sewn up. If you have small breasts, it may be necessary to graft some skin from your thigh over the cut area, because there might not be enough of a flap left to sew the wound closed. If the underarm nodes must be removed, surgical tubes will be left in place to drain lymph fluids from the surgical wound for about 4 days after the operation.

If your case is operable, the type of surgery most likely to be chosen is modified radical mastectomy. That sounds very confusing, but the procedure is fairly easy to visualize. Mastectomy literally means removal of the breast. Modified radical mastectomy refers to removal of the glands under the arm, leaving in place the chest muscles (pectoralis major and minor) that support the breast and help move the shoulder. Some modified radicals remove the minor but not the major muscle, in order to gain access to the underarm (axillary) lymph glands.

In a standard radical mastectomy both those muscles are removed, resulting in far more deformity and functional problems with the arm and shoulder.

The rationale for modified radical mastectomy is that cancer in just one part of the breast may very well be accompanied by microscopic, undetected cancer cells throughout the breast, and taking only what is seen is not wise. Also, since the underarm glands are very predictable sites for invasive-type cancers to latch onto, they should be removed. Furthermore, developing masses under the arm are not easily detectable, and they need to be examined pathologically to diagnose more exactly the extent of the disease.

There is no need to remove the major chest muscle in Stage I and II cancers because they have not reached that far. (If cancer has reached that far, it usually means it has also metastasized to distant organs, and muscle removal would be pointless from a standpoint of cure. Nonsurgical treatments, such as chemotherapy, take over for those advanced conditions.)

The advantages of modified radical over standard radical are not only cosmetic, but also functional. Retaining the major muscle avoids a concave hollow below the collarbone which would impair movement in the shoulder and very likely cause edema (swelling) in the arm.

Estimates for long-term survival are 80 to 85 percent in women who undergo modified radical mastectomy for cancer which has been detected early.

There exists a heated controversy between advocates of standard radical mastectomy and the increasing number of surgeons who now accept modified radical as adequate and effective.

The supersleuth of the breast surgery puzzle is Bernard Fisher, M.D., who pilots the NCI-sponsored National Surgical Adjuvant Breast Project, an extensive long-term study of the cure rates for all types of breast surgery and combination therapies. According to Dr. Fisher, "Standard radical mastectomies are hard to justify anymore. All our data show no difference in survival for standard versus modified radical mastectomy."

That conclusion is widely supported. A careful study by Gerald N. Robinson, M.D., and others in the departments of surgery, pathology and epidemiology at the Mayo Clinic showed no significant difference in survival of patients with identical cancers treated by either standard radical or modified radical surgery (*Mayo Clinic Proceedings,* July, 1976).

A few other surgeons advocate simple (total) mastectomy for an early, localized cancer that is smaller than a cherry pit or detectable only by mammography, provided it is not located near the nipple. That removes only the breast, leaving behind the axillary lymph glands if they appear to be cancer-free when palpated from within the surgical wound. The rationale is that the lymph glands play a big part in anticancer immunity which can theoretically block the spread of early cancer. Critics of simple mastectomy point out that those same lymph glands may eventually lose that fight and become a vehicle for the spread of the cancer. So there is no question that simple mastectomy alone will not do the job on cancer which, based on the pathology report, is prone to spread. Your surgeon must be absolutely sure that you have noninvasive (Type I) cells and no tumors in the armpit area before settling for simple mastectomy alone.

However, simple mastectomy can be combined with radiation therapy of the intact lymph glands to control spread of cancer about as effectively as either modified or standard radical mastectomy. Supplementing surgery with such nonsurgical therapy is called adjuvant, or auxiliary, treatment. Deformity is no less than that of modified radical. The major drawback is that the extent or stage of the disease cannot be determined without removal of the lymph nodes.

Very limited surgery (also referred to as partial mastectomy, lumpectomy or local excision) removes only the cancerous tissues within the breast, but not the breast itself. That is sometimes suggested for very early Type I, Stage I cancers (limited to the breast, not invasive, not metastasizing). Limited surgery by itself will cure strictly local cancer, but the hazards of cancer reappearing in other parts of the breast or launching a surprise attack on the lymph nodes is serious. By itself, limited surgery has not proved to be as effective as mastectomy (removal of the whole breast). Combined with radiation therapy, however, the results equal radical mastectomy for cancers that are definitely Stage I.

Subcutaneous mastectomy may be offered to the woman who has local, noninvasive cancer or who has already had one breast totally removed because of cancer and wants to prevent development of cancer on the opposite side. Occasionally, it is also suggested as a preventive measure in a woman who has never had true cancer in either breast but has premalignant growths or chronic, painful benign breast disease, accompanied by a strong family history of breast cancer. In other words, after a long series of biopsies and lump removals, the breast becomes scarred and deflated, and the woman may feel it is troublesome enough to warrant removal.

Aside from the fact that prophylactic removal of a breast to avoid possible future disease is jumping the gun (except in a few select cases), there are real drawbacks to subcutaneous mastectomy. These include possible excessive scar tissue buildup around the implanted capsule, infection and painful hardening of the implant into a firm, round ball. "The major objection to subcutaneous mastectomy," says Robert M. Goldwyn, M.D., professor at Harvard Medical School, "is the inability of the surgeon to remove with all certainty all the breast tissue" (*New England Journal of Medicine,* September 11, 1977).

In other words, there is no guarantee that subcutaneous mastectomy will indeed prevent cancer, and it may cause more trouble than it's worth. Careful patient screening is therefore emphasized by Dr. Goldwyn.

The mortality rate for breast removal surgery itself is relatively low, about 1 percent, primarily because general anesthesia in itself carries risks.

Although your physician can give you a fair estimate of your chances for a cancer-free life after treatment, he cannot honestly give absolute guarantees. Most patients know that and don't expect any promises. Knowing how long your physical rehabilitation will take and what you can do to speed your recovery is important to your psychological adjustment, right from the start.

The Full Recovery: Body and Soul

The road to recovery begins as soon as you wake up from the anesthesia. Taking into consideration how much tension there is in the incision, how tightly the skin pulls across your chest, and any tubes that may remain in place to drain the wound, your physician will recommend certain exercises to prevent stiffness in the shoulder and arm. You will be instructed by a nurse or physical therapist, and, perhaps, your physician who will be sure you are exercising correctly.

The easiest exercise is simply brushing your hair, which you will be encouraged to do right from Day 1. Other exercises include walking your fingers up a wall like a spider, crumpling paper into wads, squeezing a rubber ball, lowering window shades and rotating the shoulder in enlarging circles. Later, when the stitches have been removed, you will be given more vigorous exercises, which will carry over into your daily household activities after you return home.

Dozens of questions will enter your mind. Your physician will answer all of your medical questions, but will probably request that a volunteer from the Reach to Recovery Program visit you in the hospital about the fourth to sixth day after surgery. She will answer your questions about clothing and offer psychological assurance. Even if your surgeon is a woman, unless she herself has undergone mastectomy, questions about prostheses, special swimwear, going to the beach or problems with brassieres riding up can be handled most adeptly by a former breast surgery patient. Also, the shock of realizing what has happened makes it necessary to talk to someone who knows what you are going through.

Reach to Recovery is a service program of the American Cancer Society (ACS) made up of healthy postmastectomy women who have successfully adjusted to their surgery. Just talking with a former patient who is obviously well, energetic and nicely dressed is a morale boost that even the most understanding neighbor or relative cannot give. She will probably offer you a temporary, lightweight, washable prosthesis to slip into your bra. You can walk out looking the same as you did when you entered the hospital, and in a few weeks, shop for a more permanent, tailor-made artificial breast. The Reach to Recovery volunteer will also give you an informative booklet prepared by the ACS which gives exact details on such things as altering your clothing, shopping for a prosthesis and exercising at home. There is no charge for her service.

Your local Visiting Nurses Association may also provide moral support when you need it.

How long you stay in the hospital depends on your surgeon, but the average is about 7 days. You may remain hospitalized up to 14 days if you have had skin grafts, because of extra fluids which must be drained from the wound. There is also about a 10 percent chance of infection, which may delay your discharge from the hospital.

Before you go home, you will be advised to take special precautions with your affected arm. Without the lymph glands to fight infection, it will be more prone to infection and burns, including sunburn. Injections, blood tests and blood pressure checks should be done on the good arm. Edgardo Alday, M.D., associate professor of surgery at Jefferson Medical College in Philadelphia, gives his patients plenty of sage advice. "Avoid the smallest kinds of injuries to the affected arm and shoulder. Wear kitchen mitts when cooking to avoid burns, and long sleeves and gloves when gardening. (Don't get pricked by thorny roses.) Don't brush against people wearing corsages. Avoid jostling in crowds or on subways, and take care that people don't greet you with hearty slaps on the affected arm."

The most common but delayed complication after mastectomy is swelling in the arm (lymphedema). Because surgery has interfered with the lymph system, fluids can stagnate in the limb rather than recirculate to the trunk. Varying degrees of swelling show up in about one-third of postmastectomy patients, often not for a few months or even a year or more after the operation. A low-salt diet, arm elevation, an elastic sleeve prescribed by your doctor, and avoiding overweight usually help. Diuretics are sometimes prescribed. Very rarely, uncontrolled swelling requires surgical drainage of the arm.

Dr. Alday hastens to emphasize that those precautions do not imply that you will be disabled. In fact, with common sense, you should be able to resume as much activity as you feel up to.

You'll probably tire easily during your first few days at home. The change from being waited on to facing piles of laundry and empty cupboards can be discouraging, breast or no breast. Don't expect too much of yourself at first. Eventually you'll be washing windows, making beds, typing office reports, walking the dog, playing golf, putting up pictures — almost anything. One woman told us that the only thing she couldn't do was knead bread dough and that actually, the more she used the arm, the less it bothered her.

Your own recuperation will depend on your type of surgery and individual stamina. Younger women tend to bounce back more easily. Ask your doctor when you can return to work or what your limits around the house may be, if any. He'll probably tell you to do as much as you can, without straining yourself.

It is important that you continue to practice monthly self-examination on the remaining breast. Psychologically, that may be difficult, because of fear of finding a lump and once again setting off a chain of events leading to removal of your second breast. When you return to your physician for your first postoperative check of the incision, ask him to discuss that with you. Although there is a slightly increased risk of cancer turning up in a remaining breast, in most women it does not, and you are simply playing it safe by checking the breast routinely. For 3 years after mastectomy, your doctor will probably ask you to return for an office checkup every 2 to 4 months. A mammogram will be taken yearly, not only to be certain there is nothing going on in the second breast but to check for recurrence of the first cancer if you have had a partial mastectomy. Again, these checkups are sources of reassurance to the patient who has been treated for cancer diagnosed in its early stages.

Examination is then done every 6 months until 5 years after surgery, and every 6 to 12 months after that.

Choosing a breast prosthesis. When you go home, don't immediately clear your closets of all your pretty nighties and evening dresses. Having had your breast removed doesn't mean you are doomed to flannel nightgowns and shapeless smocks for the rest of your life. Most women want to face the world — and their mirror — looking their best, and breast prostheses that slip into your bra have now been perfected to the point where you can fool even your best friend. Prices and quality vary from homemade or very inexpensive dacron "falsies" or padded bras to lifelike individually fitted prostheses designed, ironically, by a postmastectomy woman who had previously designed the bosomy Barbie doll; she knew what she was talking about!

Those breast forms are made of sturdy, waterproof polyurethane, filled with liquid silicone. Some "tear-drop" styles replace only the missing breast tissue removed by simple mastectomy. Another model is molded to fill up the chest hollow and swoop under the arm, replacing everything cut out by more radical mastectomies. All models come in "rights" and "lefts," just like shoes, as well as your cup size. The artificial breast equals your own breast in contour and weight and is soft and yielding to the touch.

Obviously, the latter is the form that most closely looks — and feels — like a real live breast. It is often impossible to tell the difference, even wearing just a bra in front of the fitting room mirror. And this type is very unlikely to embarrass you by sinking or riding up.

You may have to visit more than one store until you find a satisfactory prosthesis. Good prostheses are available in specialty shops, some surgical supply houses and the intimate apparel departments of larger department stores. You will be fitted by a trained saleswoman for a properly fitting bra, because your whole chest may have changed after surgery and possible weight loss. You will then be fitted for a prosthesis just as you would be for any other special fitting problem such as wide hips, broad shoulders or a short waist, rather than for a deformity. The salespeople will also show you how to make slight alterations in your bras and swimsuits so you can wear the new breast under almost anything.

Some insurance plans pay for prostheses and some do not. Check with your insurance carrier. Medicaid will reimburse you, but the amount varies from region to region. In any case, have the salesperson write "surgical prosthesis," plus your size, on the sales slip so you may apply for reimbursement. The cost of breast forms and of fitting or altering bras is a tax-deductible medical expense.

When shopping for a prosthesis, it is a good idea to wear a close-fitting dress, sweater or clingy blouse that will give you a good view of how your bosom will look in clothing. You may wish to ask your sister or best friend to accompany you to the store, just as you may have a consultant when shopping for a gown to wear at your daughter's wedding or other special occasion.

One woman went shopping for her prosthesis just 6 weeks after her mastectomy, accompanied by two very close friends. When she modeled her prosthesis-filled bra, the artificial breast looked so natural that one friend mistakenly took it to be the real one. The woman being fitted was elated, needless to say!

Psychological effects of mastectomy. Dealing with the physical effects of breast loss is a small task compared to the psychological readjustment. Many emotions can come into play. In spite of her surgeon's reassurances, the question foremost in a woman's mind may be, "Did he get out all the cancer?" Worry over cure of a potentially fatal disease is compounded by anger and resentment that the whole nightmare has cropped up in her life. Anxiety over survival of her marriage (or future relationships if she is single, divorced or widowed) is likely to develop. Concern for her femininity develops partly because society has often stereotyped the desirable woman as one who displays a perfect set of large breasts. Even if her bosom isn't the Playboy ideal, if one breast is removed, she may wonder how her husband or companion can ever really love her again in the same way. She may fear that he will pity her or be ashamed of her.

The man who shares his life with a woman who has lost a breast to cancer has his own fears and feelings. He must be medically assured that the surgical operation itself will not affect her sexual desire or responsiveness, but that the way he and the woman *cope* with the loss can. Even such a small thing as being held and caressed may make a difference. The right attitude calls for open communication between the doctor or counselor and the woman's husband and also between man and woman. The man may be afraid he is going to hurt her during lovemaking. A simple change in position to avoid leaning on the operated side may relieve discomfort.

You may want to make love again as soon as you are physically up to it, but your husband may assume that after the operation, you don't feel like having sex, and he may avoid normal advances so as not to appear demanding. If he doesn't come up to the bedroom until after you've changed into your nightgown, he may simply be afraid that you'll be embarrassed to undress in front of him anymore. That can easily be misinterpreted by you as rejection. And if you slip into the bathroom to get dressed in the morning because you think he'll be horrified at the sight of your scar, the two of you will never adjust.

Talk about your feelings and assumptions. And remember, he married a person, not an artist's model, and he's mainly glad you're still around to cherish all the more, not less.

One postmastectomy woman, a Reach to Recovery volunteer who counsels other women, describes the readjustments very matter-of-factly.

> It's like an appendectomy scar. At first the scar is red and ugly, and you flinch when you look at it. Once you have overcome that, you don't worry about it as much. If you were relaxed about undressing in front of your husband before, it's not as much as an adjustment to face. I mean, if you've never undressed in front of him before, you shouldn't start now. Although I naturally wish I looked better, I'm not self-conscious about it, although I must admit I don't walk around the house nude.
>
> Some couples find it difficult to start making love again after surgery. Just the pressure on your chest may hurt. Or the fear of being hurt itself makes it difficult to begin. I think my advice to most women is that she must let her husband know that she's not different, because he's a little apprehensive. He doesn't want to hurt her. She must be receptive and let him know she wants to try.
>
> I must say that it was difficult and a little awkward for my husband and me at first, but we talked about it and resolved the problems.

Most men, in fact, are not horrified or repelled when their wife or lover loses a breast. Mildred Hope Witkin, Ph.D., associate director of the human sexuality program at the New York Hospital-Cornell Medical Center, emphasizes that those couples who deal with the problem immediately — from the day a woman leaves the hospital — lessen the chance of psychological trauma taking root. "It is crucial that the man display his love in very close, physical ways. It doesn't even have to be full intercourse. Otherwise, the woman will continue to feel ugly and undesirable."

Concerning the unattached woman who will worry about facing the intimate side of a future relationship with one breast, Dr. Witkin says, "Nine out of 10 men do not back away when confronted by a lover who has lost a breast. Most single patients later marry or become involved in successful, steady relationships."

Feelings of family and friends have to be dealt with, too. Having been threatened by what they see as a near tragedy may make them apprehensive. They will try to show concern without pity. You, in turn, may find yourself feeling jealous of women with 2 healthy breasts. If you have a teen-aged daughter, you may dread being confronted by her about her chances of facing the same loss. Younger children will have a lot of unanswered questions which must be answered directly in order to assuage unrealistic, imagined fears. Your actions more than words will reassure them that you are just as nurturing and maternal as you were with 2 breasts.

Some women choose to look at it this way: their breasts didn't determine their personalities, intelligence, jobs, family or social lives before surgery, so there's no reason to feel that loss of one breast is going to destroy their whole world.

You may go through a month or two of depression or withdrawal, fantasize that your husband is going to leave you, feel that friends are clamming up or worry that cancer will recur. Those reactions are not excessively morbid. But try not to prolong your emotional reaction. If it gets to the point where you are not resuming your daily activities within a few weeks, psychological counseling may be necessary.

You may be reluctant to tell your doctor that you sometimes feel sensations of itching, tingling or even pain in the "phantom breast" after mastectomy. Occasional or daily feelings that the breast is still there may begin just a few days or even a year after surgery, causing apprehension. Although it is disconcerting, you are not crazy. The "phantom limb" feeling is shared by people who have lost limbs or other body parts. Don't hesitate to discuss such sensations with your doctor.

Beyond Surgery: Keeping Cancer at Bay

For Stage I (early) cancer, no therapy other than surgery is necessary. However, breast cancer is fundamentally not a local disease. The probability that either it has spread or it might spread is the basis for adjuvant, or secondary, treatment.

Radiation therapy. If the tumor is so extensive that it cannot be completely removed surgically, or if it is located on the inner part of the breast where it is likely to spread to the lymph glands on the chest wall, radiation may be combined with surgery to control local "leftover" cancer in the region, to prevent local recurrence of the disease (Stages II and III).

Radiation therapy directs specific amounts of x-rays to the cancer cells. Because radiation alters the cells so that they cannot reproduce, the irradiated cells eventually die off, leaving no new cells behind, and the cancer is destroyed.

Radiation treatment is most effective on small cancer growths and, of course, is also capable of destroying healthy cells, so the radiotherapist uses as little radiation as possible. The surgeon first cuts out the bulk of the tumor. The sensitive tissues in the wound are allowed time to heal before radiation therapy begins. The radiation dose is tailored to the minimum effective level and concentrated on the cancerous areas. Sometimes some normal tissues adjacent to the tumor may have to be destroyed to be sure to wipe out all the cancer, but the radiotherapist tries to do only what is necessary. Treatment lasts about 4 to 5 weeks.

Scarring may be great or very little. Sometimes it is difficult for the surgeon and radiotherapist to predict the amount of scarring from radiation therapy because people's tissues react differently. Possible side effects from ill-managed radiation therapy are aggravated swelling in the arm, stiffness in the shoulder or persistent pain.

Radiation is effective in controlling local recurrence of cancer and improving quality of life for high-risk patients. It has no real effect on long-term survival. That's because neither surgery nor radiation deals with widespread cancer cells (metastases). For those distant cells, hormone therapy and/or chemotherapy is often effective in blocking systemic spread of cancer.

Hormone therapy. If the cancer has spread so far that surgery or irradiation is useless or no longer successful in keeping cancer in check, hormone therapy may be used to ease pain and prolong life. Treatment is individualized to take into consideration the age of the patient and state of the cancer. Therapy consists of cutting out certain hormone-producing glands (ovaries, adrenals or the pituitary gland), irradiating the ovaries or giving oral doses of estrogen, androgen or corticosteroids.

Hormone therapy is based on the fact that normal mammary gland cells contain specific spots which respond to circulating hormones, including estrogen, which are secreted by those glands. When the hormones hit those key spots, they trigger the cells' growth and function. If malignancy has not destroyed those spots (estrogen receptor sites), the cancer cells can be regulated by manipulating those hormones. Symptoms subside, and cancer regresses to varying degrees, adding a few months to a few years to survival, depending on the cancer.

It is strange that both *suppressing* hormones before menopause (by surgery or radiation to the ovaries) and *adding* them after menopause (by medication) result in keeping the cancer in check, and the explanation for that irony is not definitely known. But for the surgeon, having the cancer cells examined for positive estrogen receptor sites at biopsy identifies those women in whom hormone therapy is more likely to prolong life and ease symptoms. In all, one-third of breast cancer patients will respond to one or more forms of hormone therapy.

Cutting out or irradiating the ovaries suppresses estrogen activity and slows cancer growth, but either is practicable only for premenopausal women. Either technique does set off an early menopause, with its own consequences, so the patient's age and wishes should be taken into consideration.

Removal of both the adrenal glands (adrenalectomy) or the pituitary glands sometimes accentuates the results of a cut in ovarian function. In that case, corticosteroids are given to help counteract loss of adrenal secretions.

That same effect can be achieved medically instead of surgically by giving antiestrogens. Treatment with the antihormone Tamofixen and the adrenal hormone prednisone neutralizes or blocks the secretion of estrogen. While cancer remission may not last as long for that alternative, side effects are fewer and it is safer.

Estrogen therapy is appropriate only for women who are definitely past menopause (that is, who no longer show traces of ovary function on a Pap smear). Daily doses of estrogen are continued as long as the cancer is kept in check, usually several months or even years. Loss of appetite, nausea and vomiting may occur during the first few weeks and then subside. Less common side effects are fluid retention and breast enlargement, darkening of the nipple, areola and underarm skin, and the possibility of congestive heart failure. Your doctor can adjust your dose to minimize side effects.

For women who have just recently or not yet gone through menopause, an alternate hormone, androgen, is given. It may also be successful in treating women for whom estrogen therapy is no longer effective. It is also an alternative to ovary removal. Androgen therapy relieves pain in about 30 percent of the patients whose cancer has spread to their bones. It produces an increase in energy and weight gain, but causes amenorrhea (halt to menstruation). Side effects are similar to estrogen therapy, with the addition of some masculinizing effects such as acne, loss of scalp hair, growth of body hair and ruddy complexion with long-term use. For these reasons, androgen is usually given with breaks between treatments.

A subgroup of premenopausal women — those 45 years of age or more — appear to benefit from ovarian irradiation plus low doses of the hormone prednisone. In a study of 705 mastectomy patients reported by J. William Meakin, M.D., and colleagues, that combination of treatment significantly prolonged survival in that particular age group (*Canadian Medical Association Journal,* May 19, 1979).

Women who are too ill or unresponsive to other hormone therapy or who suffer severe pain and loss of appetite due to widespread cancer are given corticosteroids. The cancer subsides briefly and the feeling of well-being is boosted. Corticosteroids carry their own set of complications, including gastrointestinal ulcers and bleeding.

Chemotherapy. If a sample of cells taken at open biopsy tells your physician that cancer has invaded the lymph glands and is therefore metastatic, he may call for chemotherapy even after those nodes are removed. Chemotherapy uses highly toxic drugs to wipe out minute cancers which are likely to be lurking elsewhere in the body, far from the breast itself, in patients who are considered to be at high risk for relapse because their axillary nodes have shown evidence of cancer. Like radiation, it is most effective when begun as soon as possible after the bulk of the obvious cancer has been cut out.

Metastatic breast cancer is one of the types of cancer that is most responsive to anticancer drugs, and chemotherapy following surgery holds great promise for long-term survival. All breast cancer deaths are presumed to be due to minute, widely dispersed cancer cells far from the breast at the time of mastectomy; while surgery can remove the primary tumor and radiotherapy can control local recurrence around the breast, chemotherapy's aim is to kill any cancer cells left behind after surgery and consequently increase survival. Hormone therapy can improve survival, but only in one-third of breast cancer victims. So chemotherapy offers substantial hope.

The combined roles of surgery, radiation therapy and chemotherapy drugs in management of breast cancer are summed up by Samuel Hellman, M.D., of the Joint Center for Radiation Therapy, Boston. "A possible therapeutic approach for early breast cancer would be local removal of the tumor with sampling of the axillary lymph nodes, followed by radiation of the breast, and finally chemotherapy if the axillary nodes show cancer. This treatment plan may improve the survival of breast cancer patients and optimize both function and cosmetic appearance."

Radiation and drugs cannot be given simultaneously because the combined effect damages normal tissues.

Combination chemotherapy is more effective than any single drug used alone. Intermittent therapy is better tolerated and more effective than continuous therapy. Because cancer tends eventually to develop some resistance to the anticancer drugs, rotating different drugs delays or prevents that loss of drug power.

Some cancer cells are more sensitive to the powers of anticancer drugs during their rapid growth phases. Although it is not yet possible to determine when breast cancer cells are in those phases, chemotherapy is administered with the hope of hitting the cancer when it is more active.

Among the most common drugs used in combination chemotherapy are cyclophosphamide (C), methotrexate (M), 5-fluorouracil (F), with or without prednisone (P). A major study of 386 women in Italy has received a great deal of attention for its well-controlled trial of 12 months of CMF therapy after surgery for breast cancer with lymph node involvement versus no postoperative therapy at all. Twenty-seven months after the study began, there were 5 times as many relapses in the untreated women as those who underwent chemotherapy. Gianni Bonadonna, M.D., the oncologist who directed the NCI-sponsored study, cautions that those results are preliminary and long-term side effects are not known, but at the same time he is very optimistic about what he has seen so far (*New England Journal of Medicine,* February 19, 1976).

Another promising warrior is L-phenylalamine (L-PAM), although as a single agent it is only half as effective as CMF therapy (*Annals of Internal Medicine,* April, 1976).

All drugs are toxic, and their effectiveness against cancer depends on that toxicity. They are toxic to healthy tissues as well as malignant ones, and an overdose can be fatal. Amounts and time schedules for dosages are chosen carefully, starting low and building up to as much as the patient can stand. Oral doses of one drug may be given daily and injections of two others given at 2- or 3-week intervals. When symptoms or blood tests show toxicity, dosage is cut back. Those cycles of high doses followed by drug-free intervals of 2 to 6 weeks help to mitigate the side effects of hair loss, sore mouth, nausea, vomiting and muscle weakness, which usually subside when treatment is stopped. Unfortunately, it takes more than just a few weeks for hair to grow in again. Chemotherapy may bring a halt to menstruation. The woman's ability to fight infection, including the common cold, is lowered during chemotherapy, so theoretically drug-free intervals give the immune system a chance to recover.

Aside from the immediate side effects such as nausea, weakness and hair loss which make life miserable for the chemotherapy patient, the chances of developing serious side effects from years of chemotherapy, such as secondary cancers caused by the strong chemicals, are simply not known. Is it worth it to be kept alive, though weak and sore most the time, only to get cancer again in 20 years from prolonged use of strong chemicals in your body? How long can your body withstand the onslaught of obviously toxic drugs without becoming so run down that the common cold puts you at death's door? The aim is to prolong survival, but not at undue expense to quality of life. Dr. Fisher of the National Surgical Adjuvant Breast Project says, "The point is to find the minimal treatment that will do the job with minimal toxicity. We're putting everything we know on the line in breast chemotherapy right now. The next 10 years will be the ones that count in telling us whether we're succeeding" (*Science,* March 12, 1976).

The word "cure" has a different meaning for cancer than it does for appendicitis. Success is discussed in terms of survival rates. The 5-year survival rate is used as a rule of thumb for judging the success or failure of a cancer treatment because the majority of patients who develop recurrence usually do so within 5 years after initial treatment, which is usually surgery. During those 5 years, the chance of cancer recurring progressively decreases. At about 7 years after the surgery, the risk of death from recurrent cancer about equals the chance of death from other causes.

Reconstruction of the Breast

If you haven't already discussed breast reconstruction surgery with your physician, one of your postoperative checkups might be a good time to bring it up. Don't be disappointed if your surgeon or physician glosses over the possibility of rebuilding the breast. His word is not final. Traditionally, surgeons have felt that you should thank God for being alive, and just forget about your silly breasts. And some women do feel that way themselves, or don't want to face more surgery. Others are just too modest or embarrassed to ask about it. Still, for many women, restoration of their breasts eliminates the daily, almost hourly reminder of their loss. Psychologically, reconstruction turns the clock back to pre-breast-loss, and if reconstruction is feasible for you, you should be the one to make that choice.

Reconstruction is widely available and can be done after almost any type of mastectomy. It is even possible after the chest muscles have been removed by a standard radical mastectomy, use of skin grafts or damage to the skin by radiation therapy, although the results may not be quite as elegant as they would have been after more conservative surgery. Reconstruction is more likely to be considered when the chance of recurrence is minute (that is, early Stage I cancer). Detection of new cancer may be more difficult once the implant is in place. Safety of reconstruction from the standpoint of masking cancer recurrence is under dispute and not heavily documented, so surgeons are still cautious in selecting patients for the procedure.

Many leading surgeons, however, share the view expressed by Curtis M. Phillips, M.D., chairman of the department of surgery at Baptist Memorial Hospital in Jacksonville, Florida, regarding reconstructed breasts for women: "If we can provide a prosthesis for them, without any undue risk, why shouldn't we at least give them this option?" (*The Female Patient,* October, 1976).

A woman has only one life to live, and she very much prefers to live it with 2 breasts, in spite of cancer. Knowing that reconstruction is a possible option makes a woman less afraid of going to her doctor for early diagnosis of suspicious signs. Even if a woman must face breast removal, the prospect of reconstruction softens the emotional shock that follows mastectomy. How many women, if they lost 2 front teeth in an accident, would hesitate to get new teeth from a dentist?

Breast reconstruction is based on the surgical techniques first used for breast enlargement and is always done by a plastic surgeon. (Don't confuse the reconstruction technique with silicone injections, which are now illegal. That's a whole different — and unadvisable — ball game.) The results of reconstructive surgery are not absolutely perfect, but they are very good. Don't expect guarantees. No surgeon, plastic or otherwise, can give them. But compared to a flat or concave chest, a reconstructed breast is just dandy. You may even come through it with a new nipple.

Breast reconstruction is not usually done much sooner than 3 to 6 months after the mastectomy, so that the surgical incision can have a chance to heal, the skin to soften and stretch; also, enough time must pass to allow the doctor to check for recurrence of cancer. Reconstruction can even be done several years after mastectomy. There is also the possibility that by the time your body is ready for reconstruction, you may be so satisfied with an aesthetically pleasing prosthesis that you may no longer feel reconstruction of the breast is necessary.

Because reconstruction is an elective procedure, you will have plenty of time to choose your plastic surgeon. Write to the American Society of Plastic and Reconstructive Surgeons, Inc., 29 E. Madison Avenue, Suite 807, Chicago, Illinois 60602. They will provide names of qualified plastic surgeons in your area. You can also check the *Directory of Medical Specialists* in your local public library which lists plastic surgeons certified by the American Board of Plastic Surgery. Ask your prospective plastic surgeon if he does a lot of breast reconstruction work. Complications are minimized when the procedure is performed by a surgeon who is experienced at reconstruction.

You will visit the surgeon at his office for a consultation some time before the reconstruction operation. He will examine you, evaluate your particular case and answer your questions at that time. He will also consult the surgeon who performed your mastectomy about your eligibility for the reconstruction operation.

Reconstruction can be done in 1 operation if you have enough soft tissue left in the breast area, but is usually done in at least 2 separate operations, sometimes more if you have had skin grafts or radiation therapy. The technique is being refined so that eventually the whole job may be telescoped into 1 procedure for some patients.

The first stage is always major surgery under general anesthesia. To form the breast mound, the skin on the chest is raised to create a generous, padded skin flap, and a soft, pliable sack of silicone gel is inserted into that pocket. The opening is sewn closed and often left unbandaged for close observation. Antibiotics are routinely given to prevent infection, followed by painkillers for several days. The patient's activity will be limited during the initial week or two of healing.

Two months or more later, the second stage of surgery is done either under general anesthesia in the hospital or under local in the office operating room. The surgeon will enlarge the breast, reposition the implant, if necessary, and possibly add a nipple and aerola. Those can sometimes be fashioned from the labia (pigmented skin folds just outside the vagina) or grafted from your remaining real nipple and areola. If your nipple was saved at the time of mastectomy, it will now be removed from its temporary resting place and reapplied to the new breast.

The size, shape, position and appearance of a refashioned nipple may fall short of expectations. Restored nipples lack the sensitivity of an intact or real nipple. But many women are completely satisfied with contour restoration and are not concerned if the nipple is not restored.

You won't look like the Venus de Milo, but the implanted

breast will be rather firm and natural looking. Use of an implant limits its size, so your remaining breast may require surgical remodeling to balance it with the reconstructed breast. If your own breast is large, it will be pared down to match the new one; if it is small, it will be augmented with an implant similar to the one fit under the new breast; and if it is saggy, it will be firmed up. The goal is a new, symmetrical you.

While most women are very pleased with the results of reconstructive surgery, you should go into it knowing the minuses as well as the pluses. There are a few possible complications. The skin flap between the implant and your body is thin and its blood supply not perfectly efficient, so swelling, discoloration, infection and occasional skin breakdown may occur. Fluid may collect under the flap and persist for weeks. The implant itself can harden or shift. Dr. Goldwyn, a Boston surgeon who does a lot of breast reconstruction, feels that complications are fewer when the operation is done in 2 stages.

Fees for cosmetic surgery — which reconstruction is often considered to be — are high and depend on the extent of the surgery required. Costs may vary slightly from community to community and surgeon to surgeon. The surgeon's fee will be added to hospital costs, operating room charges and anesthesiologist fees. Costs related to breast reconstruction are not reimbursed by Medicare at this time, but the procedure is currently under review. Your private insurance carrier may reimburse you. Most Blue Cross-Blue Shield plans now cover reconstruction under Major Medical, and the trend is likely to continue. Contact your own carrier to see where you stand.

What Causes Breast Cancer, and What You Can Do about It

The question of what actually causes breast cancer is complicated, and theories abound. There is general agreement on a few main risk factors, based primarily on known links between estrogen metabolism in the body and breast abnormalities. Those risk factors do not say "you will get cancer" but are helpful in identifying women who should be especially alert.

The main risk factors seem to stem from continuous production of estrogen in the body, without pause. Such a long menstrual life may result from early start of menstruation, no childbirth, first childbirth after age 30 or late menopause.

Another recognized risk factor is the occurrence of breast cancer in a mother or sister, or prior cancer in one breast. There is only a 1 percent chance of cancer developing in both breasts at once, but a 5 to 8 percent chance of later occurrence in the second breast. That is not surprising in light of the fact that both breasts are subject to the same influences that cause cancer in the first place, whatever they may be.

Other risk factors that have been blamed are obesity, use of oral contraceptives, estrogen replacement therapy in menopause, high-fat diets and use of hair dyes. It may be somewhat reassuring to know that large breasts or injury to the breasts does not suggest any increased chance of breast cancer.

Suppose you do not have breast cancer in your immediate family but you do have a long history of benign breast problems yourself. Does that make you a more likely candidate for breast cancer? Not necessarily. While women with benign breast disease share some of the reproductive risk factors for breast cancer, the large number of cases of benign breast disease are not a prelude to breast cancer itself.

Obviously, you can't do a thing about how early you started your periods. And it's not practical to start a family just for the sake of staving off possible cancer. (However, if your mother or sister has had breast cancer and you definitely plan to have a family, getting one started in your twenties may not be a bad idea.)

If you are using oral contraceptives for birth control, an effective alternative should seriously be considered. Although not as convenient as the Pill, barrier contraceptives (diaphragm or condoms) used along with spermicidal foam approach the Pill in effectiveness when used correctly (with no risk at all to either partner).

Hair dyes? Ask your hairdresser about products derived from henna, a plant product that darkens or lightens the hair naturally, without hazardous chemicals which are absorbed through the scalp, and have been tentatively linked to cancer.

Taking estrogen for symptoms of menopause? There are so many alternatives that have worked for other women that you owe it to yourself to try them before you consent to oral or injected estrogen. Before you consider any kind of estrogen supplement, ask yourself if it's worth the risk for the 18 to 24 months or longer that menopause lasts.

Thousands of women have found that vitamin E brings relief from symptoms of menopause, hot flashes being the most frequent and bothersome. Doses of 400 to 800 International Units and sometimes higher either eliminate the hot flashes and night sweats or at least make them more tolerable. A high-protein diet, abundant in the amino acid tryptophan, often helps to lift the depression that accompanies menopause.

Stress during or after menopause can also rekindle hot flashes, and B complex vitamins, particularly B_6, cushion the effect of stress on the nervous system. If stress is a problem for you, you may need a B complex supplement that has at least 10 times the Recommended Dietary Allowance of 1.1 milligrams of thiamine (B_1), 1 milligram of riboflavin (B_2) and 2 milligrams of pyridoxine (B_6). (Be sure to look for a potency expressed in mg. [milligrams], not mcg. [micrograms]. The former unit equals one-thousandth of a gram; the latter only one-millionth.) You may need to boost the vitamin B_6 with a separate supplement to raise the total for that nutrient to 100 milligrams daily before you find a combination that works for you.

Above-average food sources of vitamin B_6 are halibut, salmon, light meat chicken, bananas and walnuts. Some foods that have been robbed of B_6 by processing are white bread, cake flour, spaghetti, French bread, crackers, canned vegetables and even canned meats.

Estrogen is often prescribed to prevent the bone demineralization (osteoporosis) that follows menopause. But calcium supplements of 1,200 milligrams a day, in the form of bone meal or dolomite, do the same thing — without the risk of cancer. To get that 1,200 milligrams of calcium from diet alone, you would have to drink at least 3 glasses of milk a day in addition to your regular diet.

Those 3 glasses are extra dietary fat, which puts you back in the high-risk category. Several studies have underlined the link between high-fat diets, hormone production and metabolism, and women at high-risk for breast cancer. Research from the Naylor Dana Institute for Disease Prevention in Valhalla, New York, shows that the breast duct fluids of high-risk women contain more hormones and circulating blood fats (lipids) than those of low-risk women. The researchers conclude the study by saying, "We propose that high fat intake, typical of the Western diet . . . promotes the growth of precancerous tumors by specifically altering the concentration of the hormones prolactin and estrogen in the breast duct fluids" (*Lancet,* October 22, 1977).

That delicate relationship between the fatty nature of breast tissues and circulating hormones makes the breasts more vulnerable to the harmful influence of cancer-causing substances (carcinogens) that enter and circulate throughout the body. Fat-soluble carcinogens are easily stored and recycled not only by breast fat but also by total body fat in general. So the fatter you are, the more likely you are to develop breast cancer.

Consequently, reducing the amount of fat in your diet helps protect you against breast cancer in 2 ways. It reduces the blood fats that end up in breast ducts, and it probably will result in overall weight loss, since the fat in foods contains more calories than protein or carbohydrates. When you consider that obesity also directly increases your chances of dying from heart disease, hypertension, diabetes, or stroke, the link between overweight and breast cancer is just one more convincing reason to get serious about controlling your weight, starting today.

In other words, keeping your weight down by exercising

more and cutting down on calories will place you at less risk for breast cancer, and reducing calories by cutting down on fats will help even more. Prime offenders to be avoided are bacon, sausage, butter, cream, ice cream, sour cream, cheesecake, cream cheese, well-marbled steaks, doughnuts and french fries. You will notice that except for those last two, the culprits are all derived from animals. Even major sources of protein which come from animals — except for fish — are higher in fat than vegetable sources (grains and legumes).

So if you must eat meat, trim the fat off that chuck roast and take the skin off that chicken. Get into the habit of choosing broiled or poached fish instead of roast beef. Spread cottage cheese on your crackers instead of Brie. Dollop yogurt onto that baked potato instead of sour cream or butter. Poach, don't fry your eggs. Make salads your main course and meat your side dish: pile lots of fresh greens, sprouts and raw vegetables into a deep bowl, and sprinkle with fat-free tarragon herb vinegar or lemon juice instead of creamy dressings. Scour your cookbooks for reduced-fat recipes. Drink your coffee without cream.

Better yet, don't drink coffee at all. Or tea. Dr. Minton, who reported complete disappearance of benign breast lumps in women who eliminated methylxanthine-containing beverages and chocolate from their diets, feels it may take some time to determine definitely whether those chemicals contained in coffee, tea, cola and chocolate influence the development of cancer. But he says, "I tell women who have a family history of breast cancer to cut out methylxanthines completely." Smart thinking!

When it comes to diet, there is one further step you can take to back yourself away from breast cancer — and even other types of cancer. Adding to the growing body of evidence in favor of dietary protection against cancer is some very encouraging news of the role of the trace mineral selenium in prevention of breast tumors. Gerhard N. Schrauzer, Ph.D., at the University of California at San Diego, added selenium to the drinking water of specially bred mice that normally develop spontaneous breast tumors. Instead of the usual cancer incidence of 80 to 100 percent, only 10 percent developed tumors.

You might think, "So what? I'm not a specially bred mouse." But the fact that breast cancer is a familial trait makes the high-risk woman very much like a specially bred mouse in that respect.

Professor Schrauzer's experiment was inspired by population data from 17 countries which showed that as levels of selenium in the blood rise, breast cancer death rates fall. In Western, industrialized countries, including the U.S., selenium was low and breast cancer mortality high.

Professor Schrauzer feels that the daily selenium intake in U.S. diets should be doubled, and to do that supplements of 150 to 250 micrograms should be added to a diet high in selenium-rich foods. Yeast supplements specially cultured to contain higher amounts of biologically active selenium are also available.

Selenium content of soils and consequently foods grown in them vary, but whole, unrefined grains are a rich source of the mineral. Professor Schrauzer specifically recommends whole wheat over white bread, wheat cereals over corn cereals, asparagus over corn and peas, and seafood and fish over beef. Garlic and mushrooms are also high on his list. He warns that "The daughter whose mother developed breast cancer, or any individual subsisting on the typical American diet should increase their consumption of cereals and seafood at the expense of meat, fat, sugar and potatoes." Those foods not only boost your selenium intake, but they coincide with your low-fat, low-risk diet.

16
Hernia

Hernia is a major surgical problem we all laugh at. No doubt this is so much whistling in the dark, because a hernia is definitely not funny: there were more than 750,000 hernia operations done in the United States last year—making it fifth on the hospital "cut-parade." It's a problem which affects an enormous number of people, and some authorities say that everyone who lives past 50 is a candidate for some form of hernia.

Hernias are so common because the forces of nature, heredity, gravity and sedentary living all attack very common anatomical weaknesses.

A hernia occurs when an organ and the tissue sheath that normally keeps it in place are allowed to move out of place by a congenital or acquired defect in the surrounding muscle walls. The energy which fuels this movement is provided by gravity or the pressure which builds up inside the body as we strain to lift heavy objects, eliminate wastes, sneeze or cough. Although hernias are possible anywhere in the body—even in the brain or the eye—they are by far most commonly in the groin and abdomen. Three out of 4 occur there, because the groin contains 2 structural weaknesses that practically invite herniation, and the normal activities mentioned above generate enormous pressures in that region even in healthy individuals. Clearly, however, as people grow older, hernia becomes more of a threat. The congenital defects that allow hernias to develop are present at birth, and many children suffer hernias in their first year of life. But childhood hernias may not present symptoms until middle age or later when tissues around the defect are also weakened, and the common medical problems of advancing age add complications.

Something that was no problem at all can suddenly become a terrible problem because of a chronic cough or repeated straining while defecating.

Unfortunately, this common problem is bewitched by controversy and disagreement in and out of the medical community. It seems to be only partially understood by surgeons and medical scientists and completely misread by laymen, victims and nonvictims alike. Doctors argue over the cause of hernia and the anatomy of the various types, and laymen puzzle over the meanings of the words "strain" and "rupture." Surgeons—dynamic and self-assured men—push favorite personal techniques as the proper corrective for a defect they alone understand, and hernia sufferers—often in pain and miserable—merely wonder how to choose a doctor and a procedure from this rowdy and aggressive assortment. They wonder whether they've suffered a "strain," which seems temporary and work related, or a "rupture," which seems permanent but somehow accidental. They wonder why the doctor called the whole unpleasant business a "prolapse," which means nothing to them but is probably the most exact term. Herniation is the falling down of a normal organ into an abnormal position, the prolapse of a perfectly healthy internal organ through a congenital defect in a muscle wall to a position outside the body cavity, to a position just beneath the skin.

Obviously, we cannot settle the squabbles that have plagued hernia repair since an Italian surgeon named Bassini described the first modern procedure in 1887. Nor can we tell you which technique by which superstar surgeon can best end your discomfort. Failure rates of between 5 and 10 percent are not uncommon in the work of even the most respected practitioners. But we can say that most authorities claim surgery is the only answer to hernias which develop uncomfortable symptons. And we can prepare you to sift through the conflicting claims and terminologies on the way to making an informed, intelligent selection of your own. We can provide accounts of the various clinical examinations for hernia and give you questions to ask your doctor. Our goal in this chapter—as in the others—is to help you find the right doctor with the right technique for your problem. With the controversy and uncertainty that surrounds hernia repair, this task is perhaps more important here than in any other case. Finally, we can provide some tips to help people who are without hernias stay that way.

First some general definitions, then some statistics. The pouch or envelope of intra-abdominal lining which is pushed out and then encloses a herniated organ—most often a portion of the intestine—is referred to as the hernia sac. That sac can be the subject of much unpleasant shouting when surgeons "discuss" hernia, but we'll get to that later. A hernia in which the protruding organ itself forms one wall of the sac is said to be a sliding hernia. An organ and its sac which return to their normal positions when the patient lies down or when pressure is applied with the fingers or a truss is a reducible hernia. An irreducible hernia, of course, cannot be replaced and is said to be incarcerated, that is, the edges of the muscular defect capture the escaping organ and lock it fast. That usually happens when a portion of the intestine bulges through a very small tear in the abdominal wall. When the defect is so small that the trapped intestine is bent back upon itself—like a garden hose in the hands of a child—and its blood supply is impaired or cut off, strangulation occurs. In cases of strangulation, emergency surgery is called for, because, if left alone, the condition invariably leads to gangrene and the risk of infection and death.

Hernias are most common in areas at which large structures—major blood vessels or portions of the intestine or other hollow organs—leave and enter the various body cavities. Those sites are vulnerable because they may contain loose or damaged tissue fittings around the point of entry or exit. About 75 percent of all reported hernias occur at the base of the abdomen, the groin, the point at which the legs and torso meet. Groin hernias can develop at 2 points on each side of the body, in the left and right inguinal canals and the left and right femoral canals. These canals are actually potential openings or areas of broad cross-hatching in the intermeshing muscles that make up the groin's anatomy. In the man the inguinal canals allow the testicles and spermatic cord to descend from inside the body to the scrotum outside the body cavity. In the woman, the canal provides a passageway through the abdominal wall for a minor ligament, the round ligament. In both men and women the femoral canals house branches of the femoral vessels, the chief blood suppliers of the thigh. The structural weaknesses at all these points in the groin are the windows or rings at each end of the canals. For some reason not clearly understood, they sometimes fail to close securely around the vessel or organ they carry and permit—much later—the movement of some uninvited guest into the canal. The internal ring—the opening deepest in the body—normally contains a bulge of abdominal lining pushed through by the changes in intra-abdominal pressure caused by coughing, sneezing and elimination. When extremes of these pressure variations cause a section of the large intestine, the small intestine, fatty tissue called omentum or the bladder to enter that pouch and travel down the canal, a hernia occurs. Because the femoral rings and their canal are very small, femoral hernias account for only a small number of all diagnosed cases but, because pregnancy can stretch the rings and weaken the canal, femoral hernias account for a third of all groin hernias suffered by women. In addition, because the rings are so small, femoral hernias are more apt to strangulate than other types. Men, on the other hand, are more prone to inguinal hernias than are women. This is true because the passage of the testicle out the inner ring, down the canal and through the outer ring can leave the inner ring abnormally large and the canal seriously weakened. A failure of that migration process in the unborn child can also result in a undescended testicle in the infant, a condition which may later lead to inguinal hernia in the adult. Hernias can occur on either side; bilateral hernia, that is, the herniation of both left and right canals, is quite frequent, but groin hernias of the right side are the most common.

One Hospital's Special Success in Hernia Repair

Before we try to unravel the tangle of opinion surrounding groin hernia, let's take a look at the bottom line: what's the operation like, and how much is it going to hurt me? Will I really be laid up for 3 or 4 months while recovering? Instead of examining the worst situation we came across and describing the longest convalescence imaginable, we'd like to look at the best and the shortest. We think a list of surgical conditions to shoot for is more useful than a collection of horrors to avoid.

We visited the best, the Shouldice Hospital in Toronto, Canada, which does nothing but abdominal hernia repairs, claims the lowest recurrence rate in the medical literature, and requires the shortest recovery time. Since 1945 the Shouldice surgeons have done over 116,000 hernia operations, and today they claim a recurrence rate of less than one-half of 1 percent of their cases. Shouldice patients are hospitalized for only 4 days; the average stay in a U.S. hospital for hernia repair is 5 days. Patients at Shouldice walk away from the operating room—with help—and are moving about on the afternoon of their morning surgery. They climb stairs to the hospital's dining room on their second day. Those with desk jobs often return to work immediately after the fourth day, while patients with physical labor jobs sometimes wait 3 to 4 weeks before returning to work. All are told to do whatever they wish whenever they feel up to it. Many Canadian patients of the hospital drive themselves home after release, and its numerous American customers fly back to the States without delay.

Shouldice's view is that if the operative technique is anatomically sound and the suturing is secure, the repair will be immediately as strong as it ever will be, because that strength depends on the suture material until the tissues heal. The surgeons there claim that passing urine normally puts as much pressure on the abdominal wall as lifting a 50-pound weight from the ground to shoulder height. Sneezing entails twice as much strain, and so it makes no sense to tell a patient to avoid work—according to them—unless he can also refrain from sneezing, urinating and moving his bowels. The hospital uses only stainless steel, nonabsorbable suture material and does most of its procedures with local anesthesia, which, it feels, offers fewer postoperative complications and allows patients to move about immediately after surgery.

It is that activity, as well as the specific technique, that accounts for the hospital's success, the doctors say. It promotes healing by increasing circulation and prevents the postoperative disasters that lead to recurrence. Constipation and the inability to void the bladder frequently follow abdominal surgery, and the strain they create increases intra-abdominal pressure, which, of course, can cause an inadequate repair to fail. Although early ambulation is widely practiced now and local anesthesia is gaining favor among hernia surgeons, the standard advice given to patients is that their abdominal wall will not return to full strength for at least 3 and maybe even 6 months. In fact, the recovery timetable in one manual for hernia patients warns that they should wait 3 to 5 days before bathing, 7 to 10 days before climbing stairs or venturing outside, 2 to 3 weeks before driving or working around the house, a month before resuming sexual activity and 2 months before returning to their jobs. The closest Shouldice comes to this gloomy report is its request that patients wait a week before soaking in a hot tub. The rest is really up to them.

Things start moving at Shouldice quite a while before the actual operation. The process usually begins when the patient notices a lump in his groin and goes to his family doctor for an explanation. The GP makes his initial diagnosis and recommends a local surgeon for the repair, but for any number of reasons the sufferer may decide to look elsewhere. A woman from Lakefield, Ontario, told us that she just didn't like the first surgeon her doctor suggested and that his second choice palpated her breast more expertly than her hernia. A man from Bedford, Ohio, with a bilateral hernia went to Shouldice because he couldn't wait the 6 weeks a local surgeon wanted between operations, and he couldn't afford a 4-month convalescence after the second procedure. At Shouldice his operations were separated by just one day. After a lengthy search—most people we met looked for at least 6 months—the patient finds Shouldice, usually through a friend. Another Ohio man, this one from Van Wert, heard of the Canadian hospital through its 12 "alumni" in his small town. A toolmaker from Georgetown, Ontario, went to Shouldice because his father had—30 years before—and lived to age 88 without another problem. Many who have had hernia operations elsewhere and suffered recurrences find their way to Toronto by way of what seems a hernia grapevine. The gentleman from Bedford, struggling with a third recurrence of both left and right hernias, went to Shouldice after a lot of study on the subject. He learned the anatomy involved, read up on the popular surgical techniques and took a plane to Toronto.

What doesn't happen very often is that the diagnosing physician recommends Shouldice. One patient we interviewed was even told to think twice about the Canadian hospital. "Who'll fix their work if it fails?" he was asked by his doctor. "No U.S. surgeon will touch it." Of the 2 or 3 dozen folks we talked to, only 1 had been referred to Toronto by his family physician. Many people were offered a Shouldice-type repair in a local hospital, but no one in the U.S., according to the Canadians, has been trained by them to use their techniques, and no U.S. hospital, as far as we could discover, is using the whole routine.

Things really get going at Shouldice with a physical examination to determine what indeed is what. The goal of the examination is to determine whether the patient has a hernia—as he suspects—and what kind of general health he's in. The doctors don't worry much about what kind of groin hernia it might be, because the hospital uses the same approach to repair both femoral and inguinal hernias. They also don't do a complete physical. Their tests cover the heart, lungs, blood pressure and urine, and they depend upon a thorough medical history to reveal other problems that might put off surgery. Shouldice has found that most hospital testing is defensive and unnecessary. It wastes the staff's time and the patient's money. One thing they do insist upon is a weight check. People who are overweight are required to lose at least half of their excess—both in pounds and inches. Fat people get more hernias; their hernias are more difficult to repair; and their repairs do not stand up well. The added burden of fat not only pulls down on and weakens stomach muscles, but it also increases intra-abdominal pressure, the immediate cause of most hernias. Patients who must lose weight are given instructions for the weight loss and provided with specific diet information.

The hospital finds that people who must lose weight or continue to live with a hernia are highly motivated to do the losing.

For people outside Canada, the hospital will begin the diagnostic process with a GP's report or with a questionnaire filled out by the patient himself. The medical tests are done for all patients on the day of admission anyway, and experience has shown that most groin hernias can be accurately diagnosed in this way. The questionnaire also asks for a detailed medical history and height and weight information that leads to a weight loss prescription for the mail-order patient who needs one.

All patients are told to take vitamin C to promote wound healing and given instructions to help them shave the operative area themselves before admission.

Admission day means a clinical examination to determine—if possible—what type of hernia the patient has and the battery of tests. These are done by the staff doctor who will do the surgery the next day. Once testing is out of the way, the newcomer is asked to change into a bathrobe and pajamas and is free to mingle with the "old-timers" upstairs, that is, the people who have been operated on the day before and are up and around in the hospital's many lounges. Shouldice carefully avoids looking, smelling and sounding like a hospital: there is no antiseptic smell, no rush of ventilation, no pea-green paint. Inside, the clinic looks like Holiday Inns should look, and outside like Jackie O's backyard. The point is to make patients into houseguests. The best way to rid people of preoperative anxiety, the hospital has found, is to make them feel at home. The main ingredient in this relaxing process is contact with other patients. To see someone whose present condition will soon be your fate, and to see him walking to lunch, laughing and riding an Exercycle is to build tremendous confidence in your doctor and his methods.

On the day of his operation, the patient is not processed impersonally, as is the case in many general hospitals. He is simply asked to wash his abdomen and groin with an antiseptic soap and given a special robe and trousers to wear into the operating room. He may wear his own socks and retain whatever rings he usually sports. The hospital has found that these practices do not contaminate their specialized operating rooms, in which only hernia surgery is performed and which are generally not exposed to disease, infection or trauma. Shouldice studies have shown that what little wound infection their patients suffer is caused by the doctors and the OR staff. Surgical team members are routinely checked for contamination and minor illness, and the hospital's infection rate has fallen to less than 1 percent. Patients are also spared the indignity of the preoperative enema. Surgery generally takes place in the morning, the patient having eaten no breakfast; but all patients eat an evening meal on admission day. The final step in this process of getting ready is a sedative given orally about an hour-and-a-half before surgery and a pain-killing shot about an hour later.

Neither of these drugs knocks the patients out. Patients walk—with help—from their rooms to the OR. The people we had met the day before were able to say, "Good Morning," and joke about our sudden promotion to the surgical team. They responded easily to introductions to staff members in the room, the surgeon, his assistant and the equipment nurse.

Once in the operating room, the patient is helped onto the table, draped in surgical linen and fitted with a blood pressure cuff. During the operation, his blood pressure, pulse and respiration is monitored by a second nurse sitting at the head of the table. The surgical drapes here, by the way, are reusable. Shouldice employs none of the paper drapes that many U.S. hospitals do and has cut its costs by doing so. The hospital's operating rooms, in fact, are stripped to the bare essentials as another economy. Customers here are generally in good health, and emergencies in the OR are few and easily taken care of.

Before the draping, the patient's stomach and groin are painted with an antiseptic solution, and the operation begins with the injection of a local anesthetic—generally Novocain—beneath the skin. The operation—whose technical aspects will be described later—is handled in stages. A series of incisions through the various tissue layers down to the inguinal or femoral canals in the groin is alternated with shots of anesthetic. As each new layer is reached, it is numbed with a shot of Novocain before being opened.

During all this, the patients feel nothing, at least nothing uncomfortable. Most told us that they felt a pinprick—no more—now and then, and occasionally a gentle tug or two. Some dozed during the operation and awoke to tell the surgeon of any discomfort. They were never jolted awake and often had to be asked—when a brow furrowed—if they were in pain. No one told us that being awake during the procedure distressed him. In fact, when asked, most delivered a lecture on the benefits of local anesthesia: earlier activity, hence faster healing, less lung congestion and less constipation.

After the repair, the tissue layers are closed with a suturing technique borrowed from plastic surgery. The original, undamaged, anatomy is reestablished as fully as possible, and the tissue edges are *overlapped* before being stitched with a continuous length of stainless steel wire. Stainless steel is used for the strength it provides and its nonirritating nature. This overlapping makes for extra strength in the long run, but at first it makes the repair thicker. A firm ridge of healing tissue can be felt beneath the skin incision for some time after a Shouldice operation. However, this line gradually thins out over a period of a few months and soon disappears. The stainless steel wire stays in permanently and gives no trouble. Its presence cannot be felt. The skin itself is closed with Michel clips, surgical staples actually, which are left in for 2 days and removed completely before the patient is discharged.

When the patient is unwrapped, he is helped to sit up and then to stand. With his arms over the shoulders of the surgeon and his assistant, he walks perhaps 100 feet to the recovery room, to stay for an hour or so while the sedation wears off. Everyone we saw taking this walk had color in his face and smiled broadly. The average time for a first repair at Shouldice is just over 40 minutes. The one complicated repair of a recurrent hernia we saw took about an hour.

Most people miss lunch on the day of the operation and doze

on and off until dinner, which is the first and last meal served in bed. Everyone takes himself to the bathroom; bedpans are banished. The hospital does everything it can to get its patients moving and to keep them up and around. On the day after an operation, all patients are expected to walk to breakfast, and patients are required to participate in group exercises each day at 10:00 A.M. The exercises—mild stretching, bending, and marching to peppy tunes—are intended to stimulate circulation and respiration and help to prevent blood clotting, speed healing and avoid lung congestion. The Shouldice staff also believes that the exercises help eliminate the gas pains and constipation that often follow abdominal surgery. A peripheral benefit is the confidence they build. A 73-year-old man told us that he hopped on the Exercycle each morning because it reminded him anew that his hernia was gone for good.

A Shouldice booklet called *On Your Way* warns patients that some pain, swelling and skin discoloration may follow surgery. It tells of stiffness and the pain of laughing or coughing. However, as a psychiatric social worker from Fairleigh Dickinson University pointed out, one shouldn't expect to be laughing on the morning after, and the general pain of the operation, in his case, was no worse than a paper cut—a minor, if insistent, nuisance. Many people have told Shouldice doctors in follow-up reports that the pain they felt after surgery was just like the pain they experienced in the first stages of their hernia. They feared that each twist and chuckle in the first few days would tear out their intricate needlework. As a result, hospital pep talks explain that different things are happening before and after. With a hernia, pain comes from muscle walls that are being torn. The pain after an operation, however, comes from muscle walls that have been purposely cut and then securely repaired. In both instances, nerve fibers are damaged, but in the operation, of course, the damaging process is stopped and healing has begun. In any case, the booklet prescribes nothing stronger than aspirin and for men the wearing of jockey shorts for the pain that may follow the operation—and then only for a peculiar kind of discomfort not directly associated with the incision. Generations of male patients have found the extra support offered by the snug-fitting underwear a blessing after their somewhat rough handling. Women, of course, aren't troubled by this problem.

Because certain minor blood vessels and nerves in the groin are sometimes unavoidably sacrificed in all methods of repair, the unpleasant side effects of hernia procedures are remarkably uniform. Most of them trouble men alone. The testicles and scrotum may be temporarily black and blue and swollen, and the testicle on the side where the cut was made may reduce in size because its blood supply has been diminished. This condition usually occurs only when there have been previous attempts to repair a hernia, and there is usually no functional impairment as a result. In elderly men and all patients with large or long-neglected or recurrent hernias, this testicle may have to be removed if its supplying vessels are completely lost in repairing the extensive damage. This is a rare occurrence, however. A few patients experience a tingling numbness in the upper thigh from the loss of a particular nerve in the region, but the sensation is generally mild and of no significance.

Causes and Symptoms of Hernias

Now back to the meat of the issue. Inguinal hernias can be both direct and indirect. If the protrusion pokes through a defect in the canal wall across to a point beneath the skin, the resulting hernia is called—with only a slight stretching of logic—a direct hernia. Direct hernias have long been called acquired complaints, the products of abdominal injury or the strain of heavy labor. Recently, however, it has appeared unlikely that an injury could cause so tiny a muscle tear, and direct hernias are now often labeled hereditary weaknesses or thought of as the result of some malfunction of collagen synthesis in the body, some inability—stemming perhaps from age or a wasting disease—to manufacture the protein that lends strength to connective tissue.

Four times more common than direct hernias, indirect inguinal hernias occur when the bulge of intestine follows the path of the canal to the scrotum or the skin surface. They are caused by a defect of the internal ring which is either congenital or acquired at the time of the migration of the testes out of the abdomen; they are sometimes referred to as hernias of the spermatic cord, because the protrusion follows the cord through the canal and can enter the sheath of tissue which surrounds the cord.

In addition to the difference between the paths travelled to the skin surface, direct and indirect hernias may be distinguished in the following ways: direct hernias are rare in women and are more likely to involve bilateral defects. With indirect bilateral herniation, the twin bulges appear one at a time, but with direct bilateral hernia, the protrusions commonly appear together. Incarceration is seldom a problem with direct hernia, and its bulge appears or disappears immediately upon standing up or lying down. The bulge of an indirect hernia takes time to develop and reduce.

Groin hernia of the inguinal canal is usually a man's problem. In most cases, no cause is found, but it can be caused by the growth of a tumor in the intestine, cancer of the colon or enlargement of the prostate gland. These grave conditions *can* lead to hernia because they involve displacement of internal organs or a disruption of the digestive system and chronic difficulty in elimination. In both cases—crowding or constipation—the result is a dangerous increase in intra-abdominal pressure and the threat of herniation. Groin hernias can also be caused by a lifetime of strenuous activity and heavy and improper lifting. When weights are supported or hoisted with the main burden resting on the stomach muscles—rather than the stronger arms or legs—hernia is often the upshot. Men who are promoted to supervisory positions after years in the shop are especially vulnerable; as their muscle tone slackens and their weight increases with days at a desk or on an expense account, the slightest abnormal exertion (or boast that they've still "got" it) can bring injury. An even more common cause of groin hernia is middle-age spread—no matter what the occupation or life-style of the spreader. Men 35 to 45 are the most frequent victims of hernia and nearly all of them are overweight. The extra baggage they carry around the waist exerts a downward pull on organs and muscle structures which can be more dangerous than the increased internal pressure it creates. That pull and the push of pressure from inside—plus the normal drag of gravity—puts an irresistible load on the congenitally weak spots in the groin. That same combination of evils also makes pregnant women and women who have had several children more apt to suffer femoral hernias than younger, childless women. People who are a bit more than just puffy—even without the added factor of injury or heavy lifting—are probably working on hernias all the time. In the fit and trim (and increasingly rare) adult, the balance between internal and external air pressure is regulated by respiration. As we inhale, pressure rises, and as we exhale, it falls. In the chronically tubby, there is no such regulation. The pressure is always greater inside, and the smallest exertion (like picking up a child or jumping down to a hard surface) can produce what amounts to an explosion of air within the body and lead to hernia at one of the likely spots in the groin.

Most groin hernias produce no symptoms until the patient notices a swelling or bulge in the abdomen or upper thigh. Femoral hernias are notoriously asymptomatic until the point of strangulation, and a hernia in someone who is terribly overweight may never show itself in an uncomfortable way. The layers of fat simply smother the telltale signs. Direct and indirect inguinal hernias generally appear as bulges under the skin just above and to the left or right of the pubic area. The herniating organ and sac of an indirect hernia can enter the scrotum and register as a swelling of one testicle. A femoral hernia usually shows up as a lump in the upper thigh, although such hernias often follow a J-shaped course and circle upward into the groin to be mistaken for inguinal defects.

Hernia bulges are frequently the size of a small marble when first noticed but then grow steadily larger as more and more intestine (or whatever) escapes into the sac. They may be reducible or irreducible, painful or completely painless when initially detected. If the hernia is not incarcerated, it will slip back into place more readily when the patient is lying down. If the problem is truly hernia, the bulge will transmit the jump and strain of a cough when the person is standing.

Beyond these changes in the landscape of the groin, hernias generally create no problems unless strangulation occurs. Direct hernias produce fewer symptoms than indirect ones, but both can create a dragging sensation in the lower abdomen that in men may radiate into the scrotum with indirect herniation. There may also be some nonlocalized aching pain in the area. Once the bulge appears, the patient may need to lie down to ease the pain. What he's doing is reducing his hernia. Most of these symptoms will seem to be centered in the abdomen rather than the groin. Femoral hernias are the most insidious of the groin defects. They almost never develop symptoms before strangulation, and they are the most likely to strangulate.

Many people do not react to a hernia until long after they notice a lump in the groin. They worry a little about discovery of the lump in an emergency room—the same reason your mother always wanted you to wear clean underwear—but because the bulge causes no discomfort, they ignore it. They're finally forced to seek a remedy when the hernial mass becomes incarcerated or strangulated and produces a sharp pain. In inguinal hernias, the pain is usually at the site of the bulge. With femoral hernias the pain is frequently not localized, and many victims must be hospitalized after disregarding the dull ache that signaled incarceration and impending strangulation.

In any case, once a suspected hernial mass becomes irreducible, it should not be ignored. Strangulation turns an elective repair into an emergency procedure which brings with it the threat of serious infection. Other signs which announce incarceration are also the symptoms of bowel obstruction, a by-product; they are: vomiting, nausea and colicky pain. The earmarks of strangulation are in turn the signs of systemic infection, its by-product; they are: fever, rapid heartbeat and an increased white blood cell count. The consequences of strangulation are, of course, severe and include puncturing of the entrapped organ, infection, gangrene and the bacterial contamination of the bloodstream. Strangulated hernias are life threatening.

Diagnosis of groin hernia begins with the patient's medical history as it relates to the problem. Most texts on the subject are magnanimous in their acceptance of the victim's own account of his pain. Patients, it is written in the *Brief Textbook of Surgery* (W. B. Saunders, 1976), can be trusted to note the site of the swelling and its first appearance. They are asked—in addition—if the bulge appears and disappears with any regularity, and if these comings and goings are affected by posture. Does the swelling disappear when you lie down and appear when you stand? Is the mass affected at all by coughing or straining of any kind? Do you experience pain? Is the pain "referred," that is, does it seem to travel to a spot other than the site of the swelling? Does it throb when the bulge is largest? Once this information about the primary signs of the problem is gathered, questions about its causes follow. Do you have a chronic cough, some nagging difficulty with urination or defecation? Is heavy lifting or are repeated stooping and bending part of your job? Have you ever suffered a groin injury at work or felt a sharp, tearing pain in the area? Has anyone in your family ever had a hernia? (Hernias are not inherited, but the kind of muscle structure and the anatomical weakness that allow them are passed on from generation to generation.) Finally, questions designed to measure the seriousness of the situation are asked. Can you reduce the swelling by placing your hands on it and gently pressing? Have you experienced a sharp pain in the area of the bulge? Are there signs of infection, such as raised temperature or redness around the bulge, that might indicate incarceration or strangulation?

The next step is a physical examination to confirm the patient's evaluation and to determine what kind of hernia is present. In this exam it is very important to recreate the conditions that bring on the symptoms recorded. If the bulge only appears during heavy lifting, the patient must lift something heavy; if the strain of coughing or elimination is the cause, these things must be tried—all within the proper clinical decorum, of course. In many cases these slightly embarrassing gyrations will be the only way to measure the size of the mass, its degree of reducibility and the extent of the damage it has caused. With these things out of the way, the doctor then palpates the area to assess the damage further. This is the turn-your-head-and-cough stage, famed in story and bad joke. When a physician makes this request and probes with his finger around the scrotum, he is trying to locate the external ring of the inguinal canal. Finding it blocked with a tissue mass—one that transmits a cough's jolt of air pressure to his finger—suggests that an indirect hernia is present. Finding no swelling at the external ring, he suspects either an incomplete indirect or a direct hernia. He cannot palpate the internal ring, which, if blocked, might confirm his diagnosis of indirect hernia. Yet, by manipulating the area over the inguinal canal with his fingers (while the patient strains), he may be able to distinguish direct from indirect. Direct hernias travel perpendicular to the canal, while indirect hernias follow its course. The inguinal canal can be approximated by projecting an imaginary line between the 2 bony prominences on the front surface of the pelvis, one near the top of the hip and the other down below the navel but just above the pubic area. If the suspected hernia lies considerably below that line, it is probably a femoral hernia. If the protrusion lies along the line, it is some kind of inguinal hernia. This step in the diagnosis is normally done twice, once with the patient standing and once with him lying down. The upright exam determines the size and location of the hernia, and the supine check reveals the condition of the tissue structures around the defect.

It is, to coin a phrase, a bone of contention whether all that locating and determining is necessary. Some doctors, like those at Shouldice Hospital, do not try to separate indirect from direct hernias in the initial clinical diagnosis. They have discovered, they say, that their early predictions are often wrong, and that proper dissection through a single type of incision allows them to treat all 3 problems. Other practitioners—such as disciples of Chester McVay, M.D., of Yankton, South Dakota—consider it essential to determine the type of hernia before surgery, because they advocate a different operation for each kind. In all cases, x-rays are seldom used in hernia diagnosis today. An x-ray taken with the patient lying on his side, or alternatively, a barium enema followed by an x-ray, is sometimes used to determine the contents of the hernial sac, to discover whether it contains a segment of bowel, for instance—but this information is seldom required. Surgical procedures for hernia repair have grown more precise, and the danger of accidentally damaging the entrapped organ has all but disappeared.

How Successful Is Hernia Repair?

Now we're into the messy part—both physically and philosophically. Hernia surgery is physically messy, because it fails so often. Hernias recur at the same point—or one close by—at an alarming rate. The textbooks most likely to be read to surgeons boning up on a specific repair all report a recurrence rate of around 10 percent for groin hernias. *Current Surgical Diagnosis and Treatment* (Lange Medical Publications, 1977) says that indirect inguinal hernias pop up again in 2 to 3 percent of all adult cases. Direct inguinal hernias, the book claims, return in just under 10 percent of their victims. The *Handbook of Surgery* (Jones Medical Publications, 1978) puts the inguinal figure at between 8 and an astounding 50 percent but suggests that "careful anatomical repair" can cut the rate to 5 percent. One wonders, of course, why careless repairs ever occur. For femoral hernias, *Current Surgical Diagnosis and Treatment* reports a failure rate of from 7 to 12 percent and dismally warns that a groin hernia complicated by its sliding nature, that is, when an organ forms one wall of the hernial sac, is even more likely to come back.

When writing for the general public, however, most surgeons turn these statistical tables around. Robert Rothenberg, M.D., in the *Complete Surgical Guide* (Simon & Schuster, 1973) says that groin hernia procedures are 90 percent successful—which still means that 10 percent of the operations are unsuccessful. Clarence J. Schein, M.D., sunnily says that only 1 in every 10 hernia operations is a blunder in *A Surgeon Answers* (G. P. Putnam's Sons, 1973), but even these odds are still nothing to lay yourself on the table for. A computer survey by the Harvard Center for the Analysis of Health Practices of all the medical literature published between 1960 and 1974 reports that the consensus of opinion of surgeons writing on hernia is that groin problems return at least 10 percent of the time. It added that a second repair ran an even higher risk of failure according to the doctors. Because the scar tissue which forms around the original incision brings new problems of dissection and reconstruction, operations for recurrences fail 25 to 30 percent of the time. Recurrent hernias are also more likely to strangulate and turn what may have been a minor defect—at one point—into a life-endangering complication.

Now the bad news. Surgeons do not agree on what a recurrence is. Those with large egos tend to say a recurrence is the return of the same kind of hernia to the same spot: a direct hernia in the right inguinal canal which shows up again after a period of months or years. Others with more a sense of their own fallibility allow that any hernia which occurs in the same general area is recurrence: a direct hernia which reappears as an indirect bulge in the left canal would be labeled a failure by these people. They reason that they have not corrected the anatomical weakness in the area with the first operation and so have contributed to the need to a second.

If that sounds a bit confusing, there's also no agreement on the time limit for recurrence. Many surgical texts say that another hernia in the same spot within a few months or a year of surgery is the result of surgeon error and should be called a recurrence. Reappearance within the first year means that the operating doctor missed evidence of an indirect or femoral hernia when repairing a direct bulge, that his suturing was imperfect or that tissues were stretched out of position to close the wound. Reappearance after 2 or more years, argues *Current Surgical Diagnosis and Treatment*, is the patient's fault. He's gone back to the same old bad lifting habits or continued suffering from the same chronic increases in intra-abdominal pressure. He may even have had the audacity to contract some wasting disease which impedes the proper healing of his tissues.

Hernia repair is philosophically messy, because there are no universal standards for it. Surgeons don't agree on how to fix particular defects, and in many cases they say nasty things about well-meaning folks who don't do things as they do them. As a result, there is no way for us to tell you exactly how to select the right doctor with the right remedy for your complaint. The best we can do is to offer some questions you might ask your doctor and a blacklist of medical malpractices to avoid.

Most hernia surgeons say their art has long been the stepchild of the hospital. It is deemed unglamorous and left to inexperienced surgical residents who often bungle it and learn nothing from their experiences. All of which seems rather defensive, as if surgeons who have chosen to do hernias are trying to justify their choice of a ho-hum specialty. In some cases, such as hernia of the diaphragm, there are simply not enough cases to allow our knowledge to expand and treatment procedures to be standardized. But with groin hernia, there seems to be no excuse for the high rate of failure. Of the nearly 750,000 hernia operations in this country in 1977, the vast majority were for groin hernias, and that yearly case load is large enough to provide the experience to perfect techniques.

To be fair, there are 3 reasons for hernia repair's miserable record and only one of them can really be blamed solely on surgeons. In the first place, Americans are fat. Fat people are more prone to hernias, and they recover from all types of surgery less rapidly and less well than thin people. In the second place, while most of us have health and disability insurance that pays for surgery and even provides paid time-off for convalescence, some would say that this time-off comes at the wrong end of the process. Benefits in the U.S. for hernia repair are very liberal. What these benefits don't provide, however, is time-off *before* surgery—or encouragement *before* the injury—to lose weight. Weight reduction may prevent hernia, and it surely adds to a patient's chance for a successful operation.

The complication that surgeons contribute to that muddle is their descriptions of the various methods of repair. Those descriptions don't always transfer successfully from one doctor to another. Maybe they aren't complete or clear, or perhaps our knowledge of the essential anatomy is flawed. What is clear is that descriptions of the groin which picture the major hernia sites as canals are not exact, and so repairs designed to reconstruct those canals may be misleading to newcomers. The area called the inguinal canal is actually a space where several intermeshing muscle layers are less tightly woven than elsewhere. This space allows the spermatic cord and the testicle to pass through, but it is not a cylindrical channel running across the groin. It does not take a surgeon to note that anatomical descriptions that talk of a canal could be misleading to an inexperienced surgeon, could even impede his progress in surgery. The *sine qua non* of successful hernia repair, according to Lloyd M. Nyhus, M.D., the editor of the textbook *Hernia* (J. B. Lippincott, 1964) and the journal *Current Surgery*, is the closing of the defect without tension, without stretching tissues out of their normal position. It seems likely that the surgeon thinking about a round canal while working on a flat series of layered muscle fibers might be apt to violate this cardinal rule.

Choosing Your Surgeon

All these factors, then, make the question, "How should my hernia be repaired?" impossible to answer. The question, by whom, is easier and probably more important. We don't mean that a surgeon's reputation in the community should be your sole guide, because it, after all, is made up of rather unreliable elements. If your family doctor says a particular surgeon is good, and you trust his advice, you may be safe in following it, at least as the first step in your own investigation. Keep in mind, however, that your family doctor gets his information from the surgeon and other doctors; it is unlikely that he has had contact with his recommendation's failures. But his advice will give you a good place to start asking your own questions.

After the examination and a preliminary determination of the nature of your hernia, ask what surgical technique he usually employs on such cases, why he chose it and where he learned it. You should also ask him how often he does the procedure, how many hernias he's repaired and what his recurrence rate is. If he doesn't have specific and candid answers to these questions, he's probably not a good choice. If he does very few hernias and learned his technique on the golf course or in the library, seek someone with more hands-on—or hands-in—experience. Familiarity with a particular technique seems to be the best guarantee of success.

A surgeon who spoke frankly to us (but asked not to be identified) said that techniques that worked beautifully for one man or team of surgeons might be disasters in the hands of others, simply because the second group did the operation too infrequently to learn it properly. He said that surgeons are trained in different ways and study with different masters. "They learn to do things in ways that worked for the old guy. If his methods worked clinically for him, they'll probably work for his students." Maybe, but if the surgeon you interview can't give you *his* recurrence rate—as this doctor could not—ask him why not. Since hernias reappear with dismaying regularity over long periods of time, patient follow-up should be a part of the treatment. If a surgeon doesn't know what happens to his patients after their operations, he can't know what's working for him and for them. And it's no good relying on patients to keep yourself informed. Satisfied ones will go on as if nothing had happened, and the unsatisfied and disgruntled will go off in search of another doctor. Only if they meet a malpractice lawyer on the way will the original surgeon learn about the recurrence. In the ideal situation, follow-up should be active and perpetual. Moreover, if your case is not an emergency and you are overweight have chronic pulmonary problems or trouble eliminating, your doctor should insist that you reduce and receive medical treatment before surgery. If he does not, you should look further. No matter how skillful a surgeon he is, your operation's chances of failure will be very high without these precautions.

How Surgeons Repair Hernias

What remains now are brief descriptions of the various techniques used for hernia repair and the preoperative and postoperative routines demanded by each. Of course, we won't try to rate these techniques for you, but we will quote the success statistics reported by their developers and let the records speak for themselves. With this warning: the student's skill or luck may not be as good as his master's. We will take special note of the postoperative requirements of each procedure. If nothing else, the dissimilarity of these commandments will indicate the lack of fundamental agreement among hernia surgeons. While many doctors fight with employers to gain their patients more time at home, Shouldice believers warn their patients that while the pain of an operation may resemble the pain of a hernia, they should not assume that exercise or even hard work will damage their repair.

Laurence S. Fallis, M.D., in his contribution to a standard textbook on hernia repair, says this comment was current when he went to medical school: "You can judge the worth of surgeon by the way he does a hernia!" However, Dr. McVay, the developer of one of the major groin hernia procedures, says that "in the entire history of surgery, no subject has been so controversial as the repair of groin hernias" and throws the whole issue into confusion. If surgeons don't agree on technique, if techniques often fail, how are judgments to be made? How can the surgical shopper protect himself? It is our opinion that the patient who knows the basic concepts behind the various treatments can formulate questions to gauge the skill and sensitivity of his surgeon.

The object in groin hernia surgery is to repair a break in the inguinal or femoral canal without stretching the tissues beyond their normal limits. Tissues stretched out of place, of course, can tear sutures and cause surgical failure. This goal has forced surgeons into some complicated anatomical gymnastics in reconstructing the canals. If the hernia is a simple indirect defect, most doctors perform what is called a "high ligation of the sac." They slice the hernia sac away from the internal ring, open it, clip off the section distorted by the bulge, reduce the herniated organ and sew up what remains of the abdominal lining that formed the sac. Sometimes, if the internal ring has been stretched by the hernia, it is nipped in with a suture or two. That technique is generally used in infants and children and quite often in first repairs of small, uncomplicated hernias in healthy, young adults. The tightening of the internal ring, however, is a part of most hernia operations.

If the swelling is a large indirect or almost any kind of direct or femoral hernia, more tissue maneuvering and relocation are required. The tissues that once formed the damaged canal must be manipulated so that they can be reconnected to strong, unbroken muscle or ligament and the passageway can be rebuilt. The Italian surgeon Bassini managed to do all this in the first modern hernia repair (1887), and his technique is still followed by many today. Some doctors claim, however, that in simply opening the canal, repairing the internal ring and reclosing the tissues, Bassini was inviting recurrence in all cases but the very minor. They argue that the tissues split and reconnected in the procedure have ruptured once and will do so again. Some stronger, unharmed tissue must be brought into play. One popular operation that achieves this is the Cooper's ligament technique devised by an Austrian surgeon named Lotheissen in 1898 and championed recently by Dr. McVay, from whom we've just heard. When asked, Dr. McVay refers to the operation as "the McVay method, of course," because he claims to have reestablished its anatomical correctness in a series of cadaver studies done during the 1930s. The principal behind McVay's procedure (which was first described in 1941) is the repair of the damaged walls of the inguinal canal by suturing one of the abdominal muscles to Cooper's ligament, a strong but inflexible piece of tissue located *below* the normal level of the canal and firmly attached to the pubic bone. Because tissue must be stretched to make this repair, and because the Cooper's ligament itself is rather rigid, a "relaxing incision" must be made in the muscle in front of the abdomen to allow it to move without strain to complete the repair. A variation to the Cooper's ligament technique was devised by Dr. Nyhus in 1959. Dr. Nyhus approaches the hernia from "behind" through a skin incision slightly higher than that used for other repairs. Dr. Nyhus claims that the sac and the damage it has done can more clearly be seen and safely reduced and repaired from this vantage point. Dr. McVay has graciously accepted Dr. Nyhus's suggestion for indirect and femoral hernias, but he continues to repair direct hernias from "above."

The group of surgeons which has done more hernia repairs than any other—with apparently more success—is the one found at Shouldice Surgery in Toronto, Canada. Yet, despite their vast experience and exclusive specialty, they are not mentioned in the textbook, *Hernia*, and noted only briefly in the latest edition of *Current Surgical Diagnosis and Treatment*. Why this is true is unclear. Dr. McVay told us that he considered the Shouldice technique anatomically unsound and procedurally overactive. He claims the Canadians routinely "do too much for the common indirect inguinal hernia." The Shouldice surgeons, naturally, returned the compliment by saying that his "relaxing incisions" were necessary because his operation was wrongheaded. The frank surgeon who wished to remain anonymous told me that he was impressed by Shouldice's success but uncomfortable with what he called the "public relations" aspect of their operation. The hospital does go to great trouble to make patients feel at home and secure, but if this is public relations, it's PR of a very high order. The Shouldice operation is similar to the Bassini technique in that it tries to open and close the inguinal canal with as little disruption of its normal geography as possible. The Shouldice surgeons claim that the key to this is the careful dissection and identification of tissue layers on the way in and strong suturing with stainless steel wire on the way out. They also recommend simplicity, no matter what Dr. McVay says. They do the same procedure for all inguinal hernias, direct and indirect. Femorals are repaired using a different technique. They check each common hernia site for possible defects during each operation. Missed hernias are frequent causes of recurrent hernias, they say. The Shouldice surgeons also advise a complete operation no matter how minor the problem is discovered to be. This means that they slice and reconstruct the "floor" of the canal with the techniques of plastic surgery in every case. They feel that this routine discovers developing hernias and leaves a potentially weak area of the body greatly strengthened. They do not believe in changing the groin's anatomy to employ Cooper's ligament (or any other abnormal element) to beef up their repair. To complaints from those who do that they are unnecessarily cutting and then reconnecting previously undamaged tissue to make a repair that depends on weak ingredients, they point to their success and the 4 uninterrupted lines of stainless steel sutures they alone employ. Also, they claim that their extensive dissection seldom fails to turn up tissue strong enough for a lasting repair.

Their success is formidable. From a recurrence rate of 18.1 percent in 1945, the hospital has moved into the neighborhood of perfection today; in 1976 they reported 1 recurrence in 5,736 operations—with their cases coming from all over the world and including many failures by other hands. Although the hospital claims that no one who has trained thoroughly with them is doing the Shouldice operation in the States, Edwin W. Shearburn, Jr., M.D., and his associates in Philadelphia claim a recurrence rate of 0.7 percent in 550 cases in 13 years with the technique. Dr Shearburn follows the Canadian example in his methods of dissection and suturing and his use of a local anesthetic, but he does not employ stainless steel wire, preferring an inert synthetic material instead. He also differs from Shouldice in favoring a Cooper's ligament repair for femoral hernias. In contrast, the McVay method, in the hands of Dr. McVay himself, has achieved a recurrence rate of 3.5 percent in 1,211 operations spread over 22 years, and statistical analysis of this figure says it will reach 4.2 percent after 25 years. Dr. McVay told us that his follow-up was 98 percent complete and accomplished by himself and his staff. He claims to have reexamined all those patients (still living) whose hernias he has repaired in the years between 1946 and 1968. He charges that Shouldice—which must check many of its foreign patients by mail and through the reports of their family doctors—is not thorough enough in its follow-up. If it were, its recurrence rate would climb, he contended. However, it is true that Dr. McVay checked his operations after the fact and all at once in 1967, a process repeated again in 1970, while the Shouldice method is to write to or see each patient each year for evidence of his condition.

Many surgeons like to use a synthetic mesh or screen to

repair large or recurrent hernias. Some even argue that such devices should be employed in all repairs because of their great strength. The materials commonly used in these screens are fibers like nylon, Dacron, Orlon, Teflon, Fortisan and Marlex and metal alloys like stainless steel and tantalum. The theory behind all the implants is that they will add their own toughness to the weakened area and provide a field on which fibroblasts, or scar tissue, can grow to seal the defect. The problems encountered in realizing this theory are also the same with each of the synthetics. They can be rejected by the body or simply tear out despite their reputed strength. The plastics can inspire allergic or foreign-body reactions and be rejected, and the metals often break up after the constant bending and work hardening of implantation. Once this breakup occurs, the brunt of the repair falls on the scar tissue, which is generally not up to the task. Most of the synthetics must also be removed in the presence of wound infection. Because of these liabilities, most surgeons employ such appliances only if forced to by huge defects or multiple recurrences; 1 very serious case in every 100 is a frequently cited projection of the practice.

The Truss Remedy

Trusses are devices intended to reduce the sac and entrapped organs of a hernia by mechanical means. They usually consist of a pad of firm material (such as rubber) which fits over the swelling and pushes inward. The pad is held in place by a snug waist belt made of leather and reinforced with steel. Trusses can be uncomfortable and do not always contribute to good grooming. They are embarrassing in emergency rooms, among other places. They must be put on when the patient is lying down, and the hernia is naturally reduced. They cannot be used with a hernia that does not spontaneously reduce in this way. The appliance must always be worn when the person is up and active. Trusses are only used for inguinal hernias; there is no model suitable for the lower placement of a femoral bulge, though there are girdles for use with certain incisional hernias of the abdomen.

The dangers of truss wearing are that the pad can cause abrasion of the skin over the swelling and that it cannot indefinitely prevent the growth of the hernia. Sliding hernias, especially, are resistant to the truss remedy, and many smaller hernias become sliding hernias with the help of such an appliance. Moreover, the constant pressure of a truss pad can weaken the tissues around the hernia and make surgical repair more difficult when it becomes necessary.

The dangers of the postponement or avoidance of hernia surgery are, of course, the threats of incarceration, strangulation and gangrene. In some cases, surgery on even incarcerated hernias can be safely deferred—to allow a patient to lose weight or correct a cough, for instance—by a process of mechanical reduction. He is given pain-killers and is heavily sedated to relax the muscle structures that grip his hernia. Then, his hips are elevated, and the protrusion is gently manipulated back into place. That is by no means a cure or even a long-term palliative.

Trusses—like hernias themselves—are sometimes funny. Everybody knows about them—even the youngest kids—because sleazy comic books still carry little truss ads in their back pages, for whose edification, the Lord only knows. Despite this evidence of their continued viability, the truss theory of hernia repair doesn't hold up much any more. Few doctors recommend them, and those who do offer them merely as temporary measures for patients who are not candidates for surgery because of their age or medical condition. People with serious heart diseases, tuberculosis or cancer are generally excluded from the operating room, as are people with small hernias who have 70 or 80 summers under their belts. But some surgeons—notably those of Shouldice Hospital with their success record and short recovery period—do not rule out surgical repair merely because of advanced age. The Shouldice staff feels that there is little risk even for the elderly with local anesthetic and contends that the removal of a hernia's discomfort is even more important to an older patient.

Thus, doctors recommend a truss only when a person refuses surgery or while he is waiting for surgery—say, for instance, while he is losing weight in preparation for an operation. Trusses may also be used by some physicians to control a hernia which has recurred 2 or 3 times. The only unqualified recommendation for the truss we could find was an incredibly complex statistical argument in a book called *Costs, Risks, and Benefits of Surgery* (Oxford University Press, 1977) compiled by a group at Harvard University. The book contains no clinical experience and argues solely from a review of recent medical literature on hernia. Its conclusion—based on a sophisticated computer analysis of the literature—is that there will be no real effect on the *quantity* of life lived by a 65-year-old male hernia sufferer whether he has surgery or wears a truss. In fact, he may live a bit longer if he refuses surgery. The man (being typical for the purpose of the study) has a projected 13.3 years yet to live. After weighing the chance of strangulation against the likelihood of recurrence, the computer decided that he can expect to lose 3.37 days from his 13 years if he wears a truss. If he elects surgery, he will forfeit 17.66 days. What the computer could not digest and analyze, of course, is the *quality* of this mathematical Everyman's life. Would he be more comfortable and fun loving with surgery? Would he grow to resent the sweaty embrace of the truss? Would he continue to wear it? What *can* be accomplished in 14.29 days? Most doctors say that the operation is the better bet. Most truss salesmen disagree.

Can Hernias Be Prevented?

Hernia prevention would seem a happier topic than repair, but some find it equally dispiriting. According to lots of experts, it may already be too late for us to think about prevention. People don't inherit hernias, it is claimed, but they do inherit the kind of muscle tissue or structure that gives way—so to speak—to them. We're either potential victims or we're not. If these folks are right, our only recourse is to fight hernia in our children *in utero*. A high-protein diet for the expectant mother helps to develop strong abdominal walls in the child and may insure the proper closing of the inguinal rings after the migration of the testes. Mothers-to-be should also stop smoking and avoid alcohol. Both stunt fetal growth and may make premature delivery more likely. Virtually all premature babies have inguinal hernias or their makings. Continued high protein and supplements of vitamin C lead to tightly knit muscle tissue in the growing child, and they may stave off an acquired hernia later on.

For older people the only preventive measures seem to be regular exercise—especially workouts for the abdomen such as sit-ups—and proper lifting habits. Weight must stay down within normal ranges and any chronic pulmonary or excretory conditions must be attended to. The Shouldice surgeons only half-jokingly told me that the widespread adoption of a high-fiber, high-bulk diet might put them out of business by eliminating many problems with constipation.

Proper lifting, according to the National Safety Council, involves a knowledge of the following guidelines. In lifting a heavy object, place one foot alongside the object being lifted and one behind it. Take a squatting position and keep the back straight, nearly vertical. Tucking in the chin will help keep the back in position. Grip the object with your entire hand, not just your fingers. To gain better strength and to keep your body weight centered, keep the arms and elbows tucked into the side of the body and draw the object close. Make sure the body weight is centered over the feet and start to lift with a thrust of the rear foot. Stretching far above your reach for large loads is a potentially disasterous habit, as is carrying them on the hip rather than the shoulder. No matter how good it is for your ego to be able to lug a monster box by yourself, it's murder on the groin. Always get help when you need it.

17
Varicose Veins

There is good and bad news about varicose veins. The bad news is that varicose veins can be ugly, painful and almost inevitable in some persons predisposed to them by a combination of heredity, life-style and occupation. The good news is that they can often be treated without surgery. Even when surgery is performed, the risk is low and the results often satisfying, both in improved appearance and alleviated pain.

A varicose vein is any vein that is dilated (stretched), tortuous, and elongated. Some people have tiny superficial varicosities on the face, which can be treated with plastic surgery. Men can get varicose veins in the scrotum. This painful condition is known as varicocele.

Generally, though, varicose veins refer to the saphenous veins of the leg—the long veins that snake their way down the inner side of the thigh and lower leg. These veins have to fight gravity when they send blood back up to the heart. One reason why varicose veins rarely develop in the trunk is that gravity is on their side. If the veins in the legs are damaged enough, the blood stagnates and pools around the ankles, leading to a host of woeful complications.

Veins that become varicose may look only slightly bluish and swollen. Others may thicken until they look like ropes, springing out beneath the skin like worms on a sidewalk after rain. Although a leg may seem to be covered with varicose veins, there is only one great and small saphenous vein in each leg—all the rest of the spidery offshoots are its tributaries.

Fortunately, the superficial saphenous veins don't play a

very important role in circulation. About 85 percent of the venous return of blood from the legs is accomplished by the deep, or femoral, veins. Deep veins aren't visible—they lie close to the bone and are kept in place by a muscular sheath. If you've ever skinned a chicken drumstick, you know how tight and strong the sheath is.

As long as the deep veins are working properly, they can easily take over the work of the superficial saphenous veins that become varicose and are candidates for removal. Because they lie largely unprotected except for connective tissue just beneath the skin, the saphenous veins are much more vulnerable than their protected counterparts in the deep venous system.

If only the superficial veins are diseased, the patient has primary varicose veins. Secondary varicose veins—ones that result from damage to or obstruction of the deep venous system—are much more serious. Thrombophlebitis is an example of a disease of the deep venous system that can lead to varicose veins. The clotted deep veins form new channels to send their blood to the superficial veins. Not made to take the increased flow and pressure, the superficial veins develop varicosities.

Complications of varicose veins, which include thinning of the skin around the ankle, discoloration of the skin, breaking and bleeding of the thin skin and hemorrhage that is spontaneous or occurs after a blow to the leg or ankle, are far more likely to occur with secondary varicose veins than with primary ones.

Less often, varicose veins develop neither by themselves nor as a result of a deep vein problem, but because of an abnormal communication between a vein and an artery known as an arteriovenous fistula. Such fistulas are usually brought on by an injury. Cirrhosis of the liver can even cause veins in that organ to become varicose.

Often patients with atherosclerosis or arteriosclerosis worry that their diseases could cause varicose veins. Not so. Leg veins usually don't "harden" like arteries do unless they are intentionally treated to do so (a procedure that will be explained later in the chapter).

Who Gets Varicose Veins, and Why?

According to some estimates, 10 to 20 percent of the Western world's population suffer from varicose veins. One researcher even claims they afflict 50 percent of the adult population of Europe. People of both sexes, many ages and many countries get them, but they are more common in women, elderly or middle-aged people and people in Western societies. People who suffer from diverticular disease of the colon, take estrogens and frequently wear tight clothing have an increased chance of developing varicose veins. So do women who have been pregnant, especially if they've been pregnant more than once. Certain occupations can also increase the risk of developing varicose veins. Assembly line work, waitressing and clerking are all examples of jobs that may contribute to varicose vein development because they require so much sitting and standing. Both sitting and standing for long periods of time cause the blood to pool in the legs, increasing the pressure. Consistent heavy lifting can also be a factor.

Why do varicose veins develop? Theories abound, but the most commonly cited culprit is heredity. Epidemologists (people who study the frequency of diseases) don't know if the inherited defect is the tendency for the vein walls to be weak and dilate or for the valves to break down in the veins. The saphenous veins have a series of valves in them at regular intervals, designed to assist the thrust of blood back to the heart. Each valve forms a floor for the column of blood above it, opening and closing constantly during normal muscular activity to "milk" the blood back up to the heart. When a vein stretches so much that the valve can't control the column of blood above it, the blood flows downhill to the valve below. The pressure of this extra blood makes the valve below work harder and stretches the varicose vein even more.

Other factors besides inherited defects are thought to contribute to incompetence of the valves and stretching of the veins. Pregnancy increases the flow of blood to the pelvic area. Abdominal tumors and obesity in addition to pregnancy cause the normal flow of blood to be obstructed.

Some doctors believe weak saphenous veins are caught in an evolutionary time lag—that they just didn't adapt quickly enough to man's adoption of the upright posture.

Several researchers believe varicose veins are the result of a diet high in processed foods and low in fiber. Such a diet, they say, causes constipation and overloads the colon. The pressure of the loaded colon or of straining while trying to defecate to relieve constipation increases the pressure of blood to the extremities and varicose veins result.

A well-known British physician told us he became intrigued when he noted so few cases of varicose veins during his 20 years of work in Africa. Denis P. Burkitt, who has recently been lecturing at meetings of American physicians, says the incidence of varicose veins in India and Africa is as low as 2 percent. "Rubbish" is the word he uses to describe the reasons most epidemiologists give for the development of varicose veins. He points out that in communities where women stand erect, bear many children and carry large burdens on their heads, varicose veins are least common. These facts of African life don't jibe with the ideas that varicose veins are caused by upright posture, multiple pregnancies and heavy lifting.

He told us: "Let me tell you a thing that your textbooks in America say on varicose veins. They say it [varicosity] is due to the fact that man isn't adapted to standing upright. This is absolutely rubbish. People in native communities probably stand far more than the average person does in the West. Secondly, your textbooks say varicose veins are due to pregnancy. There is an inverse relationship geographically between pregnancies and varicose veins. When we had 1,000 pregnant women at term before delivery examined in India, 11—or 1.1 percent—had varicose veins. A study of pregnant women of the same age group in North America found that 30 percent had varicose veins. In 5 surveys done on varicose veins in India, not more than 3 percent of the subjects had varicose veins. And in every one of them, varicose veins were more common in men than women. The men don't often get pregnant. So you see the idea that varicose veins are caused by pregnancy is wrong. If you have defective valves, then the pregnancy will make those noticeable. But they'll disappear again after the pregnancy."

Burkitt believes instead that varicose veins are caused primarily by constipation, which results from the Western low-fiber diet. When a person sits on an elevated toilet seat and strains to eliminate hard stools, Burkitt explains, he increases abdominal pressure in 2 ways. In a book documenting his research, he wrote:

"The contraction of abdominal muscles, including fixation of the diaphragm which accompanies efforts to evacuate firm feces [stools], causes raised intra-abdominal pressures that are transmitted to the vena cava [a trunk of veins for the lower extremities and pelvic and abdominal organs] and its tributaries and to the veins of the lower limb when the protective valves have become incompetent" (*Refined Carbohydrates, Foods and Disease: Some Implications of Dietary Fibre*, Academic Press, 1975).

An American surgeon agrees with Burkitt that constipation may be at least one cause of varicose veins. Robert A. Buyers, M.D., director of surgery at Sacred Heart Hospital in Norristown, Pennsylvania, told a group of nutritionists in a 1977 speech:

> All of us know about varicose veins. Every time one strains while defecating, the intra-abdominal pressure is increased. The pressure is transmitted retrograde in the legs through the veins, and this pressure exerted over years and decades in the constipated person produces dilation of the veins. The valves break down and with the help of gravity, incompetent varicose veins occur. In India and Africa, with patients on a high-fiber and vegetable diet, the incidence of varicose veins in pregnant women, for example, is less than 2 percent. In the U.S., on the other hand, the incidence reaches 40 percent during pregnancy. In Polynesia, people living in the traditional way of life have only 2 percent incidence of varicose veins yet the same people in the nearby Cook Islands, where they have been Americanized with Cokes, white bread and red meat, have an incidence 8 to 10 times greater.

Later when we spoke personally to Dr. Buyers, he said most of the patients who visit him with varicose veins are beyond prevention or nonsurgical treatment and require surgery. He suggests they try a high-fiber diet after surgery to help prevent recurrence, which ordinarily happens about 10 percent of the time, according to standard surgical texts.

He remarked, "Without statistics and scientifically collected data—which I don't have—it's impossible to say with certainty how the high-fiber diet works in treatment of varicose veins. The impression I get from patients, though, is that it has helped."

He suggested that a surgeon might demonstrate to a patient how high intra-abdominal pressure can go while the body strains by pumping a blood pressure cuff up to 200 on a patient's arm.

Lack of fiber has also been implicated as a cause of varicose veins by a second British physician, T. L. Cleave. Cleave, a surgeon, rejects the idea that straining during elimination produces varicose veins, pointing out that coughing—which is also a strain—does not dilate veins. He believes instead that an overloaded colon, also a result of lack of dietary fiber, blocks the blood flow from the leg by obstructing the left external iliac vein [pelvic vein that transports blood from the legs]. In his book, *The Saccharine Disease* (Keats Publishing, 1975), he advances the idea that white flour, white sugar, other carbohydrates and the glucose formed from them during digestion give rise to a variety of ailments, including varicose veins.

Do You Have Varicose Veins?

Even if you have all the predisposing factors described above and all the symptoms to be described below, don't assume you have varicose veins. And if you have been diagnosed as having varicose veins, report any leg pain or other symptoms that are different or more intense than the ones you've had before to the doctor. Many diseases have symptoms that mimic varicose veins, among them degenerative joint disease, restless leg syndrome, gout, arthritis, flat feet, neuromuscular problems and groin hernias. Not all prominent veins are diseased. Compare the veins on the back of your hands and on other people's to see widely varying degrees of prominence. Even if your veins really are varicose, a physician needs to test them to see if your problem is of the superficial venous system only or if an underlying disease is involved. If it's the latter, ignoring the diseased veins could be a fatal mistake.

It seems logical to think that the worse the veins look, the worse the symptoms they produce. Yet the most unsightly ones can produce little or no discomfort and those that are only faintly obvious may cause almost crippling pain, especially in women. The veins will probably feel soft to the touch except in the areas of the valves, which may be hard and knotty. Fat obscures varicose veins—if your legs are fat, your varicose veins could become more obvious when you lose weight. (Don't use this as an excuse not to diet, though—obesity aggravates varicose veins and complicates healing after surgery.)

Most patients who do complain of symptoms mention that their legs feel full, heavy, achy, tired and tender. Some get leg cramps during the night. The symptoms worsen as the day goes on, but are relieved by elevation of the legs in a night's sleep. The skin around the veins might be broken out, flaky and itchy, especially with secondary varicose veins. The feet and ankles may swell. Women who still menstruate may feel worse in the days just before their periods. A brownish red discoloration of the ankles can result from the stagnant blood trapped just under the skin. Clots form readily, sometimes causing an inflammation called phlebitis. Don't let the word alarm you, though. Such clots don't pose the danger that clots in the deep venous system do. It is very rare for a clot from the superficial veins to travel to the lungs or other vital organs, unlike the deep vein blood clots that are so potentially dangerous after surgery.

Varicose veins often develop over a period of years, so slowly and mildly that the symptoms are barely noticeable. Often the first symptom is a feeling of fullness in the legs after a day's work. The symptoms may be so minimal that the patient goes to the doctor only because he is worried about the appearance of the legs or their future. A diagnosis of varicose veins is often made when the patient is at a doctor's appointment for a different ailment or general physical exam.

Some varicose veins are so mild both in appearance and symptom that no treatment at all is necessary. A British doctor, Adrian Marston, responded to an article on varicose vein surgery in a medical journal with these remarks:

"Your otherwise excellent editorial on this subject omits to mention the most important aspect of treatment, which is that a large proportion of people with varicose veins do not require any. . . . It is a normal feature of the European body, considerably more common than is red hair or left-handedness" (*Lancet,* September 6, 1975).

Similarly, an American medical text points out:

"The severity and cause of the venous insufficiency determine the type of therapy recommended. About one-third of patients with simple varicose veins require no therapy at all or only commonsense advice about taking care of their legs" (*Current Surgical Diagnosis and Treatment*, Lange Medical Publications, 1977).

Several simple tests can be done to determine the presence and extent of varicose veins. First the physician will probably want to observe your bare legs while you are standing. If you are overweight or your legs are heavy, he may feel the veins or use percussion by placing his finger along the saphenous vein of the thigh and then tapping the vein at a lower point.

Most likely you will then be asked to lie down on your back and elevate the leg until the vein empties of blood. A rubber tourniquet will be tied around the elevated leg at the upper thigh and you'll be asked to stand. If the saphenous vein remains empty 30 seconds or longer, and then fills over a 1- to 2-minute period, you don't have varicose veins. If it fills very rapidly, however, the physician can assume that the veins are varicose and their valves are incompetent. You may be asked to repeat the procedure with the tourniquet tied at various places on your leg so the doctor can determine where the varicosities are.

If there is any reason to suspect that your deep veins are causing problems, you might be asked to undergo a second tourniquet test. A tourniquet will be applied to your leg while you are standing and then you will walk for 5 minutes. If the veins become painful and prominent, the deep veins are obstructed. Either test might be followed by venography—injection of a contrast medium into the vein in the foot so that x-rays can be taken of the veins. This test will help determine exactly what the deep vein problems are. Although this procedure is slightly painful—comparable to the intravenous pyelogram used to x-ray the kidney and ureters, according to one surgeon we spoke to—it's to your advantage to have it done. If your varicose veins are operated on and the main problem was really in the deep veins, you could wind up with a big, painful, swollen leg. If the injection for venography is made carefully into the foot, it shouldn't hurt too much.

How to Manage Your Varicose Veins — Without Surgery

Even if your varicose veins don't bother you with symptoms or look bad now, the following treatments might keep them from getting worse.

Bandages, stockings and support hose. Yves St. Laurent might not approve, but you'll probably feel much better if you don support elastic stockings sold in surgical supply houses. Don't prescribe elastic stockings or bandages for yourself without consulting the doctor, though. If you purchase ill-fitting stockings or wrap the bandages too tightly, you could impair circulation and make your veins worse.

Elastic stockings are often prescribed for primary varicose veins and almost always for secondary varicose veins. Usually they extend from just below the knee to the metatarsals (the long foot bones that end just in back of the toes). Occasionally they go clear up to the groin if the patient has varicose veins of the thighs. Measurements of various parts of your legs can be taken so that the stockings, which are made of elastic yarn or mercerized silk, can be made specifically for you. The stockings must exert equal pressure on the leg without cutting off the circulation at the top. Usually you will be advised to put them on before you get out of bed in the morning.

Elastic stockings may be ugly and at times uncomfortable, but they help accomplish several important goals: they prevent swelling, support the veins just as the muscles do for the deep vein system, encourage pumping action, prevent blood from flowing downhill instead of uphill, collapse the stagnant pools of blood and protect thin and fragile skin and tissue from injuries. Heaviness, aching, fatigue and swelling are often reduced by wearing elastic stockings.

Elastic bandages 4 to 6 inches wide may also be used to accomplish the same goals and relieve the same symptoms, but they are more difficult to apply since they aren't fitted for you and you have to gauge the tension yourself.

Support hose give some relief and disguise the varicosities without having the thick appearance of the elastic stockings, but 2 physicians we talked to said the sheer ones that look almost like regular nylons really aren't as effective as elastic stockings.

A San Francisco gynecologist and obstetrician who sees varicose veins in pregnant women, and often writes about women's medical problems, Lucienne Lanson, M.D., gave this advice in a telephone interview: "Supportive stockings will make the woman more comfortable—the very sheer support hose won't give much support and the heavy surgical stockings aren't that comfortable either. A good compromise is a not-too-sheer pair of support hose."

An internal medicine specialist suggested it may be necessary to make a trade-off between the importance of relieving symptoms and having attractive legs. Victor Pellicano, M.D., said:

"Support hose which are sheer are not as good as the thicker ones. Either can be used. It depends on how bad the veins are and how important the cosmetic factor is to the patient. With men, it usually doesn't matter."

Concerned women might consider wearing bandages or elastic stockings at home and on days they wear slacks, and support hose on days they wear dresses.

Avoid tight clothing. Almost as important as what to wear is what not to wear. Tight shoes or belts, girdles, clothes with elastic waistbands—anything constricting—could conceivably impair the flow of blood, especially from the waist down.

Leg elevation. Elevation of the legs is often used with elastic stockings to ease the symptoms of varicose veins. The legs should be elevated higher than the heart so that the blood can drain. For that reason, bed rest is far more effective than elevating the legs while sitting in a chair. A slant board would be ideal, but a pillow at the foot or head of the bed can also be used. It may help if you gently tense the calf muscle while you're resting, or put a pillow at the foot of the bed and "walk" against it. It's probably a good idea to ask the doctor about this—people who have certain diseases of the heart, chest and esophagus shouldn't do it.

Leg elevation combined with elastic stockings is especially good for pregnant women, people with severe symptoms who don't want surgery or are poor risks for it, and the elderly. It may be so effective that badly hurting legs may feel fine in the morning. Elevation can be done at periodic intervals during the day—particularly when alternated with exercise—as well as overnight.

Watch your diet. If you overeat, stop. Fat makes varicose veins difficult to detect and complicates surgery and wound healing. More important, it helps cause and aggravates varicose veins because as it infiltrates connective tissues, it robs veins of their support.

If your weight is normal, some recent research suggests you should consider getting more fiber in your diet, especially if you are constipated.

Even if lack of fiber is not a primary cause of varicose veins, a high-fiber diet is likely to be less fattening and certain to be less constipating than a low-fiber one. To get more fiber in your diet, eliminate white sugar and white flour and pies, cakes, cookies, pastries and pastas made from them. Use whole-grain flours and raw sugar or honey instead. Leave the jackets on your potatoes and the skins on your vegetables. Eliminate pretzels and potato chips and other high-calorie, low-fiber snacks in favor of fresh fruits and vegetables, raw or lightly steamed.

Vitamins. Standard medical texts do not mention nutritional supplementation for treatment of varicose veins. Vitamin C and vitamin E have both been mentioned as important supplements for the condition by many nutrition-oriented physicians, however.

Using evidence that comes from observation of patients in his practice rather than the rigidly controlled studies accepted by scientists, Wilfrid E. Shute, M.D., of the Shute Foundation in Ontario, Canada, concluded that vitamin E helps in treatment of varicose veins. He wrote in 1969:

> Our training was traditional. And so, of course, this explanation [of the possible causes of varicose veins listed earlier in the chapter] was accepted. Therefore, we at first paid little or no attention to the effects of alpha-tocopherol [vitamin E] on varicose veins. However, when we compared notes and found that our patients [treated with E for other ailments] were insisting that their varicose veins were getting smaller, we became interested (*Vitamin E for Ailing and Healthy Hearts*, Pyramid House, 1969).

Dr. Shute goes on to describe numerous cases where vitamin E was used successfully in varicose vein cases. Dr. Pellicano, the internal medicine specialist mentioned earlier in this chapter, reports similar results.

Dr. Pellicano believes heredity, pregnancy, obesity and, to a slight degree, constipation that causes straining are primarily responsible for varicose veins. He adds, though, that a "good, balanced nutritional diet" is essential for treatment. Based on Dr. Shute's report, he recommends vitamin E. "I also recommend vitamin C because it strengthens the collagen, or connective tissue. If there is no complication, such as high blood pressure, I recommend 800 to 2,400 units of E daily and 1,000 to 5,000 units of C," he told us. Dr. Pellicano is a member of the American Medical Association and past president of the Western New York Heart Association and Society of Internal Medicine.

Exercise. Leg exercises, such as walking, jogging, bicycling and swimming, that use the calf muscles, help to pump blood back toward the heart. The rhythmic muscle contractions counteract the effects of gravity and faulty valves that cause stagnation and pooling of blood in lower legs. As calf muscles are strengthened by daily exercise, they are better able to pump blood back up toward the heart. For best results, elastic support hose or bandages should be worn during exercise.

If that suggests too athletic a program to work into your daily office or household routine, investigate the gym and pool at your local "Y". Regular sessions there can significantly reduce the effects of long hours spent sitting at a desk or standing at a cash register.

"Pedaling" while lying on your back in bed or on the living room floor also helps to reverse blood flow by combining muscular pumping with elevation and elastic support. For someone who is not able to get outdoors for long walks or bike rides, cycling in bed for a few minutes twice a day or so may be helpful.

Hot and cold treatment. If the veins have no ulcers or the skin is not broken, alternate hot and cold packs might be soothing. They stimulate the vessels much as exercise does. Two to 3 minutes of heat expands the vessels, 2 minutes of cold contracts them. Alternation of packs twice a day for 30 minutes each time may bring you some relief.

Injection treatment. Injection treatment is slightly more drastic than the other treatments we've mentioned and slightly less drastic than surgery. In compression scleropathy, as injection treatment is medically called, short segments of affected veins are drained of blood and then injected with a sclerosing (hardening) agent. Bandages are applied and, over a period of several weeks, thick, hard, fibrous tissue forms between the walls of the collapsed veins. The injected veins wither away eventually, and the blood that used to circulate through them is rerouted through different, healthier channels.

Although it may sound superficially like the ideal treatment, your surgeon probably won't recommend compression scleropathy unless it is to be done along with surgery or you have only very few, small diseased veins. Although the procedure usually is swifter (it can be done in one or repeated visits to a doctor's office), cheaper and more cosmetically gratifying because there are no incisions, it is less effective over the long term than surgery. Recurrence rates are very high.

In a study in Britain, for example, 89 percent of 284 patients (384 legs) who underwent the procedure had successful results after 3 months; 74 percent after 1 to 2 years and only 68 percent after 3 to 4 years (*British Journal of Surgery*, May, 1974).

Other disadvantages are that compression scleropathy may stain the skin for at least a year or two and it can result in phlebitis, infection and other complications.

A few physicians use scleropathy as a primary form of treatment for varicose veins. Doctors we spoke to said it should be done daily to be done well. Except for these physicians, scleropathy is usually not done without surgery in this country unless the veins are neither deep nor superficial but cutaneous (in the skin). It's possible to have such varicosities without other vein problems. Patients who have them are usually seeking treatment more for cosmetic than for physical reasons.

During the treatment, the patient's leg(s) is first marked in an ink that won't rub off when the surgical scrub solution is applied. The patient lies down flat or elevates the affected leg. A test for allergies to the sclerosing solution should be done before the treatment is given. Injections are made at short intervals, usually about an inch, into the veins. Afterward, thick compression bandages will be applied and worn for about 6 weeks. Usually the patient will be instructed to wear elastic stockings or support hose for some time after the bandages are removed.

A few hours after the treatment, the vein will feel tender, hard and possibly painful. The tissue around it may redden and swell. Discomfort subsides within a few days. Compression sclero-pathy is rarely used at or above the knee because it isn't as successful there as in the lower leg.

What Can the Pregnant Patient Do?

Painful varicose veins during pregnancy can add a sour note to an otherwise joyous time. They occur because of the increased blood flow to the pelvic area and the expanding uterus' obstruction of the venous return to the heart. They can develop along the labia (lips of the vagina) and vulva (entire external genital area) in thick cords, as well as down the legs and thighs. The obstetrician might prescribe a pad wrapped in plastic and supported by a menstrual belt and elastic leotards to ease the discomfort in the genital area.

Inactivity and poor muscle tone make the problem worse, so you will probably be told to walk and do the exercises you learn in childbirth preparation classes.

Even the most zealous surgeon probably won't recommend surgery during this time unless an emergency arises. An emergency is unlikely since complications of varicose veins are rare during pregnancy, although not as unusual just after delivery. Medical and surgical texts echo the same theme—even elective surgery shouldn't be undertaken during pregnancy. Any purely elective surgery should be deferred until the postpartum period. Any major operation represents a risk not only to the mother but to the fetus as well.

Dr. Lanson made these remarks when asked about varicose vein development during pregnancy:

"Just guessing, I'd say about 12 to 15 percent of pregnant women develop varicose veins. Usually little spidery-looking ones begin to appear at about 5 or 6 months and worsen as the woman gets closer to her due date. The most common complaint is that the legs feel heavy and achy.

"I know of no way to prevent varicose veins from developing if a woman has a tendency toward them. One happy thing is that the veins do recede considerably after pregnancy. Certainly, I would not advise varicose vein surgery for a pregnant woman. I would say a woman should wait until things are back to normal—at least 6 to 9 months postpartum—before considering a surgical consultation. If she is planning to have more children, I would say she should postpone surgery until she is through childbearing, unless the veins are really huge and painful."

Why Surgery May or May Not Be the Answer

By now it should be clear that by no means everybody who has varicose veins requires surgery. There are several different reasons patients may want it or need it, though. If you and your surgeon decide you have one of those reasons, surgery doesn't have to be a big ordeal. Risk of death from varicose vein operations was a low 0.02 percent of 87,000 patients in one study done in Italy in the 60s.

Traditionally, varicose vein surgery required 3 to 7 days of hospitalization and 2 or 3 weeks out of work. Although that's still the case in some surgeons' practices, varicose vein surgery also has been done on an ambulatory basis with the patient home the same day, resting that night and off to work or doing normal activities the next day. In between the two extremes is a short hospital stay—2 or 3 days—with the patient returning to work as soon as he feels ready.

A surgeon who has done over 5,000 varicose vein operations on an ambulatory basis told us the risks are low and the results gratifying. Robert A. Nabatoff, M.D., who operates at Mt. Sinai Hospital in New York City, told us in a phone interview, "Practically everybody who needs varicose vein surgery can have it done on an ambulatory basis. That's because if a patient was a very bad risk, we wouldn't recommend an operation anyway. We try to send him to work the very next day. The patient feels better and heals better if he gets back on his feet right away. The reason is that the complications of surgery—phlebitis and thromboembolism—come on from lying in bed."

Surgical texts list several indications for varicose vein surgery. Some are: severe symptoms; very large varicosities, with or without symptoms; hermorrhage from ruptured varicose veins; ulcers resulting from venous stasis (stoppage of blood flow); thrombophlebitis; and the patient's dissatisfaction with the leg's appearance.

One reason that varicose vein surgery is not quite as popular as it used to be is that several types of surgery have been developed using the saphenous vein of the leg for grafting in other parts of the body. It's used in coronary bypass surgery, in surgery for peripheral arterial disease and in a brand-new experimental operation used to restore sexual potency to men with diabetes. Although enough of the vein can be left in the leg to be used for grafting later, many surgeons hesitate to operate. One British surgeon has even suggested that the surgey should not be performed if the patient with a healthy heart is a candidate for developing coronary disease later on because of risk factors such as smoking, family history and so on.

A general surgeon told us some reasons why he is doing fewer of the operations. Richard Raymundo, M.D., who practices in Zelienople, Pennsylvania, said, "Some surgeons like to avoid doing the operation because of the advent of coronary bypass surgery. They just don't want to remove that saphenous vein. I haven't done as much vein surgery in the last 10 years. My own feeling is that the operation shouldn't be done unless there are symptoms that bother the patient. Development of ulcers, of course, would be another indication for surgery."

If you want the surgery because you want your legs to look better you could be in for a disappointment. With a good surgeon, former patients and surgeons alike agree, the legs will look better than before. You still might not be a candidate for a panty hose commercial, though, especially if the tissues of your legs have already changed in appearance from the condition. If the skin has become discolored, for example, that might not go away after surgery. Prominent capillaries will still be visible and so will the small (an inch or shorter) scars from the incisions—there can be as many as 30 of them. Despite the many incisions, loss of blood is not dramatic.

No procedures have been developed that successfully repair what's thought to be the root of the problem, the incompetent valves. Usually a combination of ligation (tying off) and stripping of the veins and their tributaries is used.

Whether you are hospitalized or undergo surgery on an outpatient basis, your veins will be thoroughly examined and diagnosed before you are admitted.

Before surgery (directly before if it's going to be done on an outpatient basis and probably the night before the operation if it's going to be done in the hospital), the surgeon will ask you to stand bare-legged. Then he'll map out the areas he wants to work on in an ink that won't come off with the surgical scrubbing solution. The leg and perhaps the lower abdomen will be shaved. The mapping needs to be done while you're standing because the veins aren't as obvious when you're lying down. General, local or spinal anesthesia can be used.

Ligation alone might be done if there aren't many varicosities or if the saphenous vein must be saved, but usually a stripping operation is involved as well. Two basic incisions are made—one at the groin where the saphenous vein begins to drain into the femoral vein of the deep venous system and one at the inner ankle where the vein ends. Then a long flexible rod is threaded into the vein at the ankle all the way up to the groin. The rod has a small steel ball at the end. The top of the rod is then pulled up from the groin. As the rod is pulled up, it brings the saphenous vein along. The ball keeps the rod from sliding out of the vein. The procedure is similar to turning an inside out self-belt for a garment in sewing. While the vein is being stripped, some of its tributaries are torn out along with it. They bleed, form harmless clots and scar closed. The surgeon won't have to cut them, but they will cause some blue discoloration for a couple of weeks after the operation.

Any diseased tributaries not stripped out along with the saphenous vein must also be stripped, tied or injected with the sclerosing agent mentioned earlier. That's the reason for the multiple incisions. Sometimes the tributaries will be treated during the operation or immediate postoperative period, but sclerosing can be delayed for a subsequent office visit. The operation itself can take up to 2 hours if there are bad varicosities in both legs. Sometimes two surgeons work, one on each of a patient's legs.

Afterward the incisions are sutured and usually compression bandages are applied. The length of time you are asked to wear the bandages and perhaps later suppport stockings will depend on the surgeon, the operation and your legs.

Varicose veins recur in about 10 percent of cases, sometimes because not all the tributaries of the saphenous veins were treated or because veins that were healthy at the time of the operation later become diseased. Generally, though, relief of symptoms is complete and the legs look better. Most complications other than minimal postoperative pain can be avoided if the patient continues to elevate his legs, starts walking as soon as possible and remembers to avoid prolonged sitting and standing, especially in the postoperative period. A good surgeon tries to avoid the occasional after-effect of numbness of the legs or feet by using careful techniques.

18
Prostate Problems

In his third year of college one of the authors had to write an essay about a character in a Samuel Beckett play. Now, Samuel Beckett characters live *very* strange lives. One of them spends all his time buried up to the neck in the sand. Another has a cold water flat in a huge crockery jar. So it wasn't peculiar that the author said—somewhere in the essay—that his subject was "prostrate with grief." Except that his typewriter tapped out "prostate with grief." We bring up this embarrassing moment for 2 reasons. One is that the paper came back from the professor with the offending line heavily underscored and the comment: "Let's not add to his troubles!" And the other is that lots of people think that prostate trouble is *worse* than being buried alive or living in a walk-up flowerpot. These folks are worried, not because prostate disorders are usually life threatening, but because they're very mysterious. For one thing, no one really knows what causes this organ to malfunction. The trouble may be very hard to cure—and there are no surefire cures for some, short of surgery. And finally, prostate problems are considered very much involved with S-E-X.

Though still somewhat sketchy, the best information says that the fluid secreted by the prostate is the stuff that keeps sperm alive and is the lubricant through which they travel. That seems simple enough, except that most people believe that the prostate's role in sex is much greater and that trouble with the gland means the end of sex. Well, they're wrong, and to allay their fears immediately, we want to set down a few facts.

Many prostate surgeries cause no disruption of sexual activity at all. If there are sexual problems following prostate surgery, they are the tail ends of self-fulfilling prophecies. The patient *thinks* his operation will impair him sexually, and it does—at least in his mind. Fortunately, these psychological defects can be treated and cured psychologically. Some prostate treatments diminish or destroy only *half* a man's sex life. They steal his fertility—his ability to impregnate a women—without robbing him of his potency, his ability to attain erection and orgasm. In the case of the rare *young* man who must undergo prostate surgery, this loss of fertility can be more apparent than real. The sperm are not lost, just diverted to the bladder, and they can be recovered and used for artificial insemination. However, when *this* group of procedures attacks *potency*, it does so *only* by decreasing the size of the patient's ejaculate; it subtracts nothing from the other physical aspects of orgasm and detracts not at all from the emotional fireworks of the event. A small number of prostate correctives, unfortunately, end both halves of their victims' sex lives. We have to admit that. But we can also say that these serious disorders usually attack late in life—when desire and drive may have dropped off for other reasons—and that they do *not* have to become such dreaded thieves in the night. Most potency- and virility-robbing prostate diseases develop from milder forms which have not been properly attended to. If they are caught soon enough, they can be handled with little or no disruption of manhood. For this reason, most doctors say that men over 40 should have regular prostate exams.

What Can Go Wrong with the Prostate and Why

But first things first. Only men have prostate troubles, because only men have prostate glands. Women do have a little doohickey (also known as periurethral glands) which some doctors insist on calling a female prostate. Since many others do not use this terminology, and since this doohickey doesn't cause any particular trouble, we'll ignore it here.

The confusion over who's got what is something which will

plague us throughout this chapter. Not a whole lot is known about the prostate. We've said that its function and its cure remain mysteries for the most part, and we have to add here that its exact nature is a puzzle, too. Most people call it a "gland," which means that it is a specialized group of cells that manufactures and secretes a particular biochemical trigger to one of the body's many processes. But most authorities guess that it is a *cluster* of glands or glandlike bodies that is woven into a network of fibrous and muscular structures. This capsule of compressed tissue protects as well as contains the various glands of the prostate, and it is serviced by a series of nerves and muscles. What each of the products of this bundle accomplishes in the body, however, is not known.

This strange package is located in the pelvis near the rectum. In the healthy male adult it's about the size of a golf ball. When in a diseased state, it grows and can reach the size of an orange. Most of the symptoms associated with the various forms of prostate disease come from the rearrangement of its neighborhood caused by this abnormal growth. The word "prostate" itself comes from Latin and means "standing before" or "beside." The organ was so named because it stands immediately before the narrow neck of the bladder and at each side of—or rather *around*—the urethra, the tube that moves liquid wastes from the bladder, down through the penis and out. When the prostate begins to grow in size, it can pinch off the urethra, or even the bladder itself, causing changes in urination habits which range from pain, false starts and dribbling to the complete inability to void.

The controversies over what the prostate is get worse when what it *does* becomes the subject of conversation. We don't even have a clear picture of its physical makeup. In fact, there is currently only a *theory* about the gland's anatomy, the so-called "five-lobe concept." This description arranges its 5 sections around the urethra and starts with the posterior lobe—the one that projects backward into the rectum and can be felt by the physician's examining finger, moves on to a middle lobe of uncertain function and size plus two lateral lobes (one on each side of the middle section) and ends up with the anterior lobe, the region farthest forward and closest to the abdominal cavity. No one really knows what each of the areas contributes to the overall prostate picture, but it is known that the posterior lobe is the least likely to be involved in the common urinary malfunctions of prostatic disease but the most likely to become cancerous. When it does become malignant, of course, it can cause urinary disruption. The middle, lateral and anterior lobes are more susceptible to noncancerous enlargement, a disease called BPH, benign prostatic hypertrophy.

Before we talk specifically about each form of prostatic foul-up, we ought to speak generally about them as a group. Nearly half the men of European extraction in the world—and that means most U.S. males—will have some kind of prostate abnormality during their lives, even if these conditions cause no bothersome or debilitating symptoms. Most of the troubles that do cause symptoms occur after age 45, and one's chance of having difficulty goes up as his age does. Sixty percent of all 60-year-olds experience some kind of problem. Seventy percent of men age 70 do so, and nearly 95 percent of men 85 or older have a brush with prostatic disease. There also seems to be a connection between life-style, geography and prostatic disorders, but scientists haven't been able to identify it yet. Masses of uninterpreted figures, though, suggest that the diseases are more common in the West than in other parts of the world. There has been a sharp increase in the incidence of prostatic disease and cancer among American blacks lately, and the countries with the greatest number of deaths from prostate cancer are Sweden, Norway and Barbados, whose population is largely black. On the other hand, such prostate disasters are rare among Asians. The U.S. death rate due to prostatic cancer is 100 times that of Japan, but significantly, American citizens of Asian parentage incur the same risk as non-Asians. So, it's pretty clear that something we're doing (and the Japanese are avoiding) is contributing to our prostate failures. But again, no one knows what it is.

Another thing we can say about all forms of prostate disease is that the same symptoms usually announce their arrival. These common denominators are easily recognizable as changes in urination habits or abilities. A burning sensation in the urethra after urination (or ejaculation) can be a sign of coming prostate woes, although that symptom is also associated with kidney or bladder infection. The need to urinate frequently is a surer sign, as are repeated, sudden urges toward the bathroom and early rising, morning after morning, with the same object in mind. The occasional nighttime trip to the toilet is probably meaningless, but a consistent progression from once-a-night up to twice-a-night and finally 3 or 4 times down the hall is a pretty good sign that something is wrong. Other indications that you should see a urologist —a doctor who specializes in such problems—are repeated difficulty in starting to urinate, a weak and halting stream once you're going and the inability to empty the bladder coupled with lots of dribbling after—that unshakable feeling that you always have to go. Of course, any sign of blood in the urine should send you to the doctor, but that symptom does not necessarily mean that there is trouble with your prostate.

Prostate Surgery and Your Sex Life — A Better Story Than You'd Think

The other blanket statements we can make about prostate disorders involve the effect of their treatments on patients' sex lives. Although we broached this subject briefly at the opening of the chapter, it bears repeating here, because the good news it contains cannot be stressed too heavily. Prostate surgery is as loaded with fear and emotion for men as mastectomy and hysterectomy are for women—and it is just as as mysterious. Men don't know what their prostates do for them, but they assume an operation will rob them of these hazy benefits and that they will miss them terribly when they are gone. The truth is that the various prostate operations differ so much that a loss of either potency or fertility cannot be accurately predicted before most of them. What's more, the overall statistical picture is fairly cheering.

In one series of operations studied by Harold A. Lear, M.D., of the Mount Sinai Medical Center, only 14 out of 100 men undergoing the TUR, a procedure which removes the overgrowth of the prostate without removing the gland itself, suffered impotence. Dr. Lear also found that no more than 25 percent of the men who had had prostatic growths removed in his hospital by 2 of the 4 methods available—the suprapubic and the retropubic—became impotent. In fact, even the third method (the removal of a growth from below and just in front of the anus, the so-called perineal route), the method thought to be the most damaging, normally causes impotence only because the nerve and muscle fibers which control erection are unavoidably cut in getting to the prostate. The loss of prostatic overgrowth itself apparently leaves sexual abilities unscathed. And even this operation may not be as damaging as was once thought. Some doctors claim that 70 percent of their patients with this type of treatment recover full sexual activity. Other doctors don't believe them, but the message here is clear. Although the kind of surgery you get will be controlled by the nature of your complaint and your doctor's experience, you can help yourself by finding out how good your surgeon is, asking him what method he plans for you and learning what his results have been in the past. And relax—most correctives for benign prostatic enlargement, the most common disorder, have little or no effect on potency. And when impotence does follow prostate surgery, it's usually for nonsurgical reasons. One study of prostatic surgery patients we saw said that impotence normally followed the removal of a cancerous organ. But when cancer was not a factor, these doctors found that the age of the subject was the most important causal factor; sexual ability was dwindling in many patients before their operations. The second consideration was a man's sexual record prior to going to the hospital. If his interest was on the wane before surgery, it certainly wouldn't be spruced up by the procedure. Finally, and most significantly, these researchers found that the type of operation performed was the *least* important contributor to a patient's sexual problem.

The 2 physical things that probably will happen to a man's sex life after most forms of prostatic surgery are a loss of fertility and a diminishing of ejaculate at orgasm. In every procedure but the TUR the patient can usually expect orgasm after his recovery but no discernible discharge at climax. This development can bother his partner, but he may not notice it at all. It occurs because some of the nerve fibers which control erection, prevent urination during orgasm and funnel the product of the ejaculatory ducts to the urethra have been cut in the operating room. Frankly, the "loss" of ejaculate—actually it's diverted to the bladder—seems the least serious thing that could go wrong at this point. But when the ejaculate is short-circuited, the sperm goes with it, and that means infertility, of course.

Putting Out the Fire of Prostatitis

Although not the most common, the prostate disease everyone knows about is infectious prostatitis, probably because it's so hard to cure. Infections of the prostate are most often seen in young adults and come in 2 types, acute and chronic. Both kinds can be severely debilitating and intensely painful, but an acute infection, with its short life and sharp symptoms, is often less of a problem than a chronic case which may persist for years and be punctuated by numerous remissions and sudden flare-ups. So little is known about either form of the disease that the label "chronic" may even be a misnomer. It is unclear whether the repeated attacks of the disease are caused by the same set of germs which have (for some reason) lain dormant for a time or by a new group of bacteria. Contrary to certain bits of men's room gossip, most prostatic infections are not caused by venereal microbes. Eighty percent of them come from *Escherichia coli*, the most common of the colon bacteria and several skin microbes. They can enter the body when defective sewage systems contaminate pools, or water supplies (though this is rare), or more commonly from careless toilet habits, or through certain sexual practices. But the most frequent source of prostate infection is the body itself. The microbes travel to the prostate through the bloodstream or lymphatic system from other trouble spots in the body or from infections in the urethra, where they find perfect conditions to grow in the warm, sealed climate of the prostate which, by the way, is closed to many germ-killing drugs. Most sulfa and many other antibiotic, antiseptic and antimicrobic drugs are either too acidic or so insoluble in body fats that their potency is lost before they reach the prostate. The problems caused by the relative seclusion of the prostate are compounded by the peculiar give-and-take relationship that develops between bacteria and antibiotics. Drugs that immediately kill the germs responsible for acute forms of the disease often bounce off chronic cases. And almost all bacteria implicated in prostate infection eventually grow resistant to the antibiotics used against them. That means when one medicine loses its effect on a patient's condition, a new one must be tried, and a process of trial and error ensues that can be lengthy and frustrating.

The symptoms of infectious prostatitis are the signs of urinary disruption we've mentioned plus a few earmarks of systemic infection: pain in the lower pelvis between the anus and scrotum, perhaps even the lower back, alternating chills and fever, and aching muscles and joints throughout the body. If these complaints come on suddenly, an acute case of the disease is likely. If, however, the changes in urination pattern appear slowly, if the patient gradually learns to live with them and if the signs of infection—fever, chills and pain—are mild and intermittent, then a chronic case is suspected. When a chronic case has been in remission and abruptly becomes active again, its physical symptoms are often accompanied by, first, a here-we-go-again shock and, then, a fairly serious depression.

The first step in diagnosing a suspected case of prostatitis is the taking of the patient's related medical history. It's important to determine whether the symptoms are showing up for the first time, or whether they've been unwelcome guests before, because that distinction can separate a chronic condition from an acute one. The questions that are part of this history taking can be embarrassing. They involve not only the patient's bathroom practice but his sexual habits as well to determine when—exactly—the bothersome signs are occurring and to separate infection from other forms of prostate disorder.

After this grilling, a simple urinalysis will be done, which, in the presence of infection, will detect signs of pus, white blood cells and other cellular debris. Then the doctor will palpate the lower abdomen and pelvis to check for swollen organs and to pinpoint the areas of pain. And finally he will examine the rear wall of the prostate itself through the rectum with his gloved finger. That will disclose whether the gland is enlarged and be a first indication whether or not cancer is the cause of the patient's discomfort.

If all these steps suggest infection instead of benign or malignant enlargement of the prostate, the examination will move on to the 4 steps of a diagnostic procedure developed at the Stanford University Medical Center in 1965. The series of tests, composed by Thomas A. Stamey, M.D., and Edwin M. Meares, Jr., M.D., requires that the patient return to the doctor's office on a second occasion having drunk enough to be sure he is bringing a full bladder with him. When he begins to urinate (on command), 4 different samples are collected—at short intervals—for laboratory analysis. The first sample is taken immediately; the second after a considerable amount of urine has been passed; the third after the prostate has been gently massaged to expel some prostatic fluid into the stream; and the fourth just before the bladder is finally empty. All 4 samples are then sent to the lab to have the bacteria content determined. These results will tell the physician that, yes, it is a prostate infection causing the trouble, or, no, an infection of the urethra is present, but it has not yet moved up to the prostate. With any luck, they will also indicate what kind of bacteria is causing the flare-up and what sort of antibiotic should be used against it.

Yes, the stop-and-going of the Stanford test is uncomfortable. Yes, you will have to make do with medicines to reduce the *symptoms* of the disease—fever-reducers and pain-killers—until the test results come in. Yes, you will have to lay off alcohol and spicy foods while waiting. But the exam for infectious prostatitis does *not* include catheterization (the insertion of a rubber tube through the penis into the bladder to draw off retained urine), which can be much more uncomfortable. Catheterization is never used when infection is suspected, because it tends to spread the condition. It is only used when the bladder or urethra is pinched closed by an enlarged prostate and urine cannot be expelled.

And there is some even better news. Suitable samples of prostatic fluid can be obtained—nowadays—through simple masturbation and ejaculation. This has always been true, but doctors have been loath to call for the procedure, because patients have been loath to follow through with it. But since word of the clinical process that surrounds male sterilization by vasectomy has gotten around, people have grown more comfortable with such a request, and doctors are making it more frequently.

Antibiotics can help a great deal. Once the tests are in, treatment of prostatic infection is and is not easy. If the condition seems acute, the antibiotic most lethal to the germ involved is prescribed, usually a sulfa or penicillin derivative, and the symptoms normally subside rather quickly. The patient is put through the 4 Stanford tests again a few days (or up to 2 weeks) after his complaints have disappeared to check for the continued presence of infection and bacteria. In most cases, they've departed by the time of the second stop-and-going. The patient, however, must continue taking his antibiotic to guard against reinfection. How long? There is no agreement, but Dr. Meares, one of the Stanford researchers now at Tufts University Medical School, recommends 30 days.

If none of this works—or if it works for a time, only to have the infection return—the patient's prostatitis is probably chronic. Then things get tough. Some doctors try a series of antibiotics on apparently chronic cases, hoping to find a knockout punch. Before 1973, others tried surgery, hoping to remove the section of the prostate apparently harboring the resistant bacteria. (Surgery is *never* used on acute infections for fear of spreading them.) No statistics on the success of this hit-or-miss operation are available. Satisfied patients, it seems, do not call back to report their satisfaction, and dissatisfied ones go elsewhere to report theirs. Complete removal of the chronically infected prostate is sometimes done with an elderly patient, but it is avoided for most victims of the disease, because they tend to be young men, and impotence is always a risk with surgery. What happened in 1973 to focus this fuzzy picture was the development (in this country) and trial (in Europe) of a drug or actually 2 drugs, trimethoprim and sulfamethoxazole. When used together these agents proved effective against resistant infections in numerous tests. TMP-SMZ, as the tongue-twisting combo has fortunately been abbreviated, works as a one-two punch in chronically infected prostates. First, the SMZ half, a sulfa-based drug, stamps out any bacteria which may be attacking the gland from elsewhere in the body. And then the TMP, which seems able to enter the prostatic capsule more easily than other antibiotics, moves in to wipe out the trouble there. That all sounds very good, but there are 2 catches here. One is that TMP-SMZ may have to be taken by some chronic infection sufferers the way insulin is taken by diabetics: one tablet every day for the rest of their lives. And the other is that the FDA has not officially and completely cleared the drug for use in this country. The folks at the government agency say they fear *any* combination of strong drugs, because they fear the manipulation of the proportion of the ingredients; they usually insist on a fixed relationship between 2 drugs before OKing their use together. They have, however, approved the use of TMP-SMZ for treatment of urinary infection, which, according to their logic, does *not* include conditions of the prostate. But since many doctors in private practice consider prostate infection under the general heading of "urinary infection," and since urinary troubles lead to prostate troubles in many, many cases, the drug has been given widespread use in the treatment of the gland.

Enlarged Prostate: More Than Just Trouble with Urination

Now we can turn to the most common form of prostate disorder, BPH or benign prostatic hypertrophy (or hyperplasia). The thing to remember here is that first word, "benign." The prostate gland enlarges in this condition, but the growth is *not* malignant;

cancer is *not* a factor. For some reason, in something over 50 percent of all men over 50 years of age, a growth forms over the surface of one section of the organ, covering it a bit like the rind covers an orange. As far as we can tell, there is no chemical change or physical injury involved in this overgrowth. It just seems to happen, although there is no end to the theories which try to explain the phenomenon. Some scientists say that the human life span has been stretched beyond the effective age of the prostate, that after midlife it is improperly supplied with the male hormone, testosterone. But this guess seems wrongheaded, because nearly 80 percent of all men produce the hormone past age 50. Other researchers say that we continue to get the substance as we grow older, but that we lose our ability to use it, to metabolize it. Still others claim that an imbalance between the hormones estrogen and androgen in later life causes BPH, but they can't prove their contention any better than their rivals can. So we're back where we started. BPH exists, and we can't explain it. Another maddening thing about the disease is that it causes no symptoms or problems of its own. If there were room for it to grow, the benignly enlarging prostate could go ahead and do its thing. But because it lives under the neck of the bladder and around the urethra, its overgrowth can decrease the holding capacity of the former and shut down the latter.

Still another rotten thing about BPH is that its early signs can easily be ignored or rationalized away. As a result many cases are discovered by accident during examinations for other complaints. Sometimes nothing more than the occasional need to get up at night to go to the bathroom shows itself. This is true because the bladder is a very accommodating organ—as a growing prostate closes off its exit, the bladder stretches to hold more and more and builds up its muscle power to squeeze urine past the block. However, even the best of bladders can't keep this up indefinitely. Soon the symptoms get worse. The patient has difficulty starting urination; his stream is weak and hesitant once started; and he dribbles after it's stopped. He makes a great many trips to the john and yet always feels like he could use another. At this point, he might even have some pelvic pain or burning during urination. If he manages to ignore even these discomforts, and his prostate grows so large that it completely shuts off the bladder and urethra, an emergency results. He suffers severe pain from the presence of the volume of trapped urine. The bladder becomes exhausted from its repeated stretching and exertion, and may even partially rupture, producing external blowouts (or ballooning-outs) like those of diverticulitis. With the onset of this condition, called strangulation, comes the threat of infection throughout the urinary system caused by retention of stagnant urine in the bladder. The development of stones or tumors is also possible in these balloons of mucous membrane.

How Catheterization Can Bring Relief

If there's an emergency and the patient is unable to urinate, the first thing a doctor does is to catheterize the patient to release the retained fluid. This procedure is a bit painful, but so painful is a plugged bladder that the procedure is often accomplished before the patient notices. And the relief it provides is so welcome that any discomfort that comes along is a small enough price to pay.

If the worst hasn't happened, then there is a deliberate series of steps which lead to the detection of BPH. Deliberate, because it is important to distinguish BPH from infectious prostatitis. The common treatment for BPH is surgery, and—as we said—surgery spreads infection. First, the patient's medical history is examined for any pattern of the symptoms of infection. Then the size, shape and tenderness of the gland are assessed with a digital exam. During this step, the doctor gently but firmly probes and presses the prostate to force a drop of fluid into the urethra so that it may be examined along with the urine specimen taken in the next stage. If the prostatic fluid shows no signs of infection, then BPH is a good guess, because the absence of white blood cells in the liquid is characteristic of BPH. The simple urinalysis done next determines if the blockage caused by BPH's swelling has produced a bladder infection from stagnant urine. If it has, it is treated with antibiotics. After the laboratory has made its contribution to the diagnosis, a complicated series of x-rays is taken to determine how much of the urinary system is obstructed. The bladder, the kidneys and their attendant tubing are all inspected for damage and infection. Finally, if all these things point to BPH, the doctor must take a look inside for himself for the last piece of evidence. The patient is placed in the "lithotomy" position—which is similar to that for childbirth—and a cystoscope is passed through the urethra to the bladder. The tube is not a simple device like the catheter but an extremely sophisticated optical (and sometimes even a surgical) instrument which allows the physician to examine the inside of the urinary system.

OK. We know what you're thinking. This is the *worst* thing in the world, but you're wrong. Yes, the cystoscope is at least as thick as a number 2 pencil, and, yes, it must go all the way up the urethra. And yes, the tip of the penis and urethra are *very* sensitive. But no, the rest of the distance is not *that* touchy, and it is *all* remarkably flexible. The well-lubricated cystoscope passes through with nary a hitch and only moderate discomfort. How much is determined by how well the patient is prepared psychologically—the more he fears the process, the more it will hurt—and how much his doctor believes in anesthetic for the procedure. You know, after reading this paragraph, how you'll feel about this business, and if it still seems the worst thing in the world, try to persuade your doctor to use anesthesia. As in the case of simple catheterization, there is a dividend paid by cystoscopic examination. Even in moderate cases of BPH there is a good deal of urine trapped in the bladder by the prostatic swelling, and it causes low level pressure and pain. Before the exam takes place, the patient is asked to urinate as fully as he can. Then a catheter is inserted in the urethra, and it generally releases a flow of pent-up urine which comes as a great relief. This sense of relief is often strong enough to mask the removal of the catheter and the insertion of the cystoscope. At least, many people feel that the insertion of the scope is a small enough price to pay for the breaking up of the bladder's dam.

Anyway, with the cystoscope's seeing eyes and light in place, the doctor can see whether the bladder muscles have been badly stretched or even ruptured. He can tell which lobe of the prostate has become enlarged by noting where the bladder's neck has been obstructed. And he can plan his medical or surgical attack on the problem.

Unfortunately, surgery is just about the only way most doctors deal with BPH. A drug called candicidan, which was developed in the Soviet Union, has been studied by Andrew Sporer, M.D., of Newark, New Jersey; it has been observed to diminish prostatic swelling for a short time in some cases. However, it has not been cleared for general use by the FDA.

The Pluses and Minuses of Prostate Surgery

The common forms of prostate surgery are termed either "open" or "closed"; they are open if the skin must be opened to perform them and closed if it is not. The open methods are used for the removal of benign growths on the prostate and are classified according to how the gland is approached. All 3 open methods are considered major operations and are performed under either general or spinal anesthesia. The rule of thumb says that a spinal is preferable for longer procedures. The most common open type, the suprapubic, comes at the gland from above. Since the prostate lies below it, the bladder must be opened before the excessive prostatic growth can be trimmed off. Because of the bladder's involvement, this procedure leads to the most unpleasant and difficult recovery of the three. The prostatic capsule that is left must be packed to control bleeding; rubber drains or a tube is left in the bladder to allow for drainage; and the patient remains catheterized for a day or two or sometimes until he leaves the hospital. This combination of factors usually means that he needs special nursing care to tend to his morale and sanitary needs during recovery.

Neither of the other 2 open methods requires going through the bladder. One, the perineal, moves directly to the prostate through an incision between the scrotum and anus, and the other, the retropubic, works from behind the bladder. The perineal is the classic route for the complete removal of the cancerous prostate and is the procedure most often implicated in the loss of sexual potency. The retropubic is a newer way of going about the same thing. Which way your surgeon chooses to travel will be determined, in part, by the part of your prostate that has enlarged and its size. But most of his decision will be made by his experience. He'll use the method he's most comfortable and successful with. You may not be able to change methods without changing doctors, and so you should learn the pluses and minuses of the various operations and ask your surgeon to balance the pluses he sees with the minuses you'll feel. For instance, will the messy suprapubic route be justified by a better chance of complete recovery and less risk of sexual disability? Or, has the overgrowth gotten so out of hand that a TUR could not be substituted for the sexually damaging perineal passage?

The most popular surgical method among patients and doctors—and the most difficult procedure—is the so-called TUR, the transurethral resection. This fancy name means "cutting through the urethra," and that's exactly what goes on. A special cystoscope equipped with a tiny cutting device is inserted through the urethra into the bladder and pushed to the overgrown prostate. The surgery takes place without an outside incision. This method is popular, of course, because it leaves no scar, requires a shorter hospital stay and is less likely to produce sexual impotence. It's also the most kind to older folks, the very ones most apt to need surgery. It's the most complicated of the available operations and requires the most training and experience of the doctor. That's why you need a specialist.

The TUR is normally used for moderate cases of BPH, those in which the prostate has not enlarged beyond a weight of 2 ounces—the size of a chicken's egg.

No matter what type of operation your pesky prostate requires some things about your hospital experience and recovery will be the same. Your time in the operating room will run between 45 minutes and 1½ hours for all procedures. Again, no matter what kind of surgery your doctor prefers, if he's one of a fairly large group of urologic surgeons, he'll start things off with a vasectomy. This is a simple little business in which a tiny slit is made in the scrotom so that the tubes carrying sperm to the penis can be cut and tied, blocking the sperm ducts. Many surgeons feel that this step prevents complications during convalescence, but about an equal number disagree. The thing that *is* clear is that a vasectomy *insures* infertility (*not* impotency) after a surgical procedure which can produce (but does not guarantee) it. If you are of an age and have the desire and the ability to have children after your prostate troubles are over, you should tell your doctor and be sure he drops vasectomy from his routine.

What to expect after prostate surgery. If your age and general health permit, you will be up and around a bit on the day of your operation, and you will be asked to increase your activity gradually until you're moving about fairly normally by the third day. Elderly patients are usually kept quiet for a day or two before they're asked to resume anything like full activity. While you're getting your land legs back, you may not have a bowel movement for 2 or 3 days following surgery. Don't worry about it. Most patients are given enemas before their trips to the OR; they're fed very lightly after leaving it, and the absence of bowel movement is perfectly normal.

During the immediate postoperative period, urination will be handled by a catheter, which draws off urine automatically and allows the prostate and its attendant muscles—which have been battered about a bit—to rest and recover. Some people feel a strong urge to "go" while catheterized, but this is a false alarm. It is merely a sensation caused by the alien presence of the rubber tube. With the TUR, catheters are left in place from 2 to 4 days; with the various open procedures, they may remain in for a week or more. If you've had one of the open surgeries—especially the suprapubic type—you may also notice a soft rubber drain extending from the incision or a spot close to it. This tube helps remove excess fluid and blood from the surgical area and will stay in place between 2 and 4 days. The withdrawal of a catheter is usually painless, and the removal of a drain is too. It also seldom requires additional stitches. The wound simply closes by itself. Speaking of stitches, they are not a problem, of course, with the closed TUR method, and skin sutures are removed from open operations before patients are released from the hospital, about 6 to 8 to 10 days after their surgery.

When you leave the hospital, you'll probably be given antibiotics to prevent infection around the wound and speed the healing process. You may notice some burning during urination, and you may have to go more often than you think is fair—given all you've been through to correct that problem. But these are temporary setbacks stemming from the irritation of surgery and catheterization; they'll disappear in a couple of weeks. Best of all, you should notice immediately that urination is easier, more forceful and complete, and that the worst of your old symptoms have gone. You may, however, see blood in the urine or even small clots for a week or two after surgery. This also is no problem unless the amount of blood is considerable. A few TUR patients experience fairly heavy urinary bleeding *several* weeks after surgery—even if it has been clear sailing up until then. This bleeding means that scar tissue has peeled off the healing prostate. Although it's no reason for alarm, you should tell your doctor about it. He may wish to clear up the condition by rinsing the bladder with a saltwater solution for a day or two through a catheter. Sometimes this is a hospital procedure, sometimes it's not. That kind of bleeding rarely occurs with open operations.

How long will it take you to get back on your feet after prostate surgery? That depends on your age and general health before the operation. Most people have pain in the pelvic and genital areas which requires medication to live with, but it usually disappears in about a week. During this same week, most patients also tire very easily and must limit their exertions carefully. Although energy soon returns, heavy work and lifting are out for 4 to 6 weeks, and office or housework must be curtailed for 2 to 3 weeks.

Dealing with the Chance of Prostate Cancer

Before we leave the subject of prostate surgery, we've got to talk a bit about cancer. When a malignant growth is discovered on the gland, its removal is frequently the response. However, the number of cancer cases of this type is fairly small; most prostate troubles are benign. In the last few years there have been about 60,000 new cases annually, and nearly 19,000 men have died in each of the recent years for which reliable figures are available. But since there are 30 million men in the most prostate-risky age group, one's chances of having a brush with this sort of cancer are 1 in 5. Of the approximately 300,300 operations performed yearly, 80 percent of the tissue samples examined are noncancerous, according to leading urologist Irving M. Bush, M.D., of Chicago's Cook County Hospital.

Prostatic cancer is rare before age 60. Like many other disorders of the gland, its cause is not known. It is known that androgens stimulate its growth, that estrogens tend to retard it and that most malignancies arise in the posterior lobe—where BPH is very uncommon. The disease first spreads through the prostate itself, then into the attendant urinary tubing and finally into the pelvic lymph nodes and bone structure. Unfortunately, most cases of prostatic cancer are *not* detected early, because men cannot find it in themselves in the same way that women can constantly check for breast cancer. As a result, most doctors suggest an annual prostate exam for all men 50 (some even say 40) years of age. This means an assessment of the posterior lobe of the gland with the physician's finger—malignant growths tend to be stony hard—and a biopsy for lab analysis if the results of the digital exam are suspicious. For the biopsy, a tiny piece of the affected lobe is removed with a heavy needle and examined under a microscope. Biopsies are also routinely performed during all surgery for BPH conditions.

Because there is no easy check for prostate cancer, when symptoms finally present themselves, it may be too late to do much about it. These late signs are frequently identical to those of

BPH. The cancerous overgrowth obstructs the bladder neck or urethra, leds to a stoppage of urine flow and sometimes to secondary infection from stagnating waste. Such conditions are detected by the same cystoscopic means used with BPH. If the malignancy is well advanced, its movement into the lymph system may be announced by lower back pain which can also radiate down into one or both legs. When the worst happens and the pelvic bones are attacked, certain blood tests reveal the extent to which bone marrow has been replaced by tumorous growth. That replacement first produces anemia in the patient, and signs of it lead to other lab tests which disclose the various chemical and metabolic changes that come with the spread of cancer. When the symptoms indicate a very large tumor, of course, x-rays are taken to judge the extent of it.

There are many treatments for prostate cancer, and the choice of one usually depends on the age of the patient, his general health and the stage of development reached by the tumor. The complete removal of the gland cures about 70 percent of people who are fit enough for the operation and whose malignancy has not spread beyond its capsule. But major surgery is usually reserved for relatively young people. After age 70, treatments which slow the growth of the cancer normally replace surgery. This means that—technically—only 5 percent of all detected cases of prostate cancer are *permanently* cleared up. But it is also true that the palliative measures available for older, less fit patients allow them to live out longer, fairly comfortable lives. Twenty-five percent of prostate cancer cases above those permanently cleared up are controlled, allowing the patient a normal life expectancy.

The most important step in the diagnosis of prostate malignancy, once its presence is discovered, is the determination of its stage and grade, the extent to which it's spread and the activity with which it is growing. Most commonly used is the classification system for these characteristics which was modified in 1956 by Willet F. Whitmore, Jr., M.D., at The Memorial Sloan-Kettering Cancer Center in New York. Dr. Whitmore calls cancer which is confined to the prostatic capsule "stage A." "Stage B" is a tumor which has filled the capsule but gone no further. "Stage C" means that the malignancy has spread to adjacent organs (especially the seminal vesicles), and "stage D" indicates that the abberrant cells have moved through the lymphatic ducts to the pelvis and, perhaps, the lungs. Determining the *stage* reached by a patient's disease is not a difficult procedure. The problem comes in predicting how fast it will move from one stage to another, predicting its "grade," and doing it soon enough to prevent widespread damage.

Hugh J. Jewett, M.D., emeritus professor of urology at The John Hopkins University, has amended Dr. Whitmore's system to include grades 1 and 2 under the first stage of tumor growth. Grade 1 denotes a very slow moving tumor, and grade 2 refers to a condition much more likely to move onto the next level. Grades A-1 and A-2 are generally accepted as benign and malignant, respectively. Dr. Jewett doesn't bother with gradations of the later stages, because beyond the initial plateau, the determination of rate of growth doesn't help the patient much. Some time is spent separating grade A-1 from A-2, because one microscopic examination of the affected cells is not enough to classify them. Several tests and several weeks are required to tell for sure. Because prostate cancer is slow growing, this is not particularly dangerous.

Given the touch-and-go nature of diagnosis here, the choice of a treatment is sometimes difficult. With a stage A tumor, some doctors don't wait for the grading process to run its course and advise an immediate TUR, hoping that all the malignant tissue can be removed with this quick step. They, of course, keep an eye on the patient's progress after the operation for any signs that the procedure hasn't worked. Other doctors delay with a first stage growth, with the understanding that the patient will go ahead with the grading process and come in for repeated reexaminations—say every 2 or 3 months—to check for any change in the state or stage of cancer. Most of the time a stage A tumor will be picked up incidentally during a TUR for other problems, and the doctor will later go back to take more tissue.

Once the grading process is completed and a stage A-2 tumor is confirmed, many (perhaps most) urologists will suggest the complete removal of the gland. Recently, however, radiation treatment has become an option. Previous external radiation methods have been thought too unfocused for use with tightly localized tumors of the prostate, but now tiny pellets of radioactive iodine (and other substances) can actually be implanted in the diseased gland. That process, which again employs a tube not unlike a cystoscope, effectively concentrates high levels of radioactivity in a very small area. The pellets used are too small to cause discomfort when in place and have no effect on the patient's sexual abilities. After about a year, they become largely inert and can safely be left inside for the rest of the patient's life. External radiation is still used for cancers which have formed at several points in the prostate or begun to spread beyond the capsule.

For stage B cancers a prostatectomy of some kind is usually recommended. That is also true of stage C malignancies, but a subtle distinction between the "complete" removal of the gland and its "total" removal must be made here. In the stage B operation, the entire gland is often removed, but its muscular capsule is left behind. In the stage C process, the capsule is also removed. In the first case, impotency is *not* inevitable, and in the second it is.

For these more serious stages of prostatic cancer and even for the last stage of the disease—D—there are other treatments, but they are designed primarily to extend the patient's life, to slow rather than stop the progress of the cancer. One of the ancient treatments for prostatic disease was castration, and it seems to have been fairly successful. Scientists studying this phenomenon have discovered that malignancy in the gland is largely controlled by the sex hormones: growth is promoted by the androgens (the male hormones, mainly testosterone) and retarded by the estrogens (the female hormones). So, castration, in cutting off a supply of androgen, can be effective in slowing cancer's attack on the prostate. And, contrary to popular fears, it is *no* certain threat to potency. About 1 to 3 percent remain potent after castration. So, most men would rather have an alternative to castration, and Charles B. Huggins, M.D., of the University of Chicago, found one—the administration of the female hormone DES—for which he received the Nobel Prize in medicine in 1966. DES does not end the spread of cancer, but it does slow it down and can prolong lives by blocking the action of the body's male hormones on the tumor.

Beyond that step, the methods of retarding malignant growth become fairly exotic and are usually accompanied by unpleasant side effects. Often when oral DES stops working, castration can be used to supplement it. If its effect diminishes, the adrenal glands can be removed to eliminate still another source of male hormone from the body. An even more radical form of this surgical whittling is the blocking of androgen action through the removal of the patient's pituitary gland, the master control for all hormone production in the human machine. But this surgery is tedious and difficult, and removal of the pituitary can mean the disruption of crucial hormonal balances.

Because the loss of the pituitary is such an extreme step, scientists have sought *chemical* means of blocking the action of male hormones before they can spur the cancerous growth. Many doctors use "medical adrenalectomy," giving cortisone drugs which suppress androgen. Clinics across the U.S. are treating advanced prostatic cancer with the use of several other drugs which tend to disrupt the metabolism of malignant cells while leaving normal cells alone. Many drugs have been tried, some for longer periods than others, but the results are improving. The trouble with these forms of chemotherapy is that their pluses and minuses cannot be predicted. How much time they will add to a patient's life and how many good things they will take from it cannot be foretold until the treatment is complete and both the good and bad news are in.

Zinc: A Possible Role in Prevention of Prostate Troubles

One of the terrible failings of prostate research is this concentration on stalling tactics for use with advanced forms of cancer. Much more work needs to be done on the causes of the various forms of prostatic disease and their prevention. One of the reasons that more isn't being done is that the answer seems both very close and very far away. For at least 50 years we've known that there are high levels of zinc in healthy prostatic tissue and the various fluids associated with the gland, semen and prostatic fluid. A number of researchers, notably Chicago's Dr. Bush, have discovered that zinc levels drop when prostatitis and cancer strike the prostate. Dr. Bush found that patients with chronic prostatitis generally have low prostatic and semen zinc levels, though their serum (or whole body) levels are normal. He also noted that while victims of BPH display normal to high zinc concentrations in semen, people with cancer of the prostate suffer from lowered zinc in both semen and tissue tests. In fact, when cancer spreads significantly beyond the gland, serum zinc levels drop as well. Surprised and heartened by these findings, Dr. Bush started oral zinc therapy for 755 patients with various prostatic complaints.

In 1974 at a national convention of the American Medical Association, he first reported his results. Two hundred patients with infectious prostatitis were given between 50 and 150 milligrams of oral zinc sulfate (that's between 11 and 34 milligrams of zinc) per day for periods of time ranging up to 16 weeks. During the test 70 percent of the people got relief from their symptoms, and nearly all of them registered higher semen levels of zinc, which sounds good. Although similar, the results with BPH, however, weren't so terrific, maybe because men with this disease usually record normal zinc levels. Still, the findings weren't terribly discouraging either. Nineteen BPH patients were given about 35 milligrams of zinc a day (as zinc sulfate) for 2 months and then placed on a long-term maintenance program of about 10 to 20 milligrams daily. Lab tests done with these people showed no change in serum zinc levels during supplementation, but they did reveal some gains in semen levels of the mineral. More important, all 19 patients reported an easing of their symptoms, and x-rays and endoscopy (a look-see with a rectal telescope) showed decrease in prostate size in all but 5 of them. That sounds great. But despite what look like positive findings to us, Dr. Bush is careful about saying what can be concluded from his work—perhaps because zinc therapy is not ready to replace conventional means of treatment for established cases of most prostate disorders. Dr. Bush told us, "We have continued to use zinc in treatment of BPH and prostatitis with similar success. [That is, in the range of 70 percent.] And though we don't know why zinc therapy works, it is my general impression that more and more patients are getting beneficial effects from zinc therapy."

So what to do? The answer to at least some prostate trouble seems to be supplementary zinc. Unfortunately, at this stage of the game, we don't know enough about how the mineral's metabolized to ask the right questions *once a disease gets a start*. However, Dr. Bush's work suggests to us that zinc supplements might play a role in the prevention of prostate woes. According to most experts 30 milligrams a day is a good place to start. And, according to Gary W. Evans, Ph.D., a biochemist for the USDA, there is something you can do to make sure this zinc gets right to work. In experiments with animals, Dr. Evans found that much more—1½ times more—of a zinc supplement was absorbed into the body when his subjects also got large doses of vitamin B_6 (or pyridoxine). He told us that he wasn't sure why this occurred, but that he was convinced a zinc supplement would be more effective if taken along with B_6. Dr. Evans also didn't know how much B_6 was enough (who does?), but we think that if 10 milligrams is the normal maintenance dosage for the vitamin, 50 milligrams should be the right amount to bump the zinc into your system.

There may be a more certain note to be struck on prostate cancer. As we've noted, many forms of prostate disease are thought to stem from an imbalance of male and female hormones, androgens and estrogens in the system. Peter Hill, Ph.D., of the American Health Foundation, knew that black South African men have a much lower rate of prostatic cancer than North American men, and he wondered why. He didn't think the South Africans could have hormone profiles different from most Americans. But when he examined urine samples taken from both groups, he found great differences. The rural, largely vegetarian blacks excreted far less of both hormones than the Americans, urban *and* rural, and Dr. Hill guessed it was because the Africans' diet contained about half the total fat of the Westerners' diet. To test his hypothesis, he had selected groups switch diets for 3 weeks. The Americans ate low-fat vegetarian fare, and the Africans tried lots of meat and other rich, fatty stuff. Even in this short time, Dr. Hill found, a change in diet meant a reverse in hormone level, too. Hormone content went up in the Africans' urine and down in the Americans', down to a point where it resembled the original low-risk figure of the native population.

What does that mean? Probably that a switch to a low-fat, high-vegetable-protein diet can—over the course of an adult life time—considerably lower your chances of prostate cancer. There's certainly no harm in trying, for as Dr. Bush points out, similar population studies have shown that the incidence of prostate cancer goes up when a fatty Western diet is adopted by Japanese and Chinese men moving to the U.S.

19
Coronary Bypass

The number of coronary bypass operations increases by thousands each year. In some cities, it's the most frequently performed operation—and the most expensive, at an average cost of $10,000 to $15,000. If such an operation saved lives, no one would blink at the cost and everyone would praise medical science.

But medical science itself says the coronary bypass may not save—or even prolong—lives. Ninety-eight times out of 100, it's done only to relieve a symptom, angina pectoris, a very common chest pain caused by a very common disease, hardening of the arteries.

Although the causes of arteriosclerosis are not fully known, several risk factors are known to play a big part in developing the disease and then speeding it up: high blood pressure, high cholesterol and triglycerides in the blood, cigarette smoking, diabetes, stress and lack of regular exercise. Age, sex (men have a higher incidence) and family history of heart disease are other, uncontrollable factors.

Nearly all of the measures known to ward off angina involve controlling risk factors with changes in life-style or diet, which also prevent arteriosclerosis from getting worse. Drugs are often used when those changes alone are not enough. Surgery to relieve pain is used as a last resort, but unlike such conservative measures as getting more exercise or giving up cigarettes, *it does nothing to retard the underlying disease in any way.*

Many of us will face at least the option of coronary bypass surgery this year. Over 100,000 Americans undergo the procedure each year. Some clearly require the operation; some clearly don't. For the majority of people in between, there is great doubt as to whether or not it is really necessary.

There is no simple answer to the problem of angina—drugs, diet, exercise or otherwise. The purpose of this chapter is to help you determine, based on your doctor's evaluation and your symptoms, whether or not you clearly need a bypass, and how to relieve your angina if you don't.

Granted, angina can't be taken lightly, even if it is only a symptom. The slightest effort or emotional upset can bring on a gripping—and scary—chest pain. The discomfort goes away after a few minutes, sometimes with the help of a drug called nitroglycerin slipped under the tongue, but often it disappears by itself. (We'll discuss nitroglycerin later.)

Angina is not a heart attack, but merely a pain which signals a temporary shortage of oxygen to the heart. Here's a description of what happens:

Blood is continuously flowing through the veins and arteries of your body, picking up vital, nourishing oxygen from the lungs, delivering it to cells, tissues and organs (including the heart) and returning to the lungs for fresh oxygen.

Two of those transporting arteries branch off as soon as they enter the top of the heart at the main trunk, the aorta. Those special coronary arteries cling to the surface of the heart like vines covering a garden wall. The right coronary artery feeds the back of the heart. The left coronary artery branches into 2 main subdivisions, one to the front of the heart, the other to the side. All 3 main arteries branch still further into smaller vessels to deliver oxygen to all parts of the heart.

The rate at which oxygen-rich blood is pumped by the heart muscle is governed by the amount of work you are doing at any one time. If you work harder, you heart beats faster and stronger to pump extra oxygen into the system. You can feel that happen when you suddenly dash up a flight of stairs.

The coronary arteries aren't rigid. Rather, they stretch and widen in response to the heart's call for more blood and oxygen. Usually, arteries are about the thickness of a wooden kitchen match, open and smooth walled, to allow free flow of blood.

Some people's arteries are affected by a slow and subtle disease, arteriosclerosis, or hardening of the arteries. The many layers of paper-thin tissue which line artery walls thicken and gradually narrow the arteries over the years. By far, the most common form of the disease is atherosclerosis, which deposits globs of waxlike cholesterol, fatty plaque and calcium on the artery walls, in much the same way as rust builds up in an old pipe.

One or all main coronary arteries may be partially dammed up. As deposits grow thicker, less and less blood can get through the arteries. Gradually, blood flow to parts of the heart can slow down to a trickle.

That trickle, along with blood from remaining healthy arteries, may provide enough oxygen for most passive daily activities. But run up that same flight of stairs, and the heart literally gasps for air: the arteries are either too clogged or simply cannot widen enough to deliver the extra blood and oxygen, no matter how frantically the heart tries to pump.

A narrowing greater than 75 percent results in the tightness and pain of angina when the heart is stressed. (A narrowing greater than 90 percent may cause anginal discomfort even when you are at rest.) The pain subsides when your heart slows to its normal rate, and extra oxygen is no longer needed.

Angina discomfort ranges from a mild sensation of pressure to severe gripping pain concentrated on the left side of your chest. Very commonly, it starts as a feeling of fullness or tightness. Pain may seem to radiate to the neck, jaw, back or both shoulders or arms, because of the network of nerves connecting those areas. But it is really the portion of the heart temporarily deprived of oxygen which causes pain.

An angina attack may be triggered not only by physical effort, but anything that demands extra work of the heart. A drastic change in temperature, such as stepping from high heat and humidity outside into a chilly air-conditioned supermarket or building (or vice versa) can do it. Emotional upsets such as fear, anger, worry or grief can bring on an episode in a matter of seconds or minutes. Overeating also involuntarily forces the heart to put out extra effort. Sex combines physical effort with emotional excitement and can precipitate angina. It is not uncommon for angina to occur while you're fast asleep, because blood and body fluids normally pulled to the lower body by gravity collect in the torso while you are lying down, putting extra pressure on the heart.

Angina is labeled either stable or unstable. The medical books say that stable angina is "a predictable pattern of symptoms in relation to your activities over a period of time." That means that you are usually comfortable and can function in your normal daily activities—working, gardening and so on—with or without drugs. In unstable angina, the pain becomes more severe and frequent, to the point where you often have angina while at rest. If that change occurs gradually, over a period of several weeks or months, it's called *chronic* unstable angina. A sudden change over a period of days or hours is *acute* unstable angina.

- If you get angina more often each day, in a different place in your chest, or it becomes stronger or occurs at rest, see your doctor.
- If you suddenly experience any kind of chest pain for the first time, don't self-diagnose. See your doctor.

Angina may or may not be a precursor of a heart attack. One person may develop angina that lasts for years without ever having a heart attack. Another may have a full-fledged heart attack without ever experiencing any warning signs until the severe pain of dying heart muscle tissue sends him to the emergency room.

A heart attack (myocardial infarction) occurs when a portion of the heart dies of oxygen starvation. Supply simply falls behind demand—or demand outstrips supply—for a variety of reasons. A narrowed artery may finally become totally blocked, prolonging the shutdown of oxygen. Sometimes the rough surface of the diseased wall provides a niche where a blood clot can form. If that clot (thrombus) gets big enough, it may close off the artery (coronary thrombosis or occlusion).

The heart can survive even if some small portions of its tissue die. If the cut in oxygen supply is due to a blockage in an artery, the location of the blockage determines how much and what part of the heart is threatened. The left ventricle, the chamber of the heart which acts as the pump, however, cannot sustain much damage if it is going to continue to do its job.

A heart attack often comes on without exertion. The pain is much more severe than angina and does not let up after a few minutes. Heartbeat may be irregular and breathing labored. The victim may feel he is suffocating. Often, he feels a grave sense of doom. Weakness, sudden sweating, nausea or vomiting or both, and an urge to move the bowels comes on. Sometimes the victim passes out. Rest or nitroglycerin does not relieve symptoms.

If you have any doubt whether you are having an angina or a heart attack, stop whatever you're doing. Tell someone nearby what is happening. Call or ask them to call for emergency care at once. (911 is the emergency phone number in many communities.) Or if you can, go straight to the emergency room of the nearest hospital for immediate medical attention.

How Your Doctor Diagnoses Chest Pain

Chances are you will not be surprised by a heart attack without having some chest pain long before. Chest pain can mean nothing—or it can signal one of at least a dozen conditions, from simple muscle tenderness to hiatal hernia, among others. Don't try to diagnose it yourself. Visit your doctor to find out what's going on, advises W. Gerald Austen, past president of the American Heart Association. You'll probably want to, regardless of who says so.

Your doctor will carefully update your medical history, including such information as your age and current occupation, and ask you to describe your symptoms. You may be experiencing any or all of a number of different types of chest discomfort, from heavy, dull tightness to sharp pain. Try to describe any differences as accurately as possible. If you're not sure about any of your symptoms, don't be afraid to say so. The doctor will ask you if you smoke, how much, and if you are under stress. He or she will also want to know your family history of heart disease and diabetes.

Your doctor will probably use percussion (that's another word for tapping) to determine the approximate position, size and shape of your heart. He'll do that by moving one of his hands over your chest surface and then rapping it with the fingers of the other, listening for differences in sound much as a carpenter hammers along a wall to locate the supporting studs.

Everyone is familiar with the basic medical routine of listening to the heart's sounds with a stethoscope, which amplifies them. Variations in the normal lubb-dup, lubb-dup, lubb-dup can indicate certain irregularities.

Your blood pressure will be taken to determine how forcefully blood is being thrust through your arteries.

Blood tests can identify certain enzymes which are released into the blood when the heart muscle is injured. The presence or absence of those enzymes in your blood also helps the doctor to determine just how risky surgery might be for you.

More general tests for blood cholesterol and triglyceride (fat) levels, blood sugar and minerals, as well as for thyroid and lung function, may also be done. Angina may be worsened by other problems, such as thyroid disease or uncontrolled diabetes. Without concurrent treatment of those conditions, angina will be far more difficult to manage.

The electrocardiogram (EKG or ECG), routine in the diagnosis of heart disease, is a record of the electrical impulses sent out by your heart while you are resting, exercising or both.

Whenever any muscle contracts, it sends out an electrical charge. The current sent out by the contracting heart muscle spreads throughout your body, just like a charge passed along a power line. The electrocardiograph machine is able to sort out the heart's impulses from other muscle impulses. Those heart impulses are picked up by electrodes (little pieces of metal which the doctor has attached to certain spots on your skin) and recorded on a continuous roll of paper.

The electrocardiogram is not only a picture of what your heart is doing at the time of the test, but certain patterns can indicate if something has taken place earlier. For days or even weeks following a heart attack, the electrocardiogram will show abnormalities. (Eventually, it returns to normal in most people.)

Since a coronary artery that is severely narrowed may still be able to supply the heart with enough oxygen while you are at rest but not while you are exercising, an EKG taken at rest cannot tell if your heart can get enough oxygen under more demanding circumstances. For that, a treadmill stress test may be done. The stress test EKG shows the level at which your heart can work without distress.

The nurse or doctor will attach electrodes to your arms and legs. You will be told first to walk, then run on a 4-foot-long conveyor belt, while holding onto a bar for balance. You will be told to alert the tester at the first sign of chest pain or discomfort.

The treadmill may be gradually tilted to simulate a hill, increasing the workload on the heart. The belt may be speeded up to 4 mph or faster. The entire test takes from 20 to 40 minutes.

The test will be stopped either when you begin to get chest pain or when there is a change in the EKG reading. Maximum heart rate is 220 beats per minute minus your age. If you can reach that without chest pain or an EKG change, the doctor will assume your heart is getting enough oxygen under maximum stress; that is, there is plenty of blood flowing through your arteries and probably no significant narrowing. Some physicians shoot for a submaximal level of 80 or 90 percent of the maximum.

Other types of stress tests that may be used are a stationary bicycle, called an ergometer, or a special set of steps, the Master's two-step. Certain other heart tests are more complicated and take more time. A vectorcardiogram may be used to pick up abnormalities at the back of the heart, inaccessible to the regular EKG. Other tests are used to detect faulty valves or enlarged areas.

Your doctor may be able to make a diagnosis based just on those tests we've described here and your complete medical history. If he thinks he needs more information or is considering the possibility of surgery, he will do coronary arteriography to determine not only where the artery blockages are, but how big they are and what effect they are having. An arteriogram will also show whether or not new, substitute arteries, called collaterals, have branched out to take over the job of the diseased ones, and how much damage, if any, has been done to the heart.

Should you undergo an arteriogram, it will be one of the most fascinating—and perhaps awesome—medical tests you'll ever undergo, even though it's quite routine and relatively safe, according to doctors—and painless, according to patients.

Arteriography is combined with cardiac catheterization, a method of passing a narrow, hollow flexible tube into the heart, and is often simply referred to as "catheterization." In addition to making it possible to examine the coronary arteries, catheterization can be used to measure blood pressure and oxygen in each of the heart's 4 chambers, to withdraw blood samples for tests, to identify any abnormal openings or to measure the heart's overall pumping capacity.

You will be hospitalized for the procedure. Preliminary blood tests and chest x-rays will be done. Some people are allergic to the dye used in the arteriogram, so you may be given a small test dose ahead of time to avoid a reaction, such as a skin rash or an asthma attack. If you have any allergies to drugs or food, be sure to tell the nurse or doctor.

You will be given a tranquilizer the morning of the test to help you relax, but general anesthesia will not be used and you will be awake during the test. You will be wheeled to a special lab equipped specificially for this test and staffed with nurses and technicians well trained in arteriography.

Your cardiologist will explain what he's going to do and tell you when he wants you to take deep breaths, cough and so on, during the procedure.

You will be strapped to a cradlelike table, which will be tilted to take x-rays from many different angles.

The femoral artery running through your thigh is the most common site for inserting the catheter. If you are overweight or have hardening of the arteries of the leg, a main artery in one arm may be used. Either entry site provides a direct route to the heart.

An injection of local anesthesia will numb the site where the needle is to be inserted. Through that needle, a small guide wire is put in place and a long tube is passed into the artery, up into the chest and into the aorta, the main trunk artery at the top of the heart. The catheter is coaxed with relative ease into the heart to record the blood pressure there.

A cylindrical apparatus called a fluoroscope lowers an x-ray camera from the ceiling, which is positioned over your chest. An image of the catheter's progress is projected onto a nearby closed-circuit TV screen so the doctor can watch what's going on. An EKG monitor displays your blood pressure and heartbeat at all times.

After catheterization, a thick opaque dye is injected through the catheter and into the coronary arteries—the first step of the intriguing part of the procedure called coronary arteriography. (Other terms are often used: venography refers to x-rays of veins alone; angiography applies to either veins or arteries.)

The catheter is maneuvered first into the opening of the left coronary artery, then into the right. In each position, the doctor will inject a small amount of dye into the tube—and your arteries—with a syringe. Each time he will ask you to take a deep breath and then to lie very still. Several x-ray pictures will be taken while the dye is flowing through each artery. The special nontoxic dye silhouettes any blockages and pinpoints their location on the x-ray films.

A larger injection is then made into the left ventricle, the heart's pumping chamber, to see how it is working and to determine if there's any scar tissue, if you had a heart attack some time before. After each injection, you'll be asked to cough forcefully, to help flush the dye out of the arteries.

The result of the test is a motion picture cassette film of your heart and arteries in action.

The dye has a tendency to widen or dilate the arteries, so be prepared for a warm sensation after each small injection. With the larger injection, a true hot flash is sometimes felt, perhaps lasting up to a minute. Doctors report that occasionally a person may have a headache or feel queasy for about 30 seconds, but the procedure is basically only slightly uncomfortable.

When all the injections have been made, the catheter is withdrawn and pressure is applied to the leg or arm near where the artery was entered. Some antibiotic cream and a Band-Aid will be placed over the puncture site on your leg. If your arm was used, the incision will be sewn up.

How long the test takes depends on how easily the doctor can manipulate the catheter through your arteries. A simple catheterization should take 45 minutes or so; a more complicated one, up to as long as 4 hours.

You'll be back in your room in about 30 minutes afterward, able to eat or drink and visit with family. You'll probably be advised to stay in bed for at least 6 hours, to prevent bleeding from the catheterization site on your leg.

The films take some time to develop, and will be reviewed by more than one doctor before you're told what they show.

Some patients are understandably afraid of catheterization and arteriography. Having your heart poked with tubes and pumped with dye is worrisome. Doctors reassuringly say that even though the test does put stress on the heart, death from heart attack and severe complications afterward are rare. Even if a problem should arise, all the vital equipment and personnel are right there for instant rescue. Those small risks, we are told, are balanced against the cardiologist's need to know exactly what he is treating. No other test can give the information that arteriography gives.

We spoke to some patients who'd had at least one catheterization. They said it was no big worry to them. One man told us:

> It's neither painful nor dangerous, at least from my point of view. You can feel them move the catheter back and forth, into each chamber of the heart, but there's no sensation of actual pain. If you're in the right position on the table, you can even watch the catheter's progress on the screen.
>
> I never feared catheterization and I don't think anyone should. I think it's one of the best and most extraordinary diagnostic tools they use.

Another man said:

> Angina pains are a lot worse than any catheterization going. The first catheterization I had took 2½ hours, the second 45 minutes. I was a little bored, but there was no more pain after 2½ hours than after 45 minutes.
>
> I went down at 10:15 A.M. and was back in my room by 11 o'clock. By 3:00 in the afternoon the doctors were in my room telling me what they thought should be done.

Not everyone with coronary disease needs a catheterization/arteriogram. Many doctors feel it is valuable in helping to decide what treatment to prescribe, even if you don't need surgery. But doctors are divided as to its effectiveness and actual safety. Some recommend it to all their angina patients (unless another serious condition prevents it) and feel it identifies those patients who are headed for a heart attack. Others use it much more selectively. Whether or not you have an arteriogram will depend on your doctor.

Should you have an arteriogram, that does not automatically mean you will need surgery. The test may show that nature has provided its own relief system: when one coronary artery begins to clog up, new collateral blood vessels may form to connect the choked-off portion of heart muscle to a remaining healthy artery. Because they provide a detour around a blocked artery, collaterals may lessen or even eliminate angina altogether.

Unfortunately, not everyone with arteriosclerosis forms collaterals. Doctors don't know why some people do and some don't. Some believe their growth may be encouraged by exercise and hampered by smoking.

Collaterals or not, treatment of angina deals with the basic problem of oxygen supply and demand within the heart's less-than-perfect pipeline system. Your doctor may first try to help you with nonsurgical treatment. That consists of 2 major approaches: changes in one or more living habits, and administration of drugs. Let's look first at what can often be done *without* drugs.

Thirteen Natural Remedies for Angina

Before you start to rely on drugs, be sure you have tried the following:

Lose weight. Carrying around extra fat forces your heart to work harder, constantly aggravating normal oxygen demands.

Eat smaller meals. Meal-induced angina is a common phenomenon. It is not fair to ask your heart to help digest a heavy, greasy meal at the end of a weary day when your heart is semistarved (for oxygen) itself. A habit of eating smaller, lighter, frequent meals, with a small snack at bedtime, more evenly distributes the day's digestive chores.

Cut down on fat. There's plenty of well-publicized evidence that dietary fat contributes to arteriosclerosis. A neglected study done 25 years ago strongly suggested that the fat content of a meal may be the direct cause of the angina attack that so often follows. In 6 tests, a group of 14 patients at the Hospital of the University of Pennsylvania in Philadelphia were fed fatty meals at some times, ordinary meals at others. Fourteen separate attacks of angina were precipitated, all between 3 and 5 hours after fatty meals only. The level of fat in the blood rose in each patient after each fatty meal. Four of those patients who suffered fat-induced angina also showed irregular EKG changes. Researchers Peter T. Kuo, M.D., and Claude R. Joyner, Jr., M.D., remark, "This observation would, therefore, provide another rationale for the use of a low-fat diet in patients with angina of effort" (*Journal of the American Medical Association*, July 23, 1955).

Try a meatless diet. Meat and dairy products are a major source of dietary fat. An English pathologist who did several studies of diet in heart disease patients feels that a diet free of meat and dairy products "could well exert beneficial effects on subjects suffering from angina pectoris. . . . There is a considerable body of evidence to suggest that a diet devoid of animal products may have certain advantages in the prevention and possible treatment of . . . heart disease and angina pectoris" says F. R. Ellis, M.D., at Kingston Hospital in Surrey, England.

The vegan diet of which Dr. Ellis speaks is adequate if it includes a good mix of cereal grains, beans, nuts, fruits and vegetables, and is supplemented with vitamin B_{12}.

The success of the vegan diet in 4 patients exemplifies Dr. Ellis's conviction. One angina patient in particular who tried the vegan diet showed dramatic improvement: a 65-year-old man whose severe angina prevented him from walking more than 9 or 10 steps without feeling pain was mountain climbing after 6 months of not eating meat or dairy products, reports Dr. Ellis (*American Heart Journal*, June, 1977).

Bulk up on fiber. Fiber can help "scrub" waxy cholesterol and fatty deposits out of arteries and reduce angina. One medical scientist has reported that a number of patients taking wheat bran daily enjoyed a reduction in the number of angina attacks. Renzo Romanelli, M.D., professor of gerontology and geriatrics at the University of Pisa, Italy, reported to a conference of the International College of Surgeons in the U.S. that he saw actual improvement in the clinical signs of heart disease in patients taking supplemental fiber. In 5 patients over 70 years old, Dr. Romanelli said tests showed improvement in heart efficiency, and EKG signs of oxygen lack in the heart muscle were diminished.

Lower your blood pressure. Blood being pushed through your heart at unnecessarily high force, day in and day out, adds to the problem of reduced flow through already clogged arteries. Losing weight often brings blood pressure down in itself; cutting out salt and salty foods and getting more exercise also does it.

Go easy on the alcohol. A couple of drinks can furtively reduce the amount of exertion you can stand, in spite of the initial effect alcohol has of numbing angina pain. And that goes for such customary efforts like walking to your car after a business lunch or trying to make love after an evening of wining and dining with your mate.

Two to 5 ounces of 100-proof vodka significantly reduced the amount of exercise tolerated before an angina attack came on in a study of 12 men with classic stable angina, according to researchers Joan Orlando, M.D., Wilbert S. Aronow, M.D., and others at the Long Beach Veterans Hospital and University of California at Irvine. Each of the 2 amounts of vodka tested (about the amounts of alcohol a social drinker might consume at a party or watching an afternoon ball game) increased the heart's demand for oxygen by speeding up the heart rate and raising blood pressure. Drinking rounds were compared to control periods during which the same men drank unspiked Fresca only. The researchers note that the effect of drinking alcohol is similar to what happens after an angina patient eats a big meal. "On the basis of these data . . . we believe that . . . [alcohol] aggravates exercise-induced angina pectoris" (*Annals of Internal Medicine,* June, 1976). A few cocktails *and* a big meal is an open invitation to angina!

Take an easy approach to sex. Speaking of romantic evenings, the prospect of pain can make even the most amorous sweethearts shy away from sexual activity. Some simple precautions can help keep your love life lively.

Avoid sex for a least 2 hours after eating a meal or drinking alcohol. Always wait until you feel rested and relaxed. Avoid unfamiliar surroundings. Don't wander from your customary partner. Keep the room temperature comfortable. (As one doctor put it, "Do not make love out-of-doors in a blizzard after a 7-course steak dinner at the end of a hard work day.")

Exercise. With angina pain lurking around every corner, it's easy to see why many angina sufferers shun any kind of exercise. While sudden bursts of effort in an untrained body are almost certain to bring on an attack, a steadily graduated exercise program can actually improve your tolerance of such efforts as a brisk walk to the corner store. You can even look forward to enjoying sex with less fear of angina pain.

"People medically capable of exercise who can overcome their fears and actually exercise *more* stand a better chance of relieving their angina," says cardiologist Richard Stein, M.D.

"In our studies with over 60 patients either on home bicycles or in a community exercise program, we've found reduced frequency and intensity of angina pain in the majority of patients experiencing the training response," said Dr. Stein. What Dr. Stein calls "the training response" refers to the ability to exercise or perform a task at a reduced heart rate, thereby lowering the heart's oxygen requirement. Such a response is achieved by gradually intensifying exertion, causing the heart muscle to beat at 75 percent of its maximum rate for brief periods of 4- to 5-minutes each.

Dr. Stein, director of the exercise laboratory and the coronary heart disease treatment and prevention program and assistant professor at New York's Downstate Medical Center in Brooklyn, explained the process to us:

"The physiological basis for these effects is well known and observable even in healthy individuals. For example, if you were able to run up a flight of stairs today and then take your pulse, it might be 150 beats per minute. But keep doing this for several days or weeks and take your pulse again. You'll find that it is considerably lower.

"The same principle works with angina patients who may start with fairly light exercise and progress slowly to more demanding tasks. Doing such exercises over and over keeps lowering the pulse so that the heart doesn't have to work as hard or require as much oxygen."

Of course, Dr. Stein's patients don't start by running up flights of stairs. After careful stress testing, each is given a personal exercise program tailored to his or her own capabilities and limitations. "You must constantly upgrade the exercise program, based on the participant's improvement in fitness, or you will fail to progress," Dr. Stein points out.

Other researchers are reporting equally encouraging results. Writing in *Mayo Clinic Proceedings,* April, 1976, Charles C. Kennedy, M.D., and 5 colleagues describe a one-year graduated exercise program involving 8 men—ranging in age from 45 to 50—all of whom had mild angina. Four of them had previously had heart attacks.

The men met at a local YMCA 3 times a week for 45-minute exercise sessions tailored to their individual needs. They walked, jogged, did some stretching exercises and then finished off with swimming or a game of volleyball. When the 12 months were up, all 8 showed remarkable gains. Two had considerably less angina, and 6 were completely symptom-free.

"The psychological improvement experienced by each patient was perhaps the most striking aspect of the exercise program; they became much more positive in their attitude toward work, family and hobbies," added the authors.

Other doctors agree. "Exercise should not be overlooked as a prime mode of angina therapy," says Thomas A. Preston, M.D., at the University of Washington School of Medicine, and Thomas E. Richtsmeier, M.D., formerly at that school and now director of coronary care at Idaho Falls Hospital. Drs. Preston and Richtsmeier offer the following advice: "Unsupervised exercise should be at a low level and should not be strenuous or unduly fatiguing. Daily or at least every other day . . . exercise for 20 or 30 minutes is effective. The best activities are walking, swimming and bicycling. Overexertion should be avoided, but a gradual increase in activity is desirable. If more vigorous exercise is planned, such as jogging or long-distance swimming, a preliminary . . . treadmill stress test and formal [medical] supervision of the activity are advisable" (*Postgraduate Medicine,* November, 1977).

Quit smoking. That means cigarettes, pipes and cigars. Many studies link smoking with hardening of the arteries. And there's a good chance smoking stunts the growth of helpful collateral arteries.

As far as angina goes, the accumulation of carbon monoxide and other compounds sucked into your lungs from cigarettes displaces some of the available oxygen. If the small amount of blood that makes it through already narrowed arteries has less oxygen than usual due to inhaled carbon monoxide, you're all set for an angina attack. The least amount of physical or emotional stress can set off pain.

"Anginal patients who stop smoking experience fewer anginal episodes and can exercise more before developing an anginal attack," says Dr. Aronow, chief of cardiovascular research at the University of California, Irvine (*Journal of the American Medical Association,* September 23, 1974).

Avoid smoke-filled rooms. Even if you don't smoke, wallowing in the smoke of those who do can have the same effect as having a cigarette yourself. Ten nonsmoking angina patients lost 38 percent of their normal tolerance to exercise after sharing a room with 3 smokers who each smoked 5 cigarettes in 2 hours. The test simulated smoky situations such as cocktail parties, committee meetings or commuter car rides. Heart rates and blood pressures of the angina patients rose in both ventilated and nonventilated rooms. An editorial in a widely read medical journal echoed the study's obvious conclusions: "Passive smoking aggravates angina" (*Lancet,* August 19, 1978).

Be kind to your body thermostat. Be wary of extreme changes of temperature. Leaving your warm and cozy living room to run out and check the mail during a February freeze inflates your heart's energy needs. Similarly, exertion in the cold makes your heart do double duty. One doctor writes of a plant foreman who could walk all day overseeing his work at the factory with no angina trouble, but often suffered pain during the short but wintry walk from the bus stop to his front door on his way home after work.

Use common sense. Don't dash outside in your shirt sleeves if you need a jacket. After stepping into the cold, pause briefly to allow your body to adjust to the temperature change before you start to walk. Take it slow, or stop to rest for a minute or so along the way to your destination.

Don't let anxiety get the best of you. Anger, fear and excitement stimulate your glands to produce more adrenalin, a hormone which speeds up the heartbeat and raises blood pressure, increasing your need for oxygen. Since you absolutely cannot avoid some unforeseen upsets, taking all the above steps can put you at your best for weathering those that do come up. In addition, plan several small relaxation breaks a day, to prevent a crescendo of stress from building up to an angina attack. Be sure to get enough rest. Some people get emotionally upset only when they're tired.

You'll find that many of these important anti-angina steps overlap: cutting down on fat and alcohol, eating smaller meals, and exercising all help you to lose weight. Losing weight, in turn, often automatically reduces blood pressure and blood fats, especially triglycerides.

Drugs: Another Approach

If controlling the supply-and-demand of oxygen by all those means does not relieve your angina, or if it's quickly growing worse, your doctor will probably suggest adding 1 or 2 drugs to the management of your trouble. Anti-angina drugs—primarily nitroglycerin and propranolol—do not cure angina or prevent further hardening of the arteries, but simply enable the angina patient to withstand more exertion than he could without the drugs. *We wish to emphasize that drugs, when absolutely necessary, are used in addition to, not in place of, the previously discussed means of relieving angina.*

Nitroglycerin has been the mainstay of angina treatment for years. Either in real life or in the movies, you've probably seen an angina victim pop a tablet of nitro under his tongue for prompt relief at the first inkling of chest discomfort. Nitroglycerin may be taken 5 to 10 minutes ahead of time when you know that an event likely to trigger angina—such as a sexual encounter or an important business meeting—lies ahead of you, or anytime you feel an angina attack headed your way. Nitroglycerin has helped many patients continue normal daily activities. Some people can get along without it except on rare occasions. Others must take it in combination with larger doses of other drugs, which we'll discuss shortly.

Nitroglycerin may work in either of 2 possible ways. One theory says that although nitroglycerin cannot widen those arteries already narrowed by disease, it helps to redistribute blood through other, healthy main vessels and possibly collateral blood vessels. The other says that nitroglycerin lowers oxygen requirements by lowering blood pressure in the heart's pumping chamber and smaller, minor arteries.

Nitroglycerin taken sublingually (under the tongue) takes effect after only a minute or two and its effect lasts 15 to 30 minutes or so. Attacks often run their course with rest alone, before the drug has a chance to take effect, so there is some question about what may *really* relieve the angina in some patients—a halt in the aggravating effort, or the drug. For many patients, nitroglycerin combined with good sense is the most effective way to forestall or relieve predictable, stable angina.

Exactly when you take your nitroglycerin depends on when you seem vulnerable to attacks: walking from your car to your office, after the evening meal, during sex and so forth. The standard advice is to place one tablet under your tongue a few minutes before you plan on activity that you know from past experience will precipitate angina. Some doctors tell their patients that a second or third tablet may be taken during a bout of angina, but that they should get medical attention as soon as possible for any discomfort that lasts more than 20 minutes.

Indiscriminate use of nitroglycerin throughout the day is not a good idea. Some researchers say that your blood vessels may develop a tolerance to the drug, lessening its effectiveness. Regardless of those claims, why take more than you need?

A nitroglycerin cream applied topically to the skin has been in and out of favor over the past few years as a possible way to relieve nighttime or round-the-clock episodes of angina. The drug is slowly absorbed through the skin, prolonging relief for up to 6 or 8 hours. Time-release oral nitroglycerin has also been tried.

You may get throbbing headaches when you first start taking nitroglycerin. In a way, that effect indicates the drug is working. The headaches may disappear with continued use. Other side effects may be a feeling of mild fullness, warmth, weakness or slight dizziness. Mention any of those effects to your doctor. He may want to reduce the dosage, although that also reduces the beneficial effect of the drug.

Be careful to store nitroglycerin tablets in an airtight amber glass bottle, for the drug deteriorates when exposed to heat, moisture, air or light over a period of time. To be safe, discard any unused pills after 6 months. Carry daily doses with you and store the rest in the refrigerator.

If you unexpectedly run out of tablets or are caught without your nitroglycerin, it is all right for you to use someone else's tablets. (That is true *only* for nitroglycerin and no other drug.) The rationale is that any nitroglycerin is better than none at all.

In contrast to the fleeting effects of nitroglycerin, related nitrate drugs, such as isosorbide dinitrate (ISD), may protect against angina pain for up to 2 hours. Under-the-tongue doses are usually prescribed to be taken 3 times a day, after meals and before exertion or excitement, and take effect in about 5 minutes. Patients with severe and frequent angina may be told to take ISD or a related drug as often as every 1 to 2 hours during stretches of physical activity.

The reputed advantage of the nitrate drugs over nitroglycerin is their prolonged effect—2 to 3 times longer than equal doses of nitroglycerin. Possible side effects are about the same as for nitroglycerin. Nitrate drugs are more stable than nitroglycerin and don't have to be stored as carefully, so they are more convenient—but more expensive.

Other long-acting variations of nitroglycerin may be considered. Taken orally before meals, they are weaker than under-the-tongue tablets because they're broken down in the liver before they reach the heart. They may also be inadequately absorbed. Those drugs are sometimes only effective if used at high doses and are not widely favored.

Propranolol (Inderol) is entirely different from nitroglycerin or other nitrates and is used to relieve angina either from the onset or when nothing else seems to work. Propranolol is a beta-blocking drug, which means that by blocking certain nerve impulses, the drug decreases heart rate and blood pressure, reducing the heart's oxygen needs. Most patients respond to 40 milligrams, 3 or 4 times a day, but dosage needs are highly individualized.

Propranolol takes about a half-hour to take effect and lasts for 4 or 5 hours, compared to 1½ to 2 hours for nitrates. Beta-blockers are especially effective in patients who need to lower their blood pressure.

The most common side effects of propranolol are weakness, shortness of breath or bronchial spasms, impotence and stomach upsets. Some patients may suffer minor visual problems or some depression. As with any drug, there is a trade-off: patients are often willing to put up with mild side effects in exchange for angina relief.

Fluid retention at high doses may be treated by adding diuretics or digitalis, 2 other drugs commonly used in the management of heart disease. All in all, dosage should strike a balance between the most relief and the least unpleasantness.

Any patient started on propranolol should be warned against stopping it suddenly on his own. A few cases have been reported of unstable angina, heart attack or sudden death upon abrupt discontinuation of propranolol. If time allows, the dosage should be tapered by about 50 percent a week over at least 2 weeks. If you run out of medication, decrease your activity until you can get your prescription refilled.

Some patients need to take either nitroglycerin or other nitrate plus propranolol—one for its immediate effects, the other for its long-lasting effects. Your doctor will prescribe a drug or combination in amounts for you, depending on how active you are. Angina is a highly variable condition. It often seems to grow better or worse of its own accord, for no clear-cut reason. The effects of any treatment—drugs or other therapy—must take that into consideration.

Both you and your doctor must have patience in working out the medical treatment that works best for you. Carefully combined propranolol and the nitrate IDS, as part of complete medical management, benefitted more than 90 percent of 133 patients who suffered severe, intractable angina in one study; the treatment made surgery unnecessary. "Failure to prescribe these drugs or to do so [prescribe them] ineffectually has frequently led physicians to abandon medical therapy and advise surgical intervention," admonishes Henry I. Russek, M.D., research professor in cardiovascular disease at New York Medical College, who conducted that study (*Medical World News,* May 26, 1975).

When Your Doctor Suggests Surgery

With angina, the key word is relief. If you've lost weight, cut down on fat, heavy meals and alcohol, quit smoking, and tried drugs, yet your angina just won't quit—or is getting much worse—your doctor may feel it's time to suggest a coronary bypass graft procedure. He'll base that recommendation on all of the facts in your medical history, your symptoms, your physical exam, treadmill test, lab reports and arteriogram. It is quite likely that more than one cardiologist (heart specialist) will review your condition.

There may be a delay of a few weeks between the time you agree to the operation and the time it's actually done. Bypass surgery must be done in a cardiac operating room, a costly package of specialized equipment. Heart surgery facilities, because of their high cost, aren't lined up like dental exam rooms, and must be reserved well ahead of time. A bypass also requires the coordinated services of many specially trained people, whose schedules must be coordinated.

The finely turned teamwork involved in every open heart procedure is remarkable. The surgeon in charge performs the actual heart surgery, while directing the assisting surgeon and working closely with the anesthesiologist, nurses and technicians. Almost every other department in the hospital—laboratory, x-ray, EKG, respiratory, blood bank and intensive care—plays a vital part.

During one phase of the operation, your heart will be stopped, and a "heart-lung machine" will take over for both those organs, pumping the proper amounts of blood and oxygen at the proper rate to the rest of your body. Without that machine, bypass surgery would be impossible.

A coronary bypass graft procedure is technically quite simple, as operations go. The saphenous veins from one of your legs (probably your left) is removed. That nonessential vein is then attached at surgically created openings—one at the aorta and one below the blocked or narrowed portion of a diseased coronary artery—to provide a new route for blood flow to the area of the heart that disease has deprived of oxygen. You can imagine the process as a detour which routes traffic around a highway construction site.

The underlying disease which narrows one artery quite often narrows one or two others, and multiple bypasses are frequently done at the same time. About 90 percent of angina patients who have the operation experience relief of pain, presumably because of their improved blood supply.

Bypass surgery is referred to as open heart surgery, even though the heart is not opened, just exposed. After general anesthesia put you under, the surgeon makes 2 incisions. To open your chest, one incision is made along the breastbone (sternum), beginning an inch or two below the neck and reaching at least 12 inches toward your stomach. Then the breastbone is separated to gain access to the heart.

The second incision is made on the inside of your leg where the assisting surgeon will remove the vein or veins that will be used to bypass arteries of your heart.

You will be in the operating room for anywhere from 3 to 6 hours. Your family will no doubt want to be close by. They may wait in the Intensive Care waiting room, probably not far from the cardiac OR. They'll be told as soon as the surgery is over and will be allowed to visit you in the Intensive Care recovery room shortly afterward.

Should those hours of restless waiting be prolonged for no apparent reason, there's usually no real cause for alarm. Delays occur. The OR team may have gotten a late start, or the surgeon may be sticking close by you in Recovery for a while, checking on your vital signs—heart rate, breathing, blood pressure—before he reports to your family.

You'll wake up in the Intensive Care recovery room, wired to various sophisticated, but very routine pieces of equipment that monitor your condition. Nurses skilled in caring for postop cardiac patients will carefully watch over you. Both your surgeon and cardiologist, too, will continue to direct your care throughout your stay.

Don't let "intensive care" scare you. Every heart surgery patient is taken there for 2 or 3 days before going back to a regular hospital room.

You'll feel almost paralyzed for several hours until the anesthesia wears off. An endotracheal tube, passed down your windpipe, is uncomfortable, but absolutely necessary for the respirator to continue to help you breathe regularly for a few hours until you regain enough strength to breathe on your own again, and to prevent pneumonia. You cannot speak with the tube in place. All bypass patients go through this. Don't mistakenly conclude you are in some kind of danger because of the heart monitors and respirator.

Nutrients and drugs are fed via an IV tube in your arm. Tubes drain fluid from the chest cavity, to reduce pressure on the heart, and will be removed after 2 days or so.

The stitches from your incisions will be removed during recuperation leaving a scar that looks like a long zipper. The thin sterile wires holding your breastbone back together will remain, unless they cause irritation. The pain of the chest incision is much less than you might imagine, thanks to pain-killers. (Antibiotics will be given to protect you against infection in the wound.) Pain fades into tenderness over the next several weeks. Both chest and leg scars will be red for 3 to 6 months, then blanch to thin white lines within a year or two.

Possible postop complications, although relatively few, do sometimes occur and are usually directly related to your overall health when you go into the operation.

Sometimes the heart can't pump well enough after the bypass grafts are attached. When that happens, it's usually because the heart did not pump well before the surgery, and death may follow. The mortality rate is less than 2 percent. Such patients, we're told, have a short life expectancy even without surgery. Patients with hearts that pump well rarely die from surgery.

Patients with badly diseased arteries may possibly have a heart attack during the operation or the immediate postop period, but all the right people and lifesaving equipment are there to control the problem, and death from postop heart attack is very preventable.

The heart rate may speed up, slow down or become irregular. Those problems are controlled with either medication, a brief, mild electrical shock or a temporary pacemaker hooked up to the heart by a thin wire.

A blood clot in the lung (pulmonary embolism) is possible after any surgery. A small number of patients, perhaps less than 1 in 1,000, may suffer a stroke during or after the surgery from a blood clot traveling to the brain, resulting in permanent paralysis of an arm or leg. Anticoagulants (blood thinners) will reduce clot size and formation.

Less critical is blood loss; any loss of blood is replaced by an immediate blood transfusion. Any allergic, itching skin reaction to transfused blood is controlled with medication.

A small number of patients may lose the benefits of surgery because one of the replacement veins suddenly and unexpectedly closes up.

Those complications are not listed to scare you. Your doctor will discuss them with you as you weigh benefits against risks. The same goes for survival rates.

The danger of having the surgery is weighed against the consequences of not having the surgery. Survival rates for persons with coronary heart disease treated medically are predicted on the basis of how many arteries are narrowed and by how much—as shown on the arteriogram. Probability of eventual death from coronary heart disease is also determined by the health of the heart muscle and nature's own bypass procedure, the formation of collateral blood vessels, if the body has the ability to form them.

Those same factors are weighed against the estimated success rate of the surgery in judging the safety and effectiveness of bypass surgery in your particular case. Most important is the condition of the heart muscle and the state of the coronary arteries beyond the major blockage that is to be bypassed. If the heart muscle and those arteries are in good shape, the operation can be executed with relative safety, say doctors. If the heart muscle is damaged or the arteries beyond the major blockage are very narrow, the hazards go up and chances of improvement diminish.

What Can Coronary Bypass Surgery Do for You?

It would be logical to expect that with improvement in the blood supply, death from an eventual heart attack in the years following a bypass operation would surely be averted—or at least delayed for a long, long time. Unfortunately, that has not always proved to be the case. "With the exception of patients with left main coronary artery disease [disease in the vessel which supplies the left, pumping ventricle of the heart with oxygen], a number of studies over the past decade have failed to show a difference in mortality [death] between the operated and nonoperated group of patients," state Bernadine H. Bulkley, M.D., and Richard S. Ross, M.D., 2 prominent cardiologists at The Johns Hopkins University School of Medicine, in an editorial (*Annals of Internal Medicine,* June, 1978).

For the overwhelming majority of bypass patients, the surgery is done not to prolong life, but to make life more bearable by relieving angina. Many people are so distressed by angina that they are willing and *eager* to undergo surgery for that reason alone. The decision to operate for such reasons becomes a highly individual matter—and a very subtle one. Many people are falsely allowed to assume that an expensive operation that relieves most of the symptoms of a disease must cure it—and prolong life. Despite great proclamations of near universal success by doctors and patients alike, there is a great deal of controversy over surgery's proper use.

Only 20 percent of bypass operations done in the U.S. in 1977 were for the more severe, unstable angina; the rest were for mild to moderate angina. That report comes from a survey by the National Heart, Lung and Blood Institute. One inference that might be drawn from these data is that many of those less severe cases could have been successfully treated medically with serious changes in diet and life-style, or even drugs. Based on their 1977 survey results, the Institute is now following up hundreds of bypass patients to determine just when bypass surgery is necessary and when it isn't. That study should help sort out the definite advantages. (Results will not be available until 1983.)

"There definitely is a place for bypass surgery. It's clear that it is of great value to certain patients. We have to identify who those patients are," explains Michael B. Mock, M.D., director of the ongoing Institute study.

Take a person who has severe blockage of all 3 major coronary arteries, one whose heart muscle is not severely damaged. Based on research statistics, he theoretically has an 8 percent chance of dying within 5 years without a bypass operation. At the same time, he has roughly a 4 percent chance of dying from the hazards of surgery itself. So his long-term chances are about twice as good if he has an operation.

A second patient, on the other hand, with only 1 severely blocked coronary artery and fairly good heart muscle, has a 5 percent chance of dying within 5 years while on medical treatment alone—not much different from the chance of dying due to the operation itself. For that person, a bypass operation would be difficult to justify.

Few cases are so cut and dried, however. "There are those who clearly need bypass surgery, and there are those who clearly don't. In between, there are a great number of cases we aren't sure about," says Adolph M. Hutter, Jr., M.D., cardiologist at Massachusetts General Hospital and a faculty member at Harvard Medical School.

Patients have been known to recover from coronary artery surgery feeling much, much better when in fact their heart function and the amount of blood their hearts were getting remained unchanged by the operation, recalls Jerome D. Frank, M.D., psychiatrist at The Johns Hopkins Hospital in Baltimore, Maryland. "The point is that all medical and surgical procedures . . . mobilize the faith that heals in the patient. The power of this faith is sharply demonstrated by studies of the results of surgical therapy for anginal pain" (*The John Hopkins Medical Journal,* September, 1975).

During the time leading up to the operation, the surgical patient is blitzed with attention and encouragement from doctors. With all that attention reinforced by elaborate tests using impressive scientific gadgetry and dread of the potentially fatal outcome of the operation, the patient wakes up primed for success.

Another psychiatrist put it this way: "Apparently the expense, pain and fear of surgery make it extremely difficult for an individual to consider the possibility that coronary bypass surgery might not have been useful."

Which means that if the patient believes a treatment will work, it probably will. That placebo effect may account for a very large part of the apparent success of bypass surgery in relieving angina, according to Thomas A. Preston, M.D., co-chief of cardiology at the U.S. Public Health Service Hospital in Seattle. "The lifetime experience of most patients is that improvement follows treatment, and administration of any treatment may be reason enough for a patient to see an improvement in his condition" (*Coronary Artery Surgery*: *A Critical Review,* Raven Press, 1977).

The placebo effect can be credited with some of the success of any approach, medical or surgical. But because of the potential hazards of surgery, it makes sense to be sure you have first tried more conservative approaches such as exercise and medication.

Without bringing forward each of the many voices in the hot debate over surgical versus medical management of angina, we think you should know that each side continues to collect data in support of its view, only to be shot down in turn by opponents with charges of improper methods, biased patient selection and so on. The only thing that has been agreed upon so far is that bypass surgery improves the survival of those patients who have disease of the left main coronary artery. Hopefully, the questions of exactly who else benefits, and how, will be resolved by the results of the ongoing study by the National Heart, Lung and Blood Institute mentioned earlier.

Until the results are in your decision as to whether or not you want to have a bypass operation should be based largely on how convinced you are that you have given everything else a fair try, and whether you absolutely cannot live with the pain any longer. That still makes it an elective operation for most people. Bypass surgery is almost never urgent. Unstable angina can be quelled with hospitalization and drugs first. Surgery has to be delayed even in those who've had a heart attack, in order for the damaged heart to heal.

Elective or not, bypass surgery is serious business, and you owe it to yourself to ask a lot of questions before signing on the dotted line. (For that matter, don't be afraid to ask last minute questions even after you sign the consent form.)

Do you as the patient have a say in whether or not you need bypass surgery?

"The answer to that is an emphatic, yes!" says W. Gerald Austen, M.D., chief of surgery at Massachusetts General Hospital and past president of the American Heart Association. "Patients should have everything to say about surgery. Most people would never dream of investing money in anything without a great deal of investigation and many questions. But patients have a hard time asking questions when it has to do with their health. Traditionally, they have a great deal of trust in their doctors. I'm not suggesting that that isn't correct. But there is nothing wrong with asking questions and making a sensible decision based on the right information."

Much of that information will come from your cardiologist and the surgeon to whom he refers you. Another source of information is the local chapter of the American Heart Association, which provides easy-to-read booklets on angina, heart disease and bypass surgery.

Each angina patient is different from the next. While we can't determine whether or not you need the operation, we can suggest some questions you should probably ask yourself and your doctor:

- Have all nonsurgical methods been tried? Have they been tried long enough? Arbitrary numbers are hard to put forth; try at least 6 months of serious medical management of your angina before you give in to surgery.
- What are the chances the operation will relieve my angina? And for how long? Ninety percent of bypass patients receive significant relief; 60 percent, total relief.
- If angina returns, how will it be handled? Will I have to face a second operation?
- How long will it be until I return to work and other normal activities? The advantage to medical treatment is that you don't need to leave your job for a long recovery; thus you are spared a major disruption in home, family and working life.
- You will want to know your chances of surviving the operation in order to enjoy its benefits. But don't expect hard guarantees. The jury is still out on the issue of whether or not bypass operations stave off impending heart attacks. The best your doctor can do is give you an educated opinion, based on his experience in the field, the size and location of blockages in your arteries, damage to other areas of the heart muscle, your general health and your living habits.

The one question *not* to ask is, "What is the mortality rate for this operation?" That depends on the difficulty of the case. Mortality rates reported in the medical literature range from less than 1 percent to slightly more than 4 percent. Those numbers can be misleading because some reporting hospitals handle only difficult cases. Their mortality rate may be higher, but they also get more experience in the art of open heart surgery than those who take only everyday cases.

In general, it may be more desirable to have bypass surgery in a major medical center than in a local community hospital. Larger hospitals usually do more operations, more often. The U.S. Department of Health, Education and Welfare sets forth a magical number of 200 heart operations per year as a rule of thumb for determining whether or not a hospital needs the expensive cardiac surgery units. Critics say that the figure has nothing to do with how good the hospital or cardiac team is; all it did was to jack up the number of procedures recommended to help justify the existence of the facilities in some hospitals. Above a reasonable number, Dr. Austen told us, the number of procedures done per year does not necessarily make a big difference in the outcome of the surgery.

- Who is going to perform the operation? Since your heart is literally in the hands of another human being, many people are justifiably concerned about who performs the bypass. Dr Austen had some good advice to offer about that, too: "My personal suggestion is that there is nothing wrong with making a call to the head of the cardiology department or a cardiovascular surgeon of a respected institution such as a university hospital or a major medical center for advice about whom you should see."

As in any major operation, the surgeon should be board-certified in cardiovascular surgery. And you are entitled to a second opinion, or even a third, especially if you have any doubts about the need for a bypass or its potential benefit.

Dr. Austen encourages people facing bypass surgery to ask anything they may be wondering about. "The patient is facing a serious operation. It's sensible to feel secure that it is required. Ask exactly what the surgeon is going to do and why, until you get satisfaction. A second opinion would not be a bad idea. Of course, if you are perfectly satisfied with the answers you get from your first doctor, you don't necessarily need a second opinion."

Getting Back to Work and Play

You'll be sent home after about 2 weeks in the hospital. As you recover, you may expect to feel soreness and discomfort around the incision, weakness, occasional muscle aches and some depression. All that is quite normal.

Any new signs of swelling, puffiness, redness or discharge at your incision should be reported to your doctor. The same goes for chest pain that doesn't quite feel like angina yet doesn't seem to come from your incision and won't go away. Any fever higher than 101° (or a lower fever that lasts longer than the first week) should also be reported.

Stop and rest if you feel short of breath, dizzy, faint or weak. Without such signs, you can begin to enjoy your renewed fitness.

Moving into action is a must if you are to bounce back to health. While it's true that your activity will be low in a few ways at first, gradually doing more of what you are able to do will prevent your muscles from becoming weak, improve your heart's efficiency and buoy your spirits. Family and friends will instinctively fawn all over you, but you can—and should—do a lot for yourself.

First of all, get up and get dressed every morning.

During the first 3 weeks, says the American Heart Association, you should be able to: shower, shave, and wash your hair; prepare meals; wash dishes; vacuum; do laundry at home; do light home repairs; ride in a car and walk on level terrain at an easy pace. In fact, you should plan at least 2 short walks a day outside when the weather is nice. You may also walk up and down stairs at a normal pace, but not too often in one day.

That doesn't mean to try all of those each day. Don't go overboard. Carry out activity at a comfortable, moderate pace. If you get tired before finishing such a project as tidying up the back porch, stop to rest for 15 minutes before finishing up. (Any time you feel chest pain other than from the incision, stop and rest.)

Don't lift anything over 30 pounds (that's a little heavier than a large bag of dog food or a small child).

Clearly, you are not an invalid, even after what your friends think is ominous surgery. The first 3 weeks at home is no time for mowing the lawn, lifting heavy objects, heavy digging, vigorous swimming, jogging, bicycling, playing tennis, golfing or bowling. Check with your doctor, during your first or second office visit after surgery, about when you can take up those activities. You'll probably also be curious about how soon you can drive a car, travel, go back to work and resume sex. If the surgery did what it was intended to do, your activity after surgical recovery should be greater than before.

Quite possibly, quality of life after your bypass depends on how you view your operation. If you say to yourself, "This operation is going to solve my problem and take me back to life as it's meant to be lived," it will. If, however, you feel that such somber treatment as open heart surgery must surely classify you as weak, helpless and sickly for the rest of your life, it can do that, too. Two studies vividly illustrate those points.

In one study of 349 men who had bypass surgery, their physical activity such as walking or hiking increased by 83 percent over presurgery levels. Light sports, such as golfing and bowling, increased by 35 percent. "Frequency of vacations, home repairs, self-education and home entertainment increased significantly. Frequency of sexual intercourse or the need for sleep did not change," report researchers Rimm, Barboriak and Anderson at the Medical College of Wisconsin in Milwaukee (*Federation Proceedings,* March 1, 1978).

Not all patients bounce back so smartly, however. To formerly active angina patients who began to see themselves as disabled by their symptoms before bypass surgery, "coronary bypass was seen not as restorative but as proof of disability," says Michael J. Gundle, M.D., psychiatrist at the University of North Carolina School of Medicine who studied a group of angina patients in North Carolina before and after bypass surgery.

"For example, we were told, 'I must be really sick if I had to have such a big operation.' . . . The experience of surgery, frightening, painful and disfiguring, then often reinforced these changes. In these cases, although the heart may have been repaired, the self remained damaged," reported Dr. Gundle at a meeting of the American Psychiatric Association in May, 1979. Dr. Gundle's study showed that those who suffered more than 8 months of angina symptoms before surgery were more psychologically disabled when it came to attitudes toward sex or going back to work than those who had suffered less than 8 months of angina before surgery.

Dr. Gundle told us that his study calls attention to the fact that how angina affects you before surgery may have some bearing on your recovery. "Some cardiologists might want to think twice before they recommend surgery, depending on how long the patient has had angina and the effect that it has had on him before surgery."

Angina does sometimes recur after surgery. The underlying arteriosclerosis plods on, arrested only by sheer good luck, prudent changes in diet and living habits—or more surgery. Most of us don't run our lives by relying purely on luck, though, and are inherently shy about more open heart surgery. It's easy to see the sense in continuing to follow through with the 13 natural anti-angina steps to help keep your arteries open and functioning after temporary salvation by surgery.

20
Cataracts

A cataract is any kind of clouding or opacity of the lens of the eye and although there are several different kinds of cataracts, by far the most common are those with the unfortunate name of "senile cataract." According to the National Society for the Prevention of Blindness, an estimated 75 percent of Americans 65 or older will develop these cataracts, a natural by-product of aging like wrinkles or gray hair. Senile cataracts can develop in people as young as 50. There's no reason to jump to the conclusion that you will lose your sight or need an operation when the doctor tells you you have a cataract. Only 15 percent of cataracts progress enough to interfere with vision, according to the society. And in less than 5 percent will surgery be needed.

Despite the low percentage of patients who undergo cataract surgery, so many people have cataracts that it is very high on the surgical hit parade — in the U.S., cataracts result in 330,000 operations a year. When surgery is needed it is painless and usually very safe and effective. Good sight is restored to 90 to 95 percent of surgical patients. One surgeon we spoke to said that percentage is closer to 98 percent when the patient has surgery for an uncomplicated cataract and has no other eye diseases.

Senile cataracts have been recognized for a long time. Treatment of cataracts has changed so rapidly in recent years that misconceptions about them abound. Here are some of the more common myths:

If one of your parents had a senile cataract, you will too. No hereditary link has been proved for senile cataracts, although many ophthalmologists believe presenile cataracts (those that occur in early or mid-life) run in families. Congenital cataracts (those present at birth) are frequently inherited.

Very old and very young people cannot tolerate cataract operations. Both 6-month-old infants and 100-year-old adults can sail successfully through cataract surgery if they are in good general health and have no other eye diseases.

It is not a good idea to have a cataract operation in the winter. That was true before surgical techniques were perfected. At that time, a patient had to lie immobilized for days after the surgery with a sandbag on either side of his head to keep the head motionless. The inactivity led to susceptibility to pneumonia. Techniques are so much better now that you can almost walk out of the operating room. Similarly, patients with allergies used to be advised not to have surgery when the allergies were most active because a good sneeze could pull a suture. Suture material has so improved that this is no longer a consideration — most sutures used in the eye are finer than human hair and stitches are minuscule.

The cataract must "ripen" before it is removed. That, too, was true before surgical techniques were perfected. Such advances as the invention of the cyroprobe, an instrument which freezes the lens and the discovery of an enzyme that dissolves the ligaments that hold the lens in place, have changed that practice. Now, waiting until the patient is completely blind and the cataract begins to liquefy can even make examination difficult and decrease the chance of successful surgery.

One eye can "catch" a cataract from the other. This idea originated because most patients with senile cataract have opacities in both eyes. Usually, one eye is much more affected than the other. The truth is that cataracts are not contagious because they are the product of a degenerative process, not an infectious one.

Laser beam surgery can be performed on cataracts. Other eye diseases can be treated with laser beams, but not cataracts. One opthalmologist's nurse said patients request laser beam surgery for cataracts so persistently that the doctor quit explaining it doesn't exist. What they are probably thinking of is phacoemulsification, an ultrasound technique that will be explained later in the chapter.

A cataract is a film growing on the eye. It may look like it and feel like it, but it isn't. A cataract forms in the lens, in the interior of the eye, so it's in the eye, not on it.

A bump on the head can cause a cataract. A direct injury to the eye itself can cause the sudden development of a traumatic cataract in a person of any age. Lumps and bumps to the head usually won't do it.

Cataracts cause pain, tearing and redness. These symptoms can coexist with cataracts but aren't caused by them. Usually, the only symptom of cataracts is painless deterioration of vision.

Surgery is performed by popping the eyeball out on the cheek, operating and then replacing it. The eye remains in its socket and the surgeon approaches the lens through a small incision in the front of the eye.

Cataracts can be caused or hastened by reading, sewing or other close work and by watching movies or TV. These activities could increase temporary eye strain but in no way cause cataracts.

Cataracts can grow back. The entire lens is removed in senile cataract surgery. There isn't any place for the cataract to grow back. In one type of operation, though, the capsule which contains the lens is left behind and can in future years cause vision problems. The problems can be corrected, though, by a procedure called a capsulotomy — so simple it can be performed in a doctor's office.

Certain drugs can prevent cataracts or halt their progress. Promising research is underway on drugs to prevent the cataracts that sometimes accompany diabetes, but no drugs are useful in treatment of senile cataract. Drops given to cataract patients merely cleanse the eye or dilate the pupils. Application of folk remedies to and other self-medication of the eye are dangerous, as they could damage the cornea. Some drugs, in fact, can cause cataract — notably cortisone and its derivatives.

Eye exercises can prevent cataracts. Exercises can be done after cataract surgery to help the patient to adjust to his new glasses, but none can prevent or halt cataracts.

How Do Cataracts Affect Vision?

If you've looked cataract up in a dictionary, you know it comes from the Latin word for waterfall — so named by ancient medical practitioners because the cataract resembled a hazy film over the eye. Though some cataracts make the eye look filmy, the real culprit is the lens, which is behind the iris (the colored part of the eye) and the pupil (its dark center). Some cataracts can't be seen at all by the naked eye.

A normal lens is about an eighth of an inch thick, egg shaped, almost crystal clear, soft and flexible. Convex on both sides and encased in a transparent capsule, it is composed of transparent fibers that have the most intense concentration of protein in the body. It looks like a clear pill. It has no nerve or blood supply but gets its nourishment from the liquid that flows slowly in back and front of it.

The aqueous humor, a salty fluid between the cornea and the lens, supplies nutrients and oxygen for metabolism. In the lens, the aqueous humor breaks down proteins, nucleic acids and other molecules.

The lens can't slough off cells as the skin does. After forming in the five-week-old embryo, it continues to grow throughout a person's life. The cells you are born with form the nucleus (center) of the lens and your newest ones continue forming on the outside like the growth rings of a tree. The lens of an 80-year-old is half again as thick as the lens of a 20-year-old.

The lens's job in vision is to focus the light rays that pass through the pupil. The sphincter muscle of the iris contracts or expands to let the right amount of light enter the pupil. The sphincter muscle of the iris contracts or expands to let the right amount of light enter the pupil. The lens receives the rays and focuses them for the retina, which is three-quarters of an inch behind it. Muscle fibers attached to the lens enable it to flatten to focus distant objects and fatten to focus near ones. It sends a sharp, upside-down picture to the retina, which in turn transmits the image to the brain. Voila! You are able to see.

But the lens tends gradually to become more rigid and less transparent with age, as does a clear egg white frying into a thicker white solid. The lens begins to lose its flexibility after about 40 years. The lens deepens in color from pale yellow to deep amber or even dark brown as the oldest cells in the nucleus harden. It is less able to fatten or flatten to focus light. That loss of transparency is due to chemical changes not yet fully understood.

As the lens's power of accommodation decreases, the eye needs more light for vision. Children's lenses can focus objects near the eye, but the focusing point moves farther and farther away with age.

Who Gets Cataracts?

These degenerative but common changes in the eye, then, account for senile cataracts. About 3 million people in the U.S. had a cataract that affected their vision in 1977, and two-thirds of them were 65 or older. Cataract is one of the leading causes of blindness among adults in the U.S. and accounts for 1 of every 7 cases of blindness in people 20 or older.

Among causes of cataracts besides aging are chemical or mechanical injuries to the eye; diseases such as diabetes, parathyroidism and neurodermatitis; rubella during pregnancy (resulting in a cataract in the infant); radiation; exposure to intense heat; other eye diseases such as glaucoma, inflammation and retinal detachment; ingestion of some drugs and poisons; Down's syndrome; and electrical shocks. If your eye could be easily injured at work or hobbies, wear protective goggles. If you have a microwave oven, follow the manufacturer's instructions on periodic checks for leaks and other hazards.

Although cataracts are far from rare in the U.S. and United Kingdom, rates are much higher in the subcontinent of India. An Indian ophthalmologist we spoke to while he was on fellowship in the U.S. rated sunlight the most important cause of cataract in his country. Cataracts are common in Israel, too, where they are more likely to affect people of non-European stock than the descendants of Europeans. Studies in the U.S. have shown that cataracts may occur with greater frequency in the Sun Belt. Another study shows that residents in the sunnier southern part of Rumania are likelier to get cataracts than those in the north.

Coupled with evidence from studies of animal and human

lenses exposed to sunlight, the greater frequency of cataracts found in sunny areas makes some researchers suspect near ultraviolet light (a certain kind of invisible light) contributes to cataract formation.

When we spoke to a biochemist who researched a possible link between near ultraviolet light and cataracts, Seymour Zigman said that although sunlight is the major source, other sources include the exceptionally high levels of ultraviolet light used by currency examiners, laundry workers, illustrators and others, the black lights used for lighting in discotheques and clubs, fluorescent lights in offices and lights used in laser technology.

Dr. Zigman, who has a Ph.D. in biochemistry and is a professor of ophthalmology and biochemistry at the University of Rochester School of Medicine, told us:

> So far the link is not proven. I'd say we have an intuition based on studies.
>
> Studies show a higher percentage of brunescent cataracts [brown senile cataracts] in the Philippines and Tampa, Florida, than in Rochester, New York. Also twice as many brunescent cataracts were found in Filipinos who work outdoors instead of indoors.
>
> There are indications from chemical, photochemical and etiological [pertaining to the cause of disease] studies that near ultraviolet light does lead to cataract formation in humans.
>
> Skin turns brown from near ultraviolet light when you're out in the sun. From the standpoint of logic, we have suspected for some time that the same wave lengths could reach the lens of the eyes and suntan them, producing brunescent cataracts. When we take an isolated human lens and put it in ultraviolet light, it does turn darker brown.
>
> Casual exposure to near ultraviolet light isn't important unless you're taking a drug [epinephrine and psoralen, for example] that makes you sensitive to it. Or if you're exposed daily to a very low amount, like the amount in general office fluorescent light. But if you are going to be exposed for hours

at a time day after day, precautions are important. Protective glasses are available to protect the eye from this light without interfering with the use of the light for work.

Symptoms of Cataracts

The 2 common types of senile cataracts are nuclear and cortical. Nuclear cataracts form in the central nucleus while cortical cataracts are star shaped opacities in the outer area of the lens.

There are several stages of development in both kinds of cataracts:

Incipient is the earliest stage. Vision probably hasn't yet begun to deteriorate.

Immature is the stage where vision has begun to deteriorate, but the cataract hasn't occupied the entire lens.

In mature cataracts, the lens is entirely opaque and the patient is blind in the affected eye.

In hypermature cataracts, the entirely opaque lens is starting to liquefy.

To some extent, the symptoms you have depend on the type of cataract and the stage it is in. Regardless of the cataract's color or location, you will have no pain. The primary symptom is deteriorating vision, which can manifest itself in several ways. If you find yourself walking with your head bent, shading your face with your hands, frequently changing your glasses' prescription and holding reading matter close to your face, you could have a cataract. It's time to visit the ophthalmologist. Some other symptoms include the following.

Second sight. As a cataract develops, the lens changes its shape. A strong curve temporarily increases the light-bending power of the lens. Although you still won't be able to see far off, you may be able to read or do other close work without glasses. That phenomenon, a symptom of nuclear cataract, gradually disappears as the cataract progresses.

Better vision in dim light. This is a symptom of nuclear cataract.

When the pupil dilates, more of the cataract-free lens is exposed and you are able to see around the cataract. That, too, is temporary.

Better vision in bright light. A symptom of cortical cataract. As the pupil dilates, the outer area of the lens is blocked out and the clear part is available for focusing.

Sensation of a film or skin on the eye. You try in vain to blink it off.

Fuzziness and blurriness. One cataract patient we talked to said the effort to see before surgery was like trying to see through a dirty window or a veil.

Difficulty in seeing lights. The moon may look double and lights may have a glare or colored halos.

Difficulty in night driving. Because the cataract scatters light, oncoming headlights may seem dazzling and starlike.

Accidents and falls. They are more frequent because you aren't seeing as well.

Colors, especially blue and violet, look green or muddy. This happens because the lens is changing color (it becomes increasingly deep yellow or even brown or black) and alters your color perception as it filters the light that enters the eye.

Loss of focusing ability. The lens isn't flexible enough to flatten and fatten.

Reliance on the stronger eye. As long as the difference in the images the 2 eyes produce is small, the brain can handle it. As the difference increases, one eye takes over the work.

The appearance of a yellowish or blue white film on the eyes. Other people will probably be able to see this better than you will.

Double vision in one eye. This symptom decreases as the cataract progresses.

Even if you have all these symptoms, don't diagnose yourself. Other eye diseases could cause them. If an initial diagnosis of cataract is made, though, keep regular appointments with the doctor so the progress can be monitored. Report any new symptoms or a sudden change in symptoms you've already reported.

Examination for Cataracts

Before you make your appointment, you should know the differences between the 3 types of specialists that examine, treat and prescribe for the eyes.

An *ophthalmologist* is a medical doctor who specializes in treating eye diseases. He or she has had 4 years of college, 4 years of medical school, a year's internship and 3 or more years of eye care training in a hospital. An ophthalmologist can diagnose and treat diseases, perform surgery, conduct vision exams and medical checkups and write prescriptions for eyeglasses and contact lenses.

An *optometrist* has gone to college for 2 to 4 years and to a college of optometry 4 years. He or she may test vision, screen patients for eye diseases and refer them to an ophthalmologist, prescribe orthoptics (eye exercises), fit contact lenses and prescribe eyeglasses.

An *optician* fills prescriptions for glasses and contact lenses from optometrists and ophthalmologists and sells glasses and other optical aids.

Usually, during a general eye exam, your eyes will be checked for signs of certain diseases, a health history will be taken and the coordination and muscle function of your eyes will be tested. Your ability to see near and far objects and the ability of your eyes to change focus will be checked.

Various instruments and pieces of equipment may be used. You will probably be examined with a slit lamp, which sends a vertical line of light into the eye. An illuminated cross section is reflected back, which the specialist examines with a microscope held inches from your face. Eye examinations are virtually never painful or traumatic, according to specialists we talked to.

Nutrition and Cataracts

The ophthalmologist you visit can best advise you on what step is next. It could be years before your cataract requires treatment — perhaps it never will. Unfortunately, the only treatment for the minority of cataracts that do progress enough to interfere significantly with vision is surgery. Everything from ox dung to honey has been smeared on the outside of the eye in hopes of halting cataract but no medical (as opposed to surgical) treatment has been effective.

Despite promising research linking the formation of cataracts to nutrition, no studies on humans have convinced most ophthalmologists that addition of a specific nutrient to the diet can halt or prevent senile cataract. Conflicting reports came from some optometrists we spoke to. They believe nutrition may play an important role in cataract formation, but agreed that nutritional therapy isn't effective on an eye already in need of surgery. After a book about nutritional prevention of cataract was published by a nonmedical writer, one concerned ophthalmologist, G. L. Spaeth, M.D. of the Wills Eye Hospital, Philadelphia, Pennsylvania, wrote in a journal:

"There is simply no evidence that cataracts can be cured by any means. To date, the only treatment, as unsatifactory as it is, is surgery . . . . I have done considerable research investigating the effects of vitamins on the physiology of the eye and believe that proper diet and proper administration of vitamins are important matters. I am distressed, I might add, that by and large the medical profession has paid less attention to these matters than may be warranted . . . . However, to hold out false hope to individuals seems to me to be a terrible thing to do when it is clear that the hope is indeed completely unrelated to reality" (*The Sight Saving Review,* Spring, 1975).

Ophthalmologists and optometrists we spoke to agreed that a well-balanced diet promotes the general health of the eye and helps patients recover after cataract surgery. They added, though, that no studies of human lenses have convinced them that addition of a specific nutrient to the diet can halt or prevent senile cataracts.

When we asked Richard C. Troutman, M.D., the chairman of the eye department at the Manhattan Eye, Ear and Throat

Hospital, about nutrition's role in cataract formation, he answered:

"Good nutrition is essential to the health of all the body's organs, including the eye. Although there is no good statistical evidence that nutrition is related to senile cataract formation, with a proper diet, you'll get a better result with eye surgery — or any kind of surgery."

A similar theme was echoed by Merill J. Allen, an O.D. (doctor of optometry) and professor of optometry at the Indiana University School of Optometry in Bloomington. Dr. Allen, who also has a Ph.D. in physiological optics, acknowledges a stronger link than Dr. Troutman does between cataracts and nutrition. But he, too, believes that overall good nutrition is more effective in promoting good vision than addition of a particular vitamin or mineral. Dr. Allen comments:

> I think a senile cataract is a nutritional cataract. In other words, it is associated with the maintenance of an inadequate internal environment for the lens. No vitamin B_2, a low intake of vitamin A, no vitamin C and an abnormal sugar metabolism can cause complications everywhere, not just in the eyes.
>
> When I see a patient with a cataract, I ask about his diet, whether he smokes, how much exercise he gets and how much alcohol he consumes. All of these could possibly be affecting his health.
>
> I suggest he clean up his living, if need be, and supplement his diet. Since it's so difficult and expensive to find out what may be missing, it's smart to go ahead and supply 10 or 20 times the amount of materials needed and let the body select what it needs. Most people that are deficient in one vitamin or mineral are deficient in others. I suggest a nutritional formula that usually contains vitamins E, C, B_6 and niacinamide, dolomite, brewer's yeast, lecithin, and very often other vitamins and minerals.
>
> No long-term, wide-scale results of this therapy have been collected. Because I work at the university now, my

> clinical experience is limited. But, based on my experiences and my colleagues' experiences with a small group of patients — maybe 20 — I'd say our impression is that it does help. It will not dramatically improve vision, however. It may bring a person with 20/40 vision down to 20/20 for example, or 20/100 to 20/80, but not much more than that.

Because of the obvious ethical problems involved, researchers can't create vitamin and mineral deficiencies in humans and see if cataracts result. Examination of human lenses must be done either in the eye, after a cataract in the lens is removed or at autopsy. Unfortunately, studies on the lenses of animals — even other mammals — don't apply very well to the lenses of humans. Investigators assumed for many years that they did, until sophisticated microscopic methods of examining lenses were developed.

A British researcher at an ophthalmology lab at the University of Oxford explained how human and other animal lenses differ in a December, 1975 *Scientific American* article. Ruth van Heyningen noted that lenses of some baboons and monkeys (which are so expensive that research on them is limited) are probably similar to human lenses. But the lenses of men are very different from those of the usual rats and rabbits used in research. While the human lens keeps increasing in weight and thickness throughout life and can accommodate its shape to send light to the retina, other animal lenses don't. The nuclei (centers) of lenses in adult humans are much softer than those of rabbits, cows or rats. While the water content of the lenses of other animals steadily increases throughout life, it tends to remain much more constant in humans.

Researchers continue to investigate cataract formation in lab animals but are very cautious about drawing parallels to humans.

Zinc. Cataracts were prevented in trout fed supplements of zinc in an experiment conducted by researchers at the Tunison Laboratory in Cortland, New York (*Federation Proceedings,* March 1, 1978). Experiments showed that cataracts in both eyes appear in trout who are fed whitefish meal instead of herring fish meal. But when a mineral mixture or zinc alone was added to the whitefish meal, cataracts did not develop.

Isolated soy protein. Other studies at the same lab show that cataracts are induced and growth is slowed down when the only protein in the diet is an isolated soybean protein. The studies indicate that when isolated soy protein is the *only* protein in the human diet, it could possibly contribute to cataract formation. A researcher from the lab, Hugh Poston, Ph.D., believes the high incidence of cataracts in some countries where people rely heavily on soy products and other legumes instead of meat should be investigated.

Vitamin E and tryptophan. Support for the idea that cataracts in animals are caused by a deficiency of two or more nutrients instead of just one was strengthened by a study on rats. When pregnant rats were deprived of both vitamin E and tryptophan, 33 percent of their offspring were born with cataracts. A deficiency of either vitamin alone, though, produced a much lower incidence of cataracts in the offspring (George E. Bunce and John L. Hess, *Journal of Nutrition,* February, 1976).

Riboflavin deficiency. Because riboflavin deficiency has been associated with cataracts in animals, 3 University of Alabama scientists decided to study 22 patients with presenile cataracts (cataracts formed before the age of 50) for a similar relationship. They found that 8 had riboflavin deficiency.

Cautioning that the riboflavin deficiency had not been proven to cause the cataracts, they concluded that the "Exploration of this possibility [riboflavin deficiency as a cause of cataract] is particularly attractive because dietary restriction of dairy products and the administration of riboflavin are easily accomplished and might lead to either prevention or regression of cataract formation" (Josef T. Prchal, Marcel E. Conrad and Harold W. Skalka, *Lancet,* January 7, 1978).

Indications for Surgery

Even those who believe that good nutrition may slow down early cataracts agree that eye surgery is the only recourse for vision so poor that the patient is unable to live as he'd like.

For example, a 76-year-old woman had a cataract for 15 years. It wasn't just a doctor's recommendation that led to its removal. When she flunked a driving test that kept her from the driver's seat of her prized silver Mercedes, she decided to have surgery. A second patient made an appointment with the surgeon when she could no longer read the want ads of the local newspaper, as did a seamstress who felt the quality of her work was beginning to suffer.

The cases illustrate an important point — there is no physiological time at which every senile cataract should be removed. According to all the ophthalmologists we spoke to, surgery is usually necessary only when the cataract interferes with the patient's vision enough that he is unable to do what he needs or wants to do comfortably. Visual deterioration that is unacceptable to a 55-year-old jeweler might be acceptable for a retired laborer who does little reading. Although the advice of your general doctor and ophthalmologist needs to be considered, your judgment is necessary to help decide when it's time for surgery.

Several different types of cataract operations are performed, but all of them involve the usual risks of surgery and the same basic procedures. As in all surgery, some sort of anesthesia is required, an incision is made (in this case, in the front of the eye) and a period of hospitalization is necessary. And no matter which specific technique is chosen, all cataract operations remove the damaged lens, replace it with an artificial implant or restore its function with glasses or contact lenses. Most cataract operations keep patients in the hospital from 1 to 5 days.

The type of surgery you choose depends on your age, preference, type of cataract, future vision requirements and surgeon's recommendations. If you have cataracts in both eyes, they will probably be operated on at 2 different times. That way, you will have some vision from the untreated eye while the eye that has undergone surgery is recovering. Usually cataracts don't progress at the same rate so the worse eye will be operated on first.

Complications occur in less than 5 percent of cases, and are even more infrequent when the eye has no disease except the cataract. The most common complications include detachment of the retina and impairment of circulation in the eye.

Conventional surgery. The standard method of senile cataract surgery involves extraction of the lens and its capsule and usually takes less than an hour. Depending on your preference, general health and the recommendations of the anesthesiologist and other doctors treating you, you can have either local or general anesthesia. With a local, you could even have surgery on an ambulatory basis — you could be in and out on the same day. Most ophthalmologists, though, insist on at least an overnight stay in the hospital.

If you are hospitalized, you may be given a sleeping pill the night before the operation. With either type of anesthesia you will probably receive medication to prevent nausea and make you drowsy before you go to the operating room. Once you are on the operating table, your body and most of your head will be draped with sterile cloths to keep the eye area clean. Probably only the area around the eye to be operated on will be visible, but you will be able to breathe normally. Then drops will be put in your eye to numb and clean it and the area of your face around it will be carefully cleaned. An instrument will hold your eye painlessly open.

The operation itself is simple. Where the white of your eye meets the clear cornea, the surgeon will make a small semicircular incision. A small wedge-shaped bit will be cut from your iris in a procedure called an iridectomy. It provides a drainage hole which keeps the iris from falling back into the wound and maintains the normal circulation of the eye. This may be barely detectable after the operation — it will probably look like a dot — and it is usually concealed by your upper eyelid.

Then the surgeon is ready to remove the lens and its capsule. The ligaments that hold the lens in place will probably be dissolved first with drops of an enzyme called chymotrypsin. Then using either a suction cup, forceps or freezing probe, the surgeon will remove the lens and capsule intact. The wound will then be closed with tiny sutures, often finer than a human hair. Some surgeons use sutures that need to be removed postoperatively; some use sutures that remain painlessly in the eye; and others use stitches that dissolve. Most surgeons now use microscopes during the operation for greater precision — the microscope is positioned just over your eye. The surgeon looks into it while he operates. The procedure is almost bloodless.

A patch and shield will be put over your eye and you will be taken to the recovery room or back to your room. You'll probably be on your feet by nightfall and will be able to resume normal mild activity.

Postoperative instructions vary depending on your surgeon, the procedures used and the health of your eye. Although the patch can be discarded fairly soon, you will probably need to wear a shield while sleeping to keep from poking your finger in your eye. You will probably be told not to shampoo your hair for at least a week or two. Showers and baths are usually OK, but for some weeks you will probably be told not to swim under water or engage in contact sports. If your eyes tear and discharge, wipe them with sterile cotton balls. Heavy lifting is out, as is bending forward from the waist. Learn to stoop correctly, putting the weight on your legs, not your back. Straining while defecating is prohibited, too, so eat a high-fiber diet or use natural stool softeners if you are constipated. You can use your eyes as much as you wish for close work.

You will probably feel no pain, but if there is any, it will probably be slight enough to be relieved by a mild pain-killer. The surgeon can supply you with instructions about eye drops and dressing.

Increased venous pressure near the eye causes local hemorrhage — that's why pressing your eye, straining and lifting are prohibited. A small local hemorrhage isn't usually serious, but may cause you to have to put off getting glasses or contact lenses.

Report pain, swelling and bleeding to the surgeon.

Alternatives to the conventional method. The 2 other types of operations are needle aspiration and phacoemulsification. Needle aspiration — in which the lens capsule is pierced and its contents sucked out through a small hollow needle — is used on children and young adults who have softer lenses than older people with senile cataract.

Phacoemulsification is a technique used mainly in patients under 45 but also in some older patients with senile cataract. It's an ultrasound technique that uses a small incision in the front of the eye. A needle tip that vibrates 40,000 times a second emulsifies (fragments) the hard lens and the fragments are sucked out with the needle. The back wall of the capsule usually remains behind.

Advantages are that it requires a smaller incision than the conventional method, which means faster healing and a shorter hospital stay. Patients have few if any postoperative restrictions and may return to work almost immediately. Disadvantages are that since it's only been in use since the 1960s, long-term results aren't in. It's no longer considered experimental but its results haven't been evaluated in large-scale controlled clinical studies. And the capsule, which is left behind to prevent certain complications, can cloud over and interfere with vision. A hole must then be made in the capsule in a procedure called a capsulotomy. The procedure is a simple and brief one that can be performed in a doctor's office.

Charles D. Kelman, M.D., the inventor of phacoemulsification, told us: "I use phacoemulsification in probably 90 percent of the cataract operations I do. The advantages are the small size of the incision (2 to 3 millimeters as opposed to 22 millimeters in the standard method), the immediate return to activity and the absence of postoperative corneal astigmatism, which is likelier to happen with a large incision. We are statistically proving that phacoemulsification results in lower incidence of retinal detachment and retinal edema [swelling]."

Dr. Kelman, who is an assistant clinical professor of ophthalmology at New York Medical College and chief of ophthalmology at Lydia E. Hall Hospital in Freeport, Long Island, New York, admits the operation is difficult to learn and requires expensive equipment. He said an ophthalmologist should do at least a few cases a month in order to do the operation well.

Critical of the technique is Dr. Troutman, Manhattan Eye, Ear and Throat Hospital's director of surgery. "Several late problems that routinely occur can make it difficult to repair other common complications, particularly with the retina. It's an excellent technique for traumatic cataract and cataract in children and young adults, but it's not my procedure of choice for adult cataract."

A pamphlet prepared by the Information Office of the National Eye Institute describes phacoemulsification and concludes: "However, the ultrasonic method is not yet as successful as conventional techniques in treating the elderly who constitute the majority of cataract patients. It is more suitable for children and young adults because their lenses are relatively softer" (*Cataract,* U.S. Department of Health, Education and Welfare Publication No. (Nth) 73-201).

Adjusting Vision after Cataract Surgery

Once you've decided when to have surgery and by what method, you still have an important decision to make — how you are going to replace the lens. Removing the cataract won't fully restore your vision. You'll be able to see after surgery and before you choose a replacement, but not too well. The operated eye is aphakic (without a lens) after surgery. It's light-refracting power is partially missing. So you must get either glasses or contact lenses after the operation or an artificial lens implant at the time of operation. Regardless of which of these replacements you choose, your vision is going to be slightly different. Light might seem brighter, and blues will appear deeper to you — the sky may even look Wedgwood blue — because you are so used to seeing colors through the yellow filter your lens created.

Registered nurse Barbara Dice, who works for an ophthalmologist and answers many postoperative telephone calls from cataract surgery patients, told us, "Some patients call in alarmed and say that everything is rose colored, especially on a bright, sunny day when there's snow on the ground. When we tell them it's nothing to be concerned about, they laugh and say they really like the idea of seeing a rosy world."

Glasses. Replacing the lens's function with glasses is the time-honored method. It's for you if you can't handle contacts and don't want to try artificial implants until the long-term verdict is in. Unfortunately, they are going to take some getting used to.

The glasses used after cataract surgery magnify your vision by about 25 to 30 percent. Things are going to appear closer to you than they are because they look larger. You may miss when you reach for your teacup or step down too soon for a curb. There will also be some distortion — for instance, door frames might seem bowed.

Most people can adjust to glasses in about 3 to 6 months. At first, though, you may sometimes feel dizzy or nauseated. You will need to learn to hold your eyes straight and look through the center of the lenses. You'll need to turn your head, not your eyes, to read or to see to the side.

If only one eye has been operated on, you can't wear glasses without blocking out the other eye. That's because the image from only one of your eyes will be 25 to 30 percent magnified. The brain can't handle the 2 different-sized images at once, and double vision will result. You'll have to use just one eye until the second operation. Many ophthalmologists will schedule the operations for the 2 eyes as close together in time as possible, so that the patient doesn't have to use only one eye for long.

The glasses can be made out of plastic now, and aren't quite as thick as the old Coke-bottle-bottom glasses postoperative patients used to wear. You'll need to get bifocals or two pairs of glasses — one for reading and close work, one for seeing at a distance. It will probably be several weeks before glasses are prescribed. In the hospital, you may be given some temporary glasses to wear in the interim.

Two postoperative patients we talked to gave us these reports about glasses:

> I adjusted to the glasses and saw much better than I did for years before the operation.

> Glasses were my last resort. I didn't like the way they looked. I only got them after I tried contacts and just couldn't get used to them.

An optometrist and an ophthalmologist we talked to gave us similarly conflicting reports.

Optometrist Dr. Allen (from Indiana University School of Optometry) said, "Some people fear using contacts like others fear flying in airplanes — they just don't want to put anything in their eyes. Once they've had surgery and take a look through those spectacles, though, they'll take anything you'll give them — some spectacles are really bad news. They magnify and distort distances, they blur when you try to look to the sides and they make you look funny. When that's all there is, though, they're wonderful."

But the Manhattan ophthalmologist, Dr. Troutman, said, "The benefits of spectacles shouldn't be overlooked. Ordinarily, the retired need good visual acuity for reading and driving, but they don't play tennis or basketball. They were very happy with glasses until very recently when ophthalmologists told people they shouldn't be happy with them. Of course, a patient can't readily wear glasses if they've only had one cataract removed. If it's an older patient who has had surgery in both eyes, though, I always recommend glasses as the safest and most optically advantageous."

Contacts. Contact lenses are inadvisable for people who have arthritis in their fingers or hand tremors from Parkinson's disease or other similar disease. Barring these and similar problems, people of any age have learned to use contacts. Ophthalmologists and optometrists have reported successful contact use in patients from 3 to 103.

Because contact lenses for use after cataract surgery only magnify the image 6 percent, the brain can simultaneously handle the images from an eye with a contact and an eye without a contact. Contacts correct only for far vision though — you'll still need reading glasses. Both can be fitted several weeks after surgery. Either hard or soft contacts may be used — the soft, which are newer, are still slightly more expensive. The type you get depends on your preference and the condition of your eyes. The special contacts used for patients after cataract surgery are different from and slightly more expensive than normal contact lenses.

Although the contacts must be kept clean and removed and inserted daily, they do not require the visual adjustments that glasses do. Because the contact moves with your eye, you don't have to turn your head to see to the side. When we spoke to postoperative patients about their contact lenses, some said it was easy to adjust to the contacts, some adjusted with daily help in removal and cleansing from a relative or friend and some couldn't adjust at all.

Whether you decide on glasses or contacts, you can save yourself some money by comparison shopping. The Federal Trade Commission has recently lifted its ban on advertising by makers of optical lenses and ruled that whoever examines the eye must furnish you a copy of the prescription so that you can comparison shop. You should ask for the name of the manufacturer of the lenses and frames you want so that you can compare prices of identical glasses or contacts at other places.

Always make sure the cost of adjustment is included in the price. Have the person who wrote the prescription test the lenses. Afterward, make the prescription a part of your permanent medical record in case you lose your glasses.

Constant-wear lenses — something new. A growing number of doctors are trying constant-wear lenses for their patients. Similar to the soft contact lens, it is placed in the patient's eye by the doctor. The patient then returns every 2 or 3 weeks to have the lens removed, cleaned and replaced. Doctors who use them feel they are safe, virtually problem-free and far more convenient for older people who cannot tolerate regular contact lenses.

Artificial lens implants. If you are over 65, don't want to wear glasses and can't handle contacts, a lens implant might be a solution. The implants have generated great excitement since the late 1960s, but unfortunately long-term follow-up results aren't available. Some cases of lost vision due to lens implants have been reported.

The plastic lenses, which are placed in the eye during the operation about the same place the patient's own lens was, frequently take away the need for heavy glasses. Depending upon your eye condition, one of several different lens types can be used, which the surgeon can show you if you decide on this procedure.

Most surgeons implant lenses only in patients who are 65 or older, because the lenses are believed unlikely to cause serious problems in the patient's remaining life span. The procedure is usually done at the time of operation — it's rarely recommended that you have it done later. It can be done in conjunction with either standard surgery or phacoemulsification. Very rarely is it done on both eyes and then only if one eye has tolerated an implant well for some time.

Three elderly postoperative patients we spoke to raved about the implants as the right solution for them. All 3 reported that their surgeons had given them a choice of procedures and didn't push them to accept the lens implant.

In its section on cataract, one current medical text has this to say about the implants:

"Intraocular lenses are being inserted by a small percentage of cataract surgeons throughout the world. The indications for this procedure are limited and the complication rate is higher than with the standard cataract operation. For these reasons, most conservative cataract surgeons believe intraocular lenses are still in the investigative stage."

A second account was written by B. Thomas Hutchinson, M.D., associate surgeon at the Massachusetts Eye and Ear Infirmary. In the Harvard Medical School's health newsletter for laymen, Dr. Hutchinson commented:

> Although the IOL [intraocular lens] has received extensive news coverage which often suggests universally good results, the fact is there are well-recognized complications attributable to the use of the artificial material within the eye. On a national average the frequency of these complications is greater than the risks and vision failures of cataract surgery alone. Although there are many "models" of intraocular lenses, none are ideal and free of complications. *In summary, when these lenses work well, they are fantastically effective — but when they work poorly, they may be catastrophic to the vision and even to the eye itself.* [italics added] Obviously, the decision for an intraocular lens should not be made lightly, either by the patient or the ophthalmologist (*Harvard Medical School Health Letter,* January, 1978).

21
Colostomy

A colostomy is a very serious operation in which a hole (or stoma) is opened somewhere in the patient's abdomen to drain off waste from the intestine, either because the intestine has been blocked or because it is incapacitated by disease. Such a procedure can be performed on any part of the intestine, anywhere along its length, in the upper regions called the small intestine or the lower lengths called the large intestine. When it is done, of course, the bowel must be fixed to the inside of the abdomen and a hole opened in it to correspond to the one in the patient's side. Colostomies are made necessary by a great many health-threatening situations that we'll run down later. However, cancer of the bowel and diverticulitis are the 2 most frequent causes of obstruction and decomissionings. A colostomy, then, is an artificial anus created by a surgeon to replace a natural one that is no longer serviceable, a detour for human by-products on their way to normal elimination.

Because the job of the colon is to absorb water from the body's wastes, the creation of a stoma causes certain problems. If it is high up in the intestine, the waste that issues from it can be largely liquid and require that the patient — or ostomate — wear an appliance (actually a plastic bag taped to his side) to collect it. Theoretically, the further down in the intestine a stoma is placed, the more solid its contents will be and the less trouble it will cause. But this cheering equation is complicated by a third factor. The more intestine a patient loses to disease, the more that has to be removed to stop cancer or diverticulitis, the less surface he has to absorb water from stool and the more trouble he has with elimination. Still, many stomas (even those in the small intestine), like their natural counterparts, can be reliably trained to perform on command. In fact, many ostomates go without bags except during this initial training period.

Traditional terminology labels colostomies either temporary or permanent and identifies temporary colostomies as replacements for sections of bowel that must be *rested,* and permanent procedures as stand-ins for lengths that must be *retired* (or removed). However, most doctors we talked to said these distinctions were more apparent than real. They claimed that as surgical procedures have gotten better and more sophisticated, the number of permanent colostomies has become fewer and fewer. Colostomies are permanent these days only when the anus and rectum are lost to disease. This means that more and more stoma operations are temporary measures, but even this term is misleading. Sections of bowel which are "rested" by the creation of a bypass for wastes are, in fact, usually removed at some later day; they cannot really be put back in service once they've been sidelined.

Many colostomies are temporary today, because they are done to buy time. In some instances, the patient has entered the hospital in an emergency, and a colostomy is performed to remove waste trapped by some form of bowel obstruction before it bursts the intestine and poisons the body. In this case the stoma will remain only until the patient has recovered from the severe symptoms of obstruction. Other colostomies are part of a staged set of procedures. A patient who is in no condition to undergo bowel removal surgery at the moment can be made comfortable (and kept safe) with a colostomy until he is strong enough for the other procedure.

In both cases — as an emergency or a staged event — the colostomy is temporary while the loss of bowel is permanent. The only difference between the two is the time when the piece is removed — which sounds worse than it is. Such have been the advances in surgery in recent years that (as we said) very few bowel-shortening operations result in the need for permanent colostomies. In all cases but those in which the anus or rectum is lost to disease, the remaining lengths of bowel can be reconnected to form a perfectly functioning intestine. What's even better, the bowel is remarkably adaptable. Even if most of the large intestine is knocked out by cancer (for instance), and the small intestine must be run on to the anus to complete the circuit, the patient is left with a smoothly functioning disposal system. The small intestine rather quickly takes over its large neighbor's water-absorbing task, and everything proceeds at a nearly normal clip.

If it's clear that a colostomy will be temporary, the colon is *not* severed, but — instead — a loop of it is sewn to the abdominal wall. Then an opening in its side is matched to a stoma in the patient's abdomen. If the colostomy must be permanent, the colon is cut in two and the end of the section ahead of the troubled area is pulled through an opening in the abdominal wall and stitched fast. In either temporary or permanent cases, the colostomy procedure will probably be only the first stage in a series of major surgeries. It may be followed by 1 or 2 or even 3 additional steps. After the stoma is formed and functioning, a second operation will be required to remove the affected section of bowel — once the patient's symptoms have subsided — if he was too sick for this during the first stage. If cancer is the culprit, of course, every effort will be made to remove the malignancy in the initial phase to prevent its spread. After this, the remaining sections of colon are reattached to form a reliable intestine. Once this is accomplished, the original stoma is removed, either in the reconnecting step, if the patient's in good shape, or later, if he's not.

How many times do such things occur each year? The United Ostomy Association, a self-help group that helps colostomy patients (and patients who've had similar procedures) to help themselves, estimates — with figures drawn from the files of 2 government agencies — that 66,000 new stomas are opened each year. Sixteen thousand of these operations are temporary procedures, which means that 50,000 ostomates are born each year. Naturally, the earlier one's problem is diagnosed, the greater will be his chances for a temporary colostomy and a permanent cure.

If you are like most people, you froze at the mention a while back of a waste-filled bag strapped to your side. The reaction most folks have to colostomy is "Oh yuk! Going to the bathroom will be disgusting!" Or, "Oh my God, there'll be a hole in my belly!" All of which are common first reactions and usually untrue. Most colostomies — after their bearers have learned to deal with them — are quite clean. When some care is taken, there is usually little odor or soiling of the skin involved. The hole in the patient's side is not particularly gruesome and looks not unlike a second belly button — according to one doctor we consulted. And these double-barreled folks are whole people in every social and emotional sense of the term. There are usually few limits to the things they can do or the places they can go. One of the major purposes, in fact, of this chapter is to reassure the reader who faces a colostomy that his life will not end with it. Quite the contrary, it will probably be renewed by the operation. Given the very serious conditions that end up in colostomies and the pain and debilitation usually associated with them, the relief provided by this detour is a godsend. Activities that were dreary or impossible immediately before the surgery often become happy commonplaces after it. After a period of physical training and psychological conditioning, what might be called a second go-round with toilet training — for colostomy is no more than a new way to go to the bathroom — ostomates lead completely normal lives.

Another thing this chapter hopes to do is help you toward the training and compassion you need to adjust to a colostomy, something which is not as easy as it sounds. It's *not* just a matter of finding a knowledgeable and agile-fingered surgeon as it is in other sections of this book, because some doctors don't think about a stoma after the surgery is done. Although the location of many colostomies is dictated by the site of colon blockage, there is some leeway in a lot of cases and even a good deal of choice in others. Unfortunately, some doctors don't exploit these margins for error — or rather success — *before* the surgery begins. They give too little thought to where the stoma's put, and this lack of concern may cause the new owner untold problems. Of course, in the many stoma operations that are done under emergency conditions, thoughts about placement are necessarily brief, but under the best circumstances, they're crucial. Proper placement, in fact, is at least half the battle in getting along with a colostomy. Colostomy appliances on certain parts of the abdomen are just plain hard to get next to. So finding the right doctor is doubly important in this case, and we'll be as much help as we can.

Unfortunately, we can only half-deal with the problem. We can give you lots of factual information, but we can't actually train you to use your novel means of elimination, and we can't smooth you over the psychological bumps that inevitably come with it. Those 2 things must be done by someone who can see your stoma, go with you to a drugstore which handles ostomy supplies to pick an appliance that fits you properly and hold your hand when things get discouraging. The best we can do is set you going in the right direction for aid and comfort. We'll give you the facts you need to ask the right questions when searching for the right surgeon and a list of places you can go for postoperative care if your doctor's helpfulness wears off with his anesthetic. We'll show you how to find a reliable counselor, usually a registered nurse, with special training in colostomy therapy.

The end of this chapter will contain some happier matters. Colostomy may be avoidable — preventable — if one starts early enough, before the things that produce it do. If your doctor's first grave word to you is "colostomy," then the operation is probably the last word in treatment for you. Your condition has gone so far that surgery is the only alternative. However, if you're healthy *now,* there are some things you can do to change your life-style — alterations in diet, certain supplements and a commitment to exercise — that will considerably *lessen* your chances of ending up with a colostomy. Some authorities would claim that, in the case of diverticulitis, these therapies will work even after symptoms of the illness have begun. Recent research has shown that a high-fiber diet, by eliminating excessive bowel contraction through the larger stools it produces, can help prevent the tiny herniations called diverticuloses and the inflammation of those herniations or sacs called diverticulitis. It has also been discovered that diets high in bulk tend to reduce a person's risk of intestinal cancer by diluting natural and environmental compounds that can cause cancer and by speeding the passage of stools so that there is less contact between these compounds — which are naturally dangerous or undergo dangerous chemical changes during the passage time — and the lining of the colon. Of course, if you swallow a rubber peg or trinket — the way some kids do — no amount of vitamins A or C or raw bran will prevent *that* bowel obstruction. But diverticulitis and even colorectal cancer *do* become less of a risk with the proper diet and supplementation. What may be even more important — especially for folks with a family history of bowel cancer or diverticulitis — is a screening program we'll describe. Most doctors suggest some form of yearly exam for both conditions after the age of 40, because early detection and treatment can mean either a cure with less than major surgery or a temporary colostomy leading to a complete recovery later.

Why and Where Colostomies Are Done

Before we talk about making sure things go right with your colostomy, we should talk a little about how the large intestine works and the things that can go wrong with it. The kind of colostomy you have — or need — and the kind of problems it may cause are largely products of where it is placed on your tummy. And where it is is determined by what it is. The large intestine is the final 5 to 7 feet — depending on how large *you* are — of the intestinal tract. The small intestine — which is closer to the stomach than its larger neighbor — often exceeds 20 feet in length, but it's called "small" because of its skinniness. The so-called large intestine is short but fat. The colon is a wanderer, it moves up one side of the abdomen and down the other. It begins at a junction with the small intestine called the cecum in the lower right corner of the abdominal cavity and travels *up* the right side for a foot-and-a-half or so; this section is called, naturally enough, the ascending colon. At a point just under the ribs and marked by the liver, it turns left and drapes across the abdomen for 2 or 2½ feet; this branch is referred to as the transverse colon. Then, after passing the spleen, it becomes the descending colon and drops under the ribs and down the left side of the torso for another 24 inches into the pelvis. There it skips up into an S-shaped curve — the sigmoid colon — and turns down again into the rectum, which is 8 to 10 inches long, and the anal region, the last 1 to 2 inches. These final sections are located within the pelvis and behind the bladder. The sausage links of the colon are more or less held in place by a series of suspenders called the mesentery. "More or less" has to be used here, because the suspenders are free-swinging and the bowel, especially the sigmoid region, is very flexible. In fact, the large intestine can become twisted in its own mesentery (a condition called volvulus), obstructed and seriously infected. In the extreme cases where gangrene sets in, volvulus can necessitate the removal of a length of bowel and a colostomy; simpler cases can be corrected by a simple surgical unraveling. Unfortunately, once twisted and undone, the colon has a tendency to try the feat again.

An ostomy — the general term applied to all surgically made intestinal (or urinary) openings in the abdomen — can be required at any point along the intestinal tract. A stoma placed in the small intestine is called an ileostomy; one at the junction of the small and large intestine is a cecostomy; and any opening in the colon is termed a colostomy. But trouble is most common in the large intestine — especially the cecum and sigmoid regions.

The function of the colon, as we suggested earlier, is to absorb water from the waste that is left after the small intestine has processed the food we eat, and it is this job as stool-shaper that *can* make living with a colostomy a messy business. As waste material moves through the bowel, it becomes drier and more formed. The further down the intestine a colostomy occurs, the easier it is to deal with. The closer to the small intestine it's located, the more liquid its output and the more numerous its problems.

By one fairly conservative count, there are 22 diseases, syndromes and serious injuries that can end in colostomy or another form of ostomy. In alphabetical order, some of them are:

Bladder incontinence

Cancer of the bladder (In cases like these, an ostomy is usually done to handle liquid wastes for a decommissioned urinary system.)

Cancer of the colon or rectum
Congenital bladder neck obstruction
Congenital exstrophy of the bladder
Crohn's disease of the colon
Crohn's disease of the small bowel
Crohn's disease of the small and large bowel
Diverticular disease
Familial polyposis
Megacolon, congenital or Huspring's
Multiple polyposis
Radiation enterocolitis or proctitis
Trauma (direct injury to abdomen)
Ulcerative colitis

Some of these conditions — for example, megacolon — are the result of congenital malformations of the large bowel which lead to its failure. In megacolon, a too narrow or malfunctioning section of the colon, a hereditary bottleneck caused by a missing set of nerves, allows a section behind the bottleneck (or closer to the rectum) to fill with waste. Some of the conditions are degenerative diseases in which an inflammatory condition slowly eats away at the large intestine until it becomes blocked or breaks open. Ulcerative colitis and the Crohn's diseases are examples of that kind of problem. And some — multiple and familial polyposis — are caused by the growth of many benign tumors or neoplasms which can narrow the colon or block it completely if they are malignant or intussusception (the telescoping of one intestinal section over another) occurs. If we were to talk about all these things — plus the 20 other conditions (like a length of bowel caught in a strangulated hernia) that *sometimes* wind up in colostomy — we could get lost in a Siberia of symptoms and surgeries.

The important thing is that just 2 of the conditions — bowel cancer and diverticulitis — together account for 85 percent of all bowel obstructions and most colostomies. So, what we'll do is talk about the general symptoms of bowel obstruction, the clinical exams these symptoms prompt and the special cases presented by colon cancer and diverticular disease before moving on to the surgeries that are used to correct them. Which aren't terribly dissimilar and won't take us very far away from our main business, that is, the description of a screening program that can detect bowel diseases before they cause obstruction, and the care and feeding of a colostomy. This screening program is our main business, because once symptoms of bowel obstruction appear, it may be too late to think about even a temporary colostomy. It may be too late to think about tomorrow. The consequences of a blocked intestine are often very serious.

Signs of Bowel Obstruction

The symptoms of most bowel obstructions are progressive; they get worse and worse as the obstruction goes from partial to complete. What might start as infrequent bouts of crampy abdominal pain — the off-and-on pain of colic — and periodic constipation can eventually become severe and constant sharp pain and the terrors of that delicate portmanteau word, "obstipation," which is a collision of "obstinate" and "constipation" and denotes the total and persistent inability to pass gas or move one's bowels. Plus nausea and vomiting. And a growing distention of the abdominal cavity as the patient gets less and less able to empty his bowel. On the other hand, the "worse" end of this progression may not be constipation. It may be what *looks* like diarrhea, and thus mislead the patient and perhaps his doctor into thinking something else is wrong. As whatever is obstructing the colon pinches off its circumference, only liquid waste can get through, giving the illusion of loose and frequent bowel movements and another kind of problem.

One thing that can make these awful conditions unbearable is a monkey wrench called the ileocecal valve, the shutoff between the small and large intestines. If the valve works, as it does in about half the population, it normally works to keep the contents of the large bowel from backing up into the small bowel. In the presence of an obstruction, the valve abnormally works to keep gas and waste bottled up in the large intestine and to prod severe pain and a dangerous emergency. It keeps the patient from the relief that vomiting can bring. The moral of this story is that when faced with bowel obstruction, hope for a faulty ileocecal valve.

If bowel obstructions are not treated quickly — once they become complete — they can and frequently do cause death. Death when the patient is overwhelmed by the poisons his system absorbs from the stagnant bowel contents. Death from a perforation of the colon and the spread throughout the abdomen of bacteria and infection. Or death from the chemical imbalance that results in the body when several of its systems are shut down by an obstruction.

If the patient has not been diagnosed as part of a routine screening program, and he's come to the doctor showing some of the signs we've described above, he's immediately hustled off to a physical examination. In the initial cursory look-see, the doctor searches for surface signs of a distended abdomen; he asks about problems with gas and constipation and can often see the rhythmic waves of the colon spasmodically reacting to the blockage, through the skin of a thin patient. Listening with a stethoscope, he can hear the high-pitched, metallic tinkles, rushes and gurgles of the bowel's irresistible force doing battle with an immovable object.

Faced with such evidence, the examiner then orders lab tests, x-rays and other diagnostic procedures. He'll want a complete blood count, urinalysis, BUN (blood/urea/nitrogen) and serum electrolyte evaluation to check the patient's general level of health. Those tests can discover the presence of anemia (due to internal bleeding) and infection in the body which may have come from a ruptured or perforated bowel, another emergency situation. We say can because the presence of these very conditions in the body can also prompt the tests to give false readings. The tests can also tell the doctor if the patient has become dehydrated, although false positive results are a danger here, too.

The next steps are a chest x-ray and 2 sets of abdominal pictures. Chest x-rays are required of most prospective surgical patients by nearly all hospitals these days as a precautionary measure — timid administrators want to know about any hidden pulmonary problems that might complicate recovery. Is that defensive medicine? Are administrators running scared? Maybe, but we are dealing with a very serious illness that can lead to major surgery, and it is important to know about any hidden health problems before confronting the bowel disease. In addition, the chest films also reveal another sign of a perforated bowel — air trapped in the abdominal cavity beneath the diaphragm. One picture of the patient's abdomen is taken with him lying on his back to disclose any loops of abnormally distended bowel. Another see-through snapshot is taken with the patient standing to record (as closely as possible) the location or level of the intestinal block. If the obstruction is very low in the colon, where its links are tightly piled upon one another, a barium enema x-ray (an enema containing an opaque substance that shows up brightly on film) is used to pinpoint the trouble in the snaky maze of intestine.

All these tests are designed to tell the physician *where* the problem is and its probable cause. To find out *what* it is exactly, the doctor uses his gloved finger to feel the area very near the rectum or, for roadblocks higher up, one of a number of devices that are all flexible little telescopes (of varying lengths) that carry their own lamps. These instruments are called sigmoidoscopes and their use, sigmoidoscopy, is the physician's most important tool in the diagnosis of bowel defects. Inserted into the patient's anus, they allow the physician actually to see the source of symptoms throughout most of the large intestine's length. Of course, if the obstruction is complete and it's obvious, an emergency results and few diagnostic measures are required. Surgery comes almost immediately. Should the problem be a few polyps impeding progress, it is even possible to fit these telescopes with ingenious little knives that snip off the growths and remove them. Such appliances are also used to take samples of a diseased bowel for laboratory analysis and the detection of cancer.

It should be noted that all these exams — the x-rays and the optical inspections — require that the bowel be empty *below* the level of the block. With a total obstruction, it naturally is. With an incomplete block, it is not and enemas must be administered. The bowel *above* the problem cannot be cleansed, because forced vomiting would be the only way to do it, and that would be neither desirable nor endurable. So, many doctors try to protect the patient before surgery from the waste trapped above the block with large doses of antibiotics. In doing so, they're trying to prevent wound infection and general internal infection from occurring due to contact with the bowel contents during the operation; they begin this treatment shortly after the preliminary stages of examination and diagnosis. They also allow the patients only clear liquids or very low-residue diets during this period. In the presence of very severe symptoms, only intravenous feedings are permitted.

Before we talk about the surgical elimination of bowel obstruction — and the colostomy that is often a part of that surgery — we should look more closely at the most common causes of obstruction, colorectal cancer and diverticulitis. They can lead to ostomies even when they do not completely block the bowel. Since they can cause blockages, their symptoms and examinations for them are remarkably similar to those of other obstructions. X-rays and sigmoidoscopy are the most reliable diagnostic tools here too, and although it is sometimes hard to tell colon cancer from diverticulitis, a distinguishing decision is rarely required *before* the initial stage of surgery. When the signs of bowel obstruction show themselves, the important thing is to relieve the pressure caused by the bottleneck. And then, with the time purchased with a temporary colostomy, to determine its cause. However, one thing that usually does set cancer apart from other forms of obstruction is the symptom of visible rectal bleeding.

Colorectal Cancer, Surprisingly Common

First, the bad news. The colon and the rectum are the most common sites of cancer in adults in the U.S.; these organs give way to malignant tumors more often than any other part of the body — with the exception of the skin — in adults in *all* Western countries. The American Cancer Society says there will be between 100,000 and 122,000 new cases of colorectal cancer in 1980 and 49,000 people are expected to die of its complications. For reasons not well understood, women are more frequently affected by cancer of the colon, and men suffer more often with cancer of the rectum. One's chances of getting these cancers of the nether regions begin to increase about age 40 and continue to go up as age does.

The causes of colorectal cancer are the causes, in turn, of much shouting at gatherings of cancer researchers. It used to be thought that malignant tumors in this area usually began as benign polyps, but recent studies have shown (to most doctors' satisfaction) that only one kind of polyp (the papillary polyp) leads to cancer and that it produces only one-third of all cases reported. There is, however, some evidence that one-quarter of all polyp sufferers eventually develop some kind of malignancy, but most physicians don't know what to make of these findings. Cancer-causing chemicals indiscriminately produce both polyps and malignancies in lab animals. People who study these carcinogenic substances say that they may be taken in *with* the foods we eat, but, on the other hand, they may also be produced by the body from the foods we eat. Doctors don't know which for sure. One current theory is that the bacteria *normally* found in the intestinal tract alter certain chemicals in the *abnormally* refined and processed and added-to food we eat and that alteration gives rise to these carcinogens — whose number is legion. This theory is actively under both study and attack.

Now the good news. Colorectal cancers have a very slow rate of growth and — with routine screening, reexaminations for blood in the stool and other measures — can be detected before they can do much damage. It takes nearly 2 years for an intestinal tumor to double in size, and during that time — a very early stage in its awful life — it may still cause symptoms of partial bowel obstruction which will lead to examination and discovery of the malignancy. Such cancers are *not* inherited defects, although they tend to run in families, because, it is supposed, families tend to eat the same things and live in the middle of the same environmental hazards — such as chemical plants and nuclear reactors. Families with familial polyposis or ulcerative colitis also are more prone to bowel cancer than others, as are those with a history of *any* malignant disease. And whole hemispheric *groups* of families, groups to whom a low-fiber, high-animal-fat diet is native — groups like us — tend to have a fairly high incidence of this kind of cancer.

Most of the late symptoms of bowel cancer are identical to those of other bowel-obstructing diseases. What differences they do present show up according to the location of the cancer, its size and its stage of spread. Bowel cancer may cause perforation, complete blockage or bleeding in the stool. Bowel cancers come in 2 types: a lump that grows on one wall of the intestine and eventually clogs it from the side and a ring that encircles the inside of the colon and slowly grows in size until it plugs the opening the way sediment builds up in a water pipe. Both kinds tend to develop in either the right (or ascending) colon or the left (and descending) colon, the sigmoid region and rectum. Growths in the right side, which is large in diameter and has thin, flexible walls, can become very large before they cause symptoms.

When symptoms arise, they often are fatigue, weakness and severe anemia. Even if there is no sign of blood in the patient's stools, it may still show up in chemical tests in the laboratory. Some vague pain — not unlike that associated with mild gallbladder attacks — can accompany these cancers. There are *few* changes in bowel habits with a malignancy of the right colon, and perhaps only the increasingly liquid nature of the feces will be noted. This is true, because as the intestine becomes increasingly more blocked, it will allow only liquid waste to pass. The left branch of the large intestine is smaller in diameter and a bit tougher. Tumors here tend to be the encircling kind, and they obstruct the bowel more quickly than do those on the other side, bringing the classic signs of colicky pain, constipation and abdominal distention. Rectal bleeding and blood-streaked stools are more frequently found with this type of tumor. Probably the first sign of a malignancy of the left side is a reduction in the size of stools, producing what medical books fastidiously call "small caliber pencil-shaped stools" issuing from a (presumably) smaller bore colon. The major symptoms of rectal cancer are periodic or chronic constipation in the middle stages and the persistent passage of blood with the stool and obstipation in the later stages.

The examination for colorectal cancer is similar to those for most bowel obstructions. It includes the same lab tests, plain and barium x-rays, and optical inspection via one of a number of snaky little telescopes. The most valuable tool is the fiberoptic colonoscope, the longest of the telescopes. Its use can be managed as an outpatient procedure and is only slightly more uncomfortable than that of the sigmoidoscope, a shorter device used in routine rectal inspections. Fortunately, about two-thirds of all colorectal cancers are at the doctor's fingertips. They can be felt as hard, flat, oval or encircling tumors by the physician's probing finger.

Diverticular Disease, a Blowout from Our Modern Diet

If bowel cancer causes a condition like clogged plumbing, diverticulitis is like a blowout in an automobile tire. Diverticular disease is caused by small fingers of the large intestine's lining which are actually blown out through weaknesses in its muscular outer layer by high air pressure inside the bowel. What causes these increases in pressure is not known. Although the process is similar to the conditions that produce a hernia, diverticulitis is *not* particularly related to constipation or lifting loads, the bugaboos in hernia. Some authorities claim that the disease is the result of the aging process and that a slackening of internal muscles produces flaws in the intestine. Others claim that the condition is congenital, that the weaknesses that permit diverticular blowouts exist at birth.

A less airy explanation comes from one of the men who did the pioneering studies of high-fiber diets in certain African countries, the British physician Neil S. Painter. Painter claims that the high pressure that causes diverticular blowouts comes from the strain it takes to move small, low-fiber stools through the colon. In 1978 he wrote in the journal, *Critical Reviews of Food Science and Nutrition,* to summarize his findings of the early '70s:

> I believe that if the colon has to propel hard stools for 40 years as opposed to soft bulky ones, it must overwork to produce abnormally high pressures. Over half a lifetime, the sigmoid [region overdevelops], its muscle thickens and is thrown into ridges between which there are gaps. This is the "prediverticular state." Finally the [intestinal lining] is driven through the muscular coat by the force of the intracolonic pressure as the colon struggles with an abnormally hard stool.

Although that theory was not enthusiastically greeted when it was first advanced, later studies — which ingeniously measure pressures inside the intestines of both sufferers and nonsufferers alike — have tended to support it. For instance, doctors at the Royal Infirmary at Sheffield, England, reported in the *British Medical Journal* in April of 1976 that a switch to a bulky diet significantly lowered these internal storms in their diverticular patients.

Whatever their cause, these bowel explosions occur singly or in clusters in about 10 percent of the U.S. population over the age of 40; more than half the Americans over the age of 80 have them. They are slightly more common in women than in men, and many of them show up low down in the sigmoid colon. In the precise language of medical textbooks, there are 2 kinds of diverticular disease, and they are distinguished by their increasing seriousness. "Diverticulosis," the word most of us know, is used by doctors only to refer to an early, unserious stage of the disease, in which the characteristic blowouts exist without complication and without symptoms. "Diverticulitis," a word few know and none can pronounce (it's die-ver-tick-you-lié-tis), is used by medical folks to refer to a more serious and painful stage in the disease in which chunks of food (or simply gastric juices) get caught in the accidental nooks and crannies (inflated by increased air pressure) and cause inflammation and swelling that eventually seal off the diversion as a separate bump on the intestine's outside surface. This condition leads to scarring on the *inside* as the inflammation heals, and that leads — when a number of bumps are involved — to a narrowing of the colonic passage and obstruction. And that's not the worst part. While all this healing over and scarring are taking place, the bit of food that originally caused the problem has decomposed, caused more inflammation, more swelling, ruptured its tiny pod on the bowel wall and — in the most serious cases — spread infection in the abdominal cavity. Diverticulosis, in the proper sense, rarely requires surgery. Diverticulitis usually does, and so it is with it that we'll be dealing here.

About half the people who develop diverticulitis suffer no symptoms at all. Symptoms occur only when inflammation occurs and only when it leads to a good deal of swelling and scarring in the outcroppings. Then, in this late stage, its signs are the signs of the bowel obstruction these things create. The colon takes on a saw-toothed look (the blowouts on the outside and their covers of scar tissue on the inside form the teeth) and becomes blocked. Diverticulitis, like other intestinal obstructions, causes considerable pain, which can be acute, persistent *and* crampy, and feel like appendicitis on either side of the abdomen. Unlike bowel cancer, it usually causes no rectal bleeding or blood in the stool.

The examination used to detect diverticulitis differs little from those already described for other obstructions. Both barium x-rays and the colonoscope pick up the telltale saw-toothed appearance of the diseased bowel and provide the diagnosing physician with reliable clues. However, since the problem with the disease is a series of tightly stretched outpouchings of the intestine, doctors are cautious with barium enema and x-ray. The outpouchings can rupture, and barium that has leaked through a perforation can cause serious body contamination. So, when perforation is suspected from blood tests and temperature readings, the barium x-ray is avoided.

This has necessarily been a bleak picture. Neither bowel cancer nor diverticulitis produces terribly uncomfortable symptoms in the early stages, and both are apt to develop into serious health threats before they do. So, in order to adequately isolate these diseases for you, we've had to concentrate on their later phases, when, unfortunately, it may be impossible to get away from them scot-free. When symptoms of bowel obstruction occur, it may be too late — already — to think of a complete recovery. But, fortunately, all is not dark; we've got something to suggest that may pick up the beginnings of bowel cancer and (to a certain extent) diverticulitis before they pick up your well-being and run away with it. What we're talking about is a screening program that is designed to detect colorectal cancer but — because it relies on optical examination of the lower end of the large intestine — can also uncover developing cases of diverticulitis.

Most authorities agree that we can get to colorectal cancer before it gets to us, that we can diagnose it at a curable stage. Sadly, they also know that we don't often take advantage of the technological means we have. Over 50 percent of these malignancies now uncovered have already spread to the surrounding lymph nodes, and 20 percent have moved into the liver. When colorectal cancers are detected and treated before they spread, nearly 70 percent of the patients involved live for at least 10 years after the diagnosis. When conditions remain hidden until after lymph node involvement, the victim's chances for 10 more years drop to about 30 percent. So, the value of a screening program to find cancers without symptoms is clear. It can more than double your option on a longer life.

The elements of the screening program we're about to describe are not new; they've been around as diagnostic tools for years and are not subjects for debate. What is being contended these days is *when* their use should begin. Although our risk of colorectal cacer goes up each year we live beyond age 40, many doctors think that testing programs begun at 40 hold few benefits for folks in the greatest danger from the disease. Researchers at the Life Extension Institute who believe that the presence of benign polyps in the colon is a fairly reliable sign that cancer may one day show up also say that polyps begin to develop between the ages of 20 and 50 in about one-third of the population. They suggest that all people undergo sigmoidoscopy for the detection of these growths between 20 and 30. For those with positive results, the doctors prescribe a yearly routine composed of some of the things we'll talk about in a minute. Those with negative results can forego further testing until age 40. In addition, other Institute findings indicate that several kinds of people should undergo yearly exams even if their early results are clear. These include: folks with a family history of cancer, familial polyposis or ulcerative colitis, and people with their own record of other forms of cancer or colitis. These 2 groups have a risk of colorectal cancer that runs 3 to 6 times greater than that of the general population.

After the initial step of testing for polyps, the screening program consists of the same progressive stages — no matter when it begins. Each positive result moves the patient on to the next examination. The first item on the annual agenda — whether it comes before or after age 40 — is the Hemoccult test, which is an examination of 6 stool samples (easily prepared by the patient himself) taken over a 3-day period. The exam, which can detect the minute amounts of blood released into the stool by a new cancer, makes no demands on the subject except for an increase in dietary fiber and a decrease in red meat while the samples are being taken. It is also a good idea to cut down on vitamin C dosages during the Hemoccult screening, because large amounts of C tend to produce falsely negative results. Along with the Hemoccult procedure, all patients should undergo sigmoidoscopy; it can discover the start of malignancies and the presence of polyps low down in the colon. In the case of polyps, it can even be used to remove them, because its telescope can be fitted with a wire cutting snare that snips them off.

If either Hemoccult or sigmoidoscopy uncovers anything suspicious or the patient is having telltale symptoms, a barium enema and x-ray should follow to paint a clearer picture of the intestine and pinpoint its invader. If the x-rays tell a dangerous story, they should be followed by colonoscopy, a telescopic look at regions higher up in the bowel. Colonoscopy can help resolve a disagreement between positive Hemoccult showings and a negative barium x-ray by uncovering something beyond the reach of an enema.

The point of all this is that cancer can be successfully eliminated with surgery, radiation or chemotherapy when its growth is localized, and so the goal of this screening program is to keep a constant watch on highly susceptible individuals to discover cancer's presence *before* it can spread. Patients suffering severe symptoms of bowel obstruction caused by cancer may already have lost their hold on a normal life. They may even be able to make their own diagnosis of their illness. The best weapon against this disaster is a knowledge of the various categories of risk and a rather constant vigil against cancer's onslaught.

Preparing for a Colostomy

We've reached a point where we *could* talk about the surgery to remove a disabled section of the bowel (and the colostomy that sometimes goes with it), but we won't, because we don't want you to be left holding *just* your little plastic bag. Instead, we're going to back up a bit — to the point where you've been told that your problem is a serious bowel disorder — and then go on from there to find the proper surgeon to fix your ailment, connect your mechanical detour and teach you to use it. If we don't backtrack in this way, all that's gone before will be for naught. Bowel removal surgery is a dangerous business, but it's normally handled without a hitch these days; except when complicated by the presence of cancer, it is no less safe than most of the procedures in this book. The rerouting of the intestine into a stoma is also a fairly routine procedure for the skillful surgeon. What isn't routine is the colostomy patient's adjustment to his new sidekick, and so we'll start at the point where later problems can be avoided early, the *very* beginning.

To find the right surgeon to clear up your bowel obstruction and fashion a smoothly functioning colostomy (if one is necessary), you should *first* do all the things one usually does to discover a careful, well-trained physician. Get a second opinion — preferably from a gastroenterologist or internist. Ask your family doctor for his recommendations, surgical and otherwise. Call the county medical board. Ask around among people with similar problems. Then, with all these things out of the way, consider yourself on square 1, and remember, finding the right doctor is a more complex problem in bowel surgery than in any other case covered in this book, even hernia. Sad but true, because the surgeon who is a technically proficient hernia mender may still be a rotten colostomy maker despite his deft fingers. The rub is that too many surgeons consider colostomy a sideline to bowel repair. They do it as a sideline — a throwaway, actually — to their main business. What's worse, even a doctor who is experienced in performing colostomies can do you wrong *if* the hospital he chooses to work in is not prepared to give you the kind of support services you need after surgery, services like proper appliance fitting and second-generation toilet training.

Your grilling of surgical candidates and members of their hospital teams should tell you how prepared they are to help you learn to live with a colostomy. Does the doctor or some staff member have the training, patience and compassion necessary to help you deal with a traumatic experience? If neither he nor anyone else nearby fills this bill, can they send you to someone appropriate? Another thing. How comfortable do you feel with these folks? If you don't relax with a particular doctor, if you can't discuss intimate problems and emotions with him (and the members of his support team), look further. However, if he does seem to have the right training and helpers, if you can talk to him and them, move to square 2. Ask your doctor if he'll get your training started before surgery; ask him if he'll help you prepare psychologically. What's even more important, ask him if he'll plan the *placement* of your stoma before you go into the OR, before you go into the hospital.

Proper placement and construction of a colostomy are crucial. While the placement of a stoma may be less crucial in the transverse or sigmoid colon than in an area closer to the small intestine, considerable thought still ought to be given to its location. Moreover, the stoma — wherever it's placed — should be well built and of the proper size. That is, it should rise high enough from the abdomen to allow for the secure attachment of the bag. A stoma of the correct size and in the correct place produces less upheaval, because it causes fewer mechanical problems. If your current first choice's attitude is, "wait and see," get up and go.

One more thing. Do you need to lose weight, and will your doctor require it before surgery — if it's *not* an emergency procedure? Obesity makes any abdominal surgery more difficult, but it's an invitation to misery with colostomy. Fat people or, rather, fat people's fat stomachs make stoma placement a very difficult problem, and they lead to many more troubles in colostomy management than flat stomachs. Does the surgeon put the opening on the up or the down side of a bulge, and how can he get the bag to lie comfortably on it? He can't. It's like trying to lay this book flat on a very round gelatin mold — impossible! If your doctor doesn't mention weight reduction to you, mention it to him. If he doesn't pick up on it, find someone who will.

The doctor you choose should have something significant and comforting to say about all the things mentioned above. If he doesn't, here are some things you can do and places you can go to get the help you need. Look in the phone book for a local chapter of the United Ostomy Association (U.O.A.), or get in touch with the national organization in California at 1111 Wilshire Boulevard, Los Angeles, California 90017, (213) 481-2811. The folks there will tell you what to read to prepare yourself, send you a helpful booklet and give you the name of the nearest trained ostomy counselor. Another place to write is the International Association for Enterostomal Therapy, 2506 Gross Point Road, Evanston, Illinois 60201. This group trains nurses to deal with colostomy patients and can provide you with the same kind of information as the U.O.A. and perhaps a larger and more up-to-date list of qualified therapists.

If neither association can help you where you live, try the pharmacy that sells ostomy supplies in your town. It may be able to send you to a local group of ostomates organized to help each other through bad times. In areas where no self-help group exists, call the Red Cross, Visiting Nurse, or Nurses' Registry for their help. At the very least, they can put you in touch with another colostomy wearer who may be willing to share his experiences.

Your insurance company should be anxious to help, too. After all, a speedy recovery and a smooth adjustment to your appliance are in their interest, too.

If none of these sources of comfort and information presents itself to you, don't panic. You can still go to the nearest large city medical center for your surgery (even if it is hours away) and then try this slightly unusual but highly reliable outlet for further help. On the say-so of the U.O.A., we went to a large drugstore in Allentown, Pennsylvania, near the headquarters of Rodale Press, and the people there put us in touch with a salesman for a firm that makes ostomy supplies. He came equipped with many of the tips you've just read and convinced us that he could both fit one of his devices to its user *and* deal with most of its minor malfunctions. As a last resort — and perhaps sooner — don't overlook this source of semiprofessional advice.

Finally, here's a list of must-do and must-have experiences that should be undertaken *before* surgery:

- Lose weight! If your colostomy can be done on an elective basis and your general health permits it, lose as much girth and bulk as you can. And firm up those stomach muscles. Your surgery will be easier, your recovery quicker and your device more efficient.
- See a stoma before you have one of your own. They are *not* nightmares, but they are not rosebuds either. Foreseen is forewarned is forearmed.
- Find a source of ostomy supplies before you need them, and make an appointment with your source to check your hospital fit after you're released.
- Make sure you have a spare appliance to carry with you at all times, even on the way home from the hospital. The disaster of a leaking appliance can be turned into a minor nuisance by the presence of a security bag.
- Learn something about the treatment of minor skin irritations around colostomy attachments. They are something every

ostomate must deal with, and they can be the quickest way to maladjustment. Stay tuned for our tips.

- Get some information about odor control in your preparation bag. Odor is another common dilemma for new baggers. Again, hang around for our suggestions.
- Do not think for one moment that colostomy will end life as you know it. Your operation will change nothing you love about the world, and it will eliminate — so to speak — certain things you've grown to hate during your illness. The only people who are guaranteed a shock with colostomy are those folks whose greatest pleasure in life is reading on the toilet.

What Happens If You Need Colon Surgery

OK, what do you get after you've turned yourself into the saint described above and found a saintly doctor? An operation to modify a section of large bowel and a colostomy, which is, again, an opening someplace on the abdomen through which *all* bowel contents are emptied. Urine, of course, will still be passed normally. This operation will probably be done with a general anesthetic, although some bowel and colostomy procedures are done with spinal anesthesia. Depending on how serious your bowel problem is — how many complications it has caused and how sick you are — the bowel cutting and stoma fashioning can take place either in one operation or more than one. For the removal of a fair number of benign polyps and the placement of a temporary colostomy to rest the abused intestine, the 2 steps are done at once, and the whole business may take between 1 and 2 hours. If the complaint is more serious but not yet life-threatening — for example, an intestine tangled in its mesentery — the surgery could take from 2 to 4 hours, but both steps would still be done at once. However, in the *worst* cases when the symptoms of bowel obstruction have themselves become lethal, the colostomy and the bowel surgery will be done separately in 2 or 3 steps, each separated by several weeks. In these cases, a colostomy (requiring 30 to 60 minutes) is performed to relieve the symptoms of bowel obstruction — pain, abdominal distention and infection — and drain the intestine of backed-up waste. Then, when the patient's condition has stabilized and his colostomy incision has completely healed, the bowel work is done — requiring another 2 to 4 hours. If the colostomy is to be temporary, a third operation some months (up to 2 years) later will be done to close the stoma, remove the diseased section and reconnect the bowel to put it back in service. If the anus and rectum must be removed, the colostomy is permanent and nothing is required after the second step, except when normal aging — or injury — demands maintenance work on the stoma, or when, for reasons of surgeon error or patient weight gain, it must be moved.

The incision for any all-in-one procedure begins over the bit of colon that will be brought to the surface to form the colostomy and moves on down or across the abdomen to expose the bowel section affected. For the step-by-step type, there will, of course, be at least 2 incisions, one over the colostomy site, and one over the intestinal links to be removed.

Most temporary colostomies are loop devices somewhere on the transverse colon — wherever disease dictates they be placed. This is so because the job is easily done there, the opening is easily closed when the time comes and it's out of the way when the bowel surgery comes up. The disadvantages of a colostomy at this point are that it opens the *right* colon, has a somewhat unpleasant look and discharges liquid material into its bag. It is also more prone to odor problems, but since it's a temporary measure, its advantages are usually allowed to sway surgical decisions. The site of a *permanent* colostomy will, of course, be determined by the troubles that lead to it; but — theoretically — the best spot for it is somewhere on the left or descending colon, because wastes discharged by this section of bowel are formed and more solid and much easier to live with. Stomas placed in this area also make bag wearing more comfortable. Fortunately, theory also meets practice here, for most serious obstruction problems occur in the sigmoid regions, that is, on the lower left side, and call for left-handed colostomies. The comfort *you* should draw from all this theoretical geography is that temporary colostomies can be harder to live with than permanent ones. If you're stuck with a messy temporary one, remember, the end is in sight. If you've got a permanent detour, remember its end products could be worse.

Let's take a time-out. You're probably thinking that the most natural spot for an unnatural anus is right next to the natural one. But if you'll sit down and think about it for a minute, you'll see that there are all kinds of pressing things wrong with this particular placement. Like sitting down and soiling and leaking and lack of control. Believe us; the experiment has been tried, and it failed.

The surgical maneuvers just ticked off, for the most part, remain unchanged when bowel cancer or diverticulitis enters the picture. Both conditions usually require the multistep procedure, but frequently, with early detection, a temporary colostomy is used. However, if the anus and rectum are lost, it is not possible to reconnect the colon; the lower terminus is gone. Then, a permanent colostomy is the upshot. Permanent colostomies are also common with bowel cancer where a great deal of tissue above and below the original tumor plus (usually) the nearby lymph nodes and even the mesentery must be cut out to stop the cancer's spread. With a malignant tumor, as with any bowel obstruction, doctors try to avoid a colostomy and retain the anus and its sphincter valve, but in a great many cases they cannot. If the growth is very low in the rectum or anus, a colostomy is almost a certainty.

How long will all these things take? It's hard to say, because so many types of illness are involved. A case of obstruction caused by surgical adhesions (which *might* require a temporary colostomy if the bowel had become badly irritated) would probably disable its victim for only a few weeks after surgery. A terrible onslaught of diverticulitis or bowel cancer, on the other hand, with its multiple operations separated by weeks or even months, would have its victim in and out of the hospital for over a year. A rule of thumb is that if your condition is serious enough to warrant a colostomy, it will require considerable recovery time and dish out a good deal of pain and discomfort during that time.

What does a stoma look like? Depends what kind it is and where it is. When it's brand-new, it will be red and swollen and appear quite large. Once it's healed, however, it will settle down in both appearance and size. One-half to 2 inches in diameter is the normal range of stoma sizes. It may be flush to the skin's surface or stick out a bit. According to one medical man, a stoma resembles a tiny, shiny volcano on the lower abdomen, because it is composed of bowel tissue which has been pulled through, turned over and remains shiny even after seeing the light of day. According to a doctor with an unusual sense of metaphor we consulted, a flush stoma looks like a second belly button, and a protruding stoma looks like "a cocktail frankfurter." We'd prefer to say that a stoma can look like either an "insy" or "outsy" belly button and leave it at that.

Where will this surplus navel be? Again, it depends on where and why you have it. But within the limits set by the disease causing the illness, your surgeon will try to place the stoma in a convenient spot. That means *away* from bony prominences in the pelvis and out of the way of sagging waistlines and spare tires of fat which can make wearing a bag uncomfortable. It should be *below* the belt line to allow for shorts and bathing suits and elastic waistbands, all of which can make bags embarrassing or painful. It should also be steered clear of the *first* belly button to prevent soiling that natural depression.

How long will you be laid up by bowel surgery and colostomy? Again, it's hard to pin down, because there are so many different conditions included under these general headings. If your case is relatively minor, with a temporary colostomy and an intestinal tract which needs some adhesions snipped, you can resume normal activities like bathing as soon as the surface wounds have healed, and restart your usual diet inside of 2 weeks. Although the colostomy will not be closed until the doctor is sure the bowel has completely healed (which could take 6 weeks or more), you should be back to full strength, doing all the work and things you always do, before a month is out. After that and until the colostomy is closed, you will experience some inconvenience but no real curb on your activities. If your case is much more serious and requires several different operations, you might not be up and going again for 3 to 4 months *after* your last visit to the operating room. It will take your body at least that long to recover from these multiple assaults.

Living with Your Colostomy

For want of a better label, this next (and nearly the last) section of the chapter could be called "the etiquette of a colostomy." It could be called the most important, too, because it concerns how you should treat your artificial exit and how it, in turn, will treat you.

The first touch you will have with your colostomy is with the bag itself, which will already be fitted in place when you awake in the hospital's recovery room. Chances are, this appliance will not be the one you will stick with, because it was chosen hastily and not fitted to an active human being. Also, because stomas shrink as healing takes place, it may take several weeks of trial and error to find the right make and model for your needs, but with the help of a properly trained counselor who knows what's available and what's happening to you, a perfect match can be made. And "perfect" is probably the right word here, because bags have improved a lot lately; they can now eliminate most problems. Once they were leaky rubber pouches. Now they are airtight plastic bags which nearly end wet spots and embarrassing odors. They used to be attached to a sweaty leather belt that had to be strapped around the patient. Now they stick to a wide piece of tape which, in turn, sticks to the patient. The tape has a hole in the center that is tailored to the size of the stoma and ensures a tight, secure hold — both to the body and to the stoma opening. There is even a brand new attachment — a magnet — which is implanted in the stoma itself to attract a metal ring sewn into the bag. And modern appliances lie flat; no bulges, no bumps in any but the tightest clothing, clothing that would give away all other secrets as well.

The first step in learning to care for a stoma is usually emptying the pouch. Modern appliances are disposable and need not be cleaned and reused. During the first few days after the operation, a nurse with special ostomy training does most things for you, such as fitting the bag and changing it. But as you get stronger and more ready for the information she has to give, she gradually turns the various tasks over to you. First, the washing of the skin around the stoma with plain soap and water. Then the placing of adhesive tape around the stoma. Then fitting the bag. And so on until you're in complete command. Many of these nurses like to involve the patient's family in this getting-acquainted stage, both to ready a back-up team for emergencies and to convince family members that their loved one hasn't changed all that much.

The next step in this shakedown cruise is learning the ways of a colostomy, and that means learning to deal with the pattern of elimination it develops for itself. Trained help and compassionate support are needed here, because each colostomy generates a different pattern and plotting it can be frustrating. This stage can turn into a breakdown cruise without the proper advice; it is a second round of toilet training, and it can be as socially and psychologically stressful as the first.

After an early period of spasmodic action, colostomies generally "learn" a cycle of elimination. They learn when to and when not to, and most can be depended upon in tightest situations. In fact, they are so reliable that many ostomates — especially those with stomas in the sigmoid region — get rid of their bags and cover their openings with just gauze bandages after the first year. Some unfortunate people, of course, never reach this stage, but a good many do. The road to this point is often paved with good irrigation. Water is allowed to flow gently into the stoma at the same time each day from a bag held at shoulder height (or below). A special cone-shaped nozzle fits snugly into the opening and prevents both leakage and injury. One timetable we read claimed that it took 3 months for most new colostomies to become toilet trained, but 6 weeks seems a more accurate figure. In the early stages of this housebreaking, the process is a bit balky, and the patient may have to replace his bag and wait for the desired results. But later on, irrigation will generally induce a fairly rapid elimination which can be deposited directly into the toilet. What may take an hour to do early in the game, will, after the proper training, soon take far less time. The thing to keep in mind during the trial-and-error stage is that the stoma wants to cooperate. A considerable number of people even develop this regularity and dependability without any pump priming at all.

OK, colostomies can usually be trained. Do they require special eating habits? No. Food must be well chewed. Lots of liquids are essential, but you can eat anything you enjoy and your nutritional conscience and your physician allow. It used to be the conventional wisdom that colostomies were prone to diarrhea, but to that we can say, "pooh!" People cause diarrhea with their eating habits, not colostomies. In general, things that were apt to cause trouble before your operation will continue to do so afterward. It was also once the accepted doctrine that roughage, nuts and seeds had to be severely limited or removed from the ostomate's diet. Now, however, it seems that this may not be the best advice in all cases — *if* one has a great deal of functioning large bowel left; that is, if his colostomy is far down on the colon. It has been learned that fiber keeps the intestine in shape and helps prevent *all* kinds of bowel diseases (more about this later). It would seem good sense, then, to eat high-fiber foods after colostomy to avoid further problems, again, if the system can tolerate them.

The subject of diet limitations naturally brings up the more general topic of ostomy handicaps. What will my condition prevent me from doing. Directly, almost nothing, except wearing a bikini. Even two-piece bathing suits are normally possible with most stomas. There are no restrictions on travel, although many patients fear traveling, because they fear being away from their doctors. But the United Ostomy Association will supply travelers with the names of appropriate medical people in whatever areas they plan to visit. Most sports are completely within the ostomate's bounds. Violent contact sports may be the exception, but that's not much of a handicap. Most ostomates are over 40 and benched by age anyway. The only aspect of either traveling or most recreational activities that is a common problem for most colostomy patients is their need for private changing and toilet facilities. These things, however, can usually be arranged beforehand like any other accommodations and with as little hassle. What about jobs? Most ostomates return to their former jobs after surgery and recovery with no problem. Very heavy lifting may be out for the patient, because he does face the danger of hernia around the stomal incision. Once again, though, the average age of most of these folks means that they will have left lugging far behind them. The real occupational hazard for ostomates comes in changing jobs. It's often very difficult. Some personnel managers have wrongheaded prejudices about the ostomate's health and strength being limited, and some insurance companies wrongly exclude them from group insurance plans. That kind of discrimination can and should be fought with medical statistics and expert testimony. Your doctor and your therapist can help you there.

The medical problems encountered with colostomy fall into 2 categories, the serious and the nonserious. The serious are quite rare, and the nonserious are easily remedied. They usually require no more than an adjustment or change of the patient's appliance. The overall rate for complications with colostomies is something like 20 percent, and only about 15 percent of these require a relook or recut by the surgeon — a good thing, because most of them are due to surgical errors in the first place. Two things, you can be pretty sure, won't happen. Infection will not enter the body through the stoma, and normal accidents and physical injuries won't hurt it. It takes a severe, direct blow to do any real damage. The kind of things that less-than-acceptable surgery causes are: hernia through the stomal incision (caused by a poor sewing job or your aging), retraction of the bowel end from the stoma (again, poor sewing) and death of the bowel end (due to inadequate circulation provided by the surgeon). The things your body can do to your colostomy which are serious are thankfully few. Surgical adhesions can stop it from functioning, and *more* bowel trouble higher up can cause it to bleed and shut down. And the things you can do to mess it up are exactly one. You can irrigate it improperly by being impatient or using a tip which is misshapen and too firm. That can perforate the bowel section which forms your stoma. All these serious complications demand surgical correction.

The nonserious things are really that. Some patients experience skin irritation around the stoma, mostly from the constant use of appliance adhesives, but also from occasional soiling of the skin. Some have skin dryness from the constant covering of the bag and its tape. A few people even develop allergies to the various materials involved. Fortunately, all these nuisances can be controlled by changing products, modifying them or simple topical balms and medications. The best tip we know about skin irritation comes from Dorothy E. Fisher, enterostomal therapist at the Pottsville Hospital and Warne Clinic in Pottsville, Pennsylvania, where she developed and extensively tested her remedy. Ms. Fisher liberally applies vitamin E oil or vitamin E succinate powder and prescribes an oral supplement at the first sign of irritation and has effectively eliminated most skin problems from her patients' worries. She reports clearing up even a badly ulcerated stoma in less than a week. Most prospective ostomates, however, don't think about skin irritation or the more serious medical emergencies of the condition when the subject of complications first comes up. They think about odor. Will I offend? No more than usual. At first, there is considerable odor with a colostomy but later that settles down until there is no more with this artificial exit than with the natural one. When odor does begin to cloud the patient's horizon, he should think of trying 2 things. The first is that he may be eating gassy foods or eating too much animal protein and causing his own problem. In these cases, he should switch diets (if he can) or investigate a new, more secure appliance (if he can't). Well-fitting bags *should* turn gas into a visual manifestation. They should trap gas, balloon up with it and then hold on until it can be discreetly released. Many modern appliances even have charcoal filters and gas-release valves. If yours doesn't, it should be replaced. The second thing that should occur to the ostomate bothered by gas and odor is the same thing anyone with that embarrassment should consider. Is there some serious medical problem that is causing your bag to swell? If the answer seems to be yes, consult a doctor. For the very timid or suspicious or insecure, there are deodorant sprays for the area and tablets for the appliance itself, which are lousy. What does work is bismuth subgallate, which is available without prescription, taken orally.

Another public problem with a colostomy is leaks. They happen, because the nature of any device is to break down. If yours does, you should have a spare handy to replace it. Most leaks, however, come from ill-fitting, not broken, bags. After a period of education and practice, you should be rid of that annoyance altogether.

One thing these 3 minor colostomy problems share is their psychological terror. To make a stink, or a wet spot, or even to suffer through itchy or sore skin does not threaten one's life. But they do embarrass the ostomate and tend to make him think of himself as an outcast. That feeling — the fear that his operation will make him unfit for work, unfit for the things he enjoys, unfit even for company — is the worst thing faced by the potential ostomate. So strong is this feeling, in fact, that it sometimes does no good to show the patient medical counterparts who are none of those things but, instead, normally functioning, happy members of his neighborhood. This psychological bugbear is all the more forbidding, because it's associated with 2 other fear-laden subjects. Colostomy *makes* us think about our rectum, the anus, about elimination and all of its unpleasant fringe benefits, and we don't like to do it. Anthropologists would call this a taboo subject, and we suppose it is. But it's also an icky subject, and *that's* probably more to the point. We refuse to deal with our colostomies, because it's unpleasant to do so, and people have become invalids to avoid relearning to do a few simple things that would make a return to normal life possible. The other factor in these psychological difficulties is that a great many ostomates have to face their tail-end problem *and* cancer in the same moment. They find they can't face a major change in life-style *and* the possibility of death in the same turn of fate, and become frozen.

OK, we've said the worst of it. Colostomy is hard to live

with, because it produces physical dislocations and physical discomforts in life, and because it results in psychological stresses at a time when most people have the least energy to cope with them — when they're sick, very sick. That means that a colostomy is not finished when the patient wakes up in the recovery room or when he leaves the hospital or *even* when he goes back to work. A colostomy is not finished until your doctor and his staff gives you the training you need, and you accept that training as a way of convincing yourself that very little has changed in your life. It may seem that *everything* has changed in *all* the worst ways. But it has not. What's good is still good. The ways of achieving those goods are still effective. And *all* of them are available to you.

Even after that outburst, we're not done with problems, but this last one has had to wait, because it's somewhere between the physical and the psychological. Unfortunately, this section might be called, "Sex and the Single Stoma." Some *men* have a potency problem after colostomy procedures. In all cases, this impotence is *not* caused by the presence of the stoma itself. Some of these men have a purely physical problem; nerves deep in the pelvis were severed during one of the several surgeries that lead to their stoma, and they were left with a handicap. They may also be unable to empty their bladders for the same reason. Fortunately, this is a very infrequent complication. If completely physical, the problem can be helped with a surgically implanted prosthesis. Most of the men who are sexually affected by their operations, however, suffer no physical damage at all. The impotence is psychological. These men may be ashamed of a changed body; afraid of offending with the ostomy appliance; convinced that their condition sets them apart and makes them unlovable. The only way out of this slough is competent, compassionate professional therapy.

Preventing Bowel Troubles

That's just about the bottom line for the end game of colostomy. But we would be doing only half our job if we ended this chapter without talking about *avoiding* bowel obstruction in the first place. "Groan," you say. "You're going to tell us how to avoid the 20-odd causes of bowel obstruction? . . . One by one?" No, we're not. We're going to tell you that both the latest scientific literature on bowel disease, diverticulosis and cancer, as well as reports presented at the National Symposium on Colorectal Cancer (held in New York in 1979) suggest there are a few good ways to fight *all* forms of bowel disorder, including cancer.

A culling of the papers read by doctors and scientific researchers at the symposium provides this list of dos and don'ts in the fight against cancer — as well as some impressive documention for them. First, don't feed on red meat! Barry Goldin, Ph.D., of the Tufts-New England Medical Center in Boston, told the New York audience that while a number of environmental pollutants, food additives and even methods of preparing food have been implicated in colon cancer, a reading of the medical literature on the subject and his own research has led him to believe that it is the amount of red meat one eats that is the crucial factor. Some things we eat are turned into cancer-causing enzymes by the benign bacteria that carry forth digestion in the intestine. Some of the worst by-products of this process are formed when the intestinal flora (as these bacteria are romantically called) work on red meat, and Dr. Goldin discovered significantly *smaller* amounts of these enzymes in the feces of vegetarians. What's more, he found that cancer was much more difficult to instigate in laboratory animals who were kept away from meat. Two other researchers reporting in New York added further information to Dr. Goldin's argument and helped to explain it. Geographical studies put together by John H. Weisburger, Ph.D., and Ernst L. Wynder, M.D., of the American Health Foundation, Valhalla, New York, have shown that colon cancer is highest in Anglo-Saxon countries and in Western Europe, where meat is the first item on every table, and lowest in Japan, Eastern Europe, and most of Latin America, where the diet is usually centered around various grains and beans. The exceptions which prove their rule are the Latin American countries Uruguay and Argentina, which *do* have a high rate of malignancy — but also a high rate of meat consumption.

The cautions that Drs. Weisburger and Wynder would add to our list are: do cut down on all forms of animal fat and don't bathe in cholesterol! People who are high cancer risks consume an average of 130 to 150 grams of fat per day, which amounts to 40 to 45 percent of their total calories. People who are low risks, on the other hand, take in only 40 to 80 grams per day or 10 to 20 percent of their caloric supply. These high-riskers, of course, are also much more prone to heart attacks and such other cholesterol-related ailments as gallbladder disease. In their laboratory, Drs. Weisburger and Wynder discovered that it is much harder to induce cancer in rats on a low-fat diet than it is in animals gorged on fatty foods. Some of the intestinal dwellers that Dr. Goldin found turning traitor and generating malignancy were the bile acids and salts produced by the gallbladder to digest fats and dissolve cholesterol. It stands to reason then, according to Drs. Weisburger and Wynder, that the more fat you eat, the more of these potential turncoats you'll produce.

Another insight offered by both the statistical and experimental work reported by these 2 scientists is that a lot of fiber in a diet can offset a number of other sins. The fat-relishing rodents they studied were much more resistant to chemically induced cancer when fed naturally bulky foods as well. And the people of Finland, who eat enormous quantities of butter, milk and eggs — in addition to a nearly American amount of meat — nonetheless enjoy a low incidence of colon cancer, because they traditionally consume lots of fiber in whole grains and root vegetables such as potatoes, carrots and turnips. This high intake of fiber, the doctors (along with many colleagues) theorize, serves to dilute the surplus bile acids from the Finns' greasy diet — to soak them up, in effect — and to push any other cancer-causing agents swiftly through the bowel with the volume of stool it creates. As we have advised throughout this book: Do add fiber to your bill of fare!

Three other areas of cancer prevention that received quite a bit of support at the symposium were programs of supplementation. Jerome J. DeCosse, M.D., of The Memorial Sloan-Kettering Cancer Center, told the group that vitamin C, ascorbic acid, has long been known for its antitumor effects in laboratory animals. Although it was supposed that the vitamin's antioxidant properties produced this benefit, he said he couldn't be sure. He was sure, however, that doses of vitamin C did retard the growth of the kind of rectal polyps that turn into cancer in a study of an experimental group of patients at Sloan-Kettering.

A man who says he is sure about the cancer-fighting properties of vitamin C is Ewan Cameron, a Scottish surgeon who is currently working at the Linus Pauling Institute for Science and Medicine in California. In 1971, Cameron reported the case of a truck driver whose cancer went into complete remission after he started taking vitamin C. Trying to explain what seemed either a miracle or dumb luck, the doctor discovered that cancer cells have 2 qualities that separate them from other body-building blocks. They have the ability to proliferate, unchecked by other cells or body systems, and the power to invade cells and structures which stand in their deadly way. Most cancer treatments try to stop proliferation with surgery or drug or radiation therapy.

Coming at the problem from the other angle, the Scot sought to discover whether there might be some way of inhibiting the blitzkrieg of malignant cells. He found that cancer eats its way through the body using a series of caustic enzymes, and that healthy individuals manufacture a chemical, called hyaluronidase, which fights off (or at least slows) these enzymes. And the raw material of that inhibitor is — ascorbic acid or vitamin C. With this knowledge he could explain why cancer victims are often found to be seriously deficient in the vitamin and why cancer often spreads more quickly after surgery, which depletes the body of C. All this led to a continuing regimen of vitamin therapy for Cameron's Scottish patients and has prompted us to add vitamin C to our list of dos and don'ts.

Morris S. Zedeck, Ph.D., also of Sloan-Kettering, in summarizing work being done on cancer in lab animals for symposium members, singled out 2 diet supplements that promise great things but need more testing. He noted that rats on high-fat diets in several studies proved resistant to chemically induced colon cancer when vitamin A was added to their food. He also described several studies that were started when geographical surveys of cancer cases showed that the incidence of bowel cancer is low in areas where there are high levels of the mineral selenium in the soil. This finding led to a discovery that cancer patients have low selenium levels in their blood and that produced several animal experiments which showed that dietary supplements of the substance lowered the incidence of both naturally arising and artificially produced tumors in rats. He was quick to add, as we are, that the true value of vitamin A and selenium in cancer prevention is not yet firmly established.

The nice thing about all this is that the surest weapon against bowel cancer is also the biggest gun against diverticulosis, the other major precursor of colostomy. The bigger, smoother stools associated with a fiber-ful diet — as we said in an earlier section of this chapter — move easily through the colon. Their progress does not require the straining that can produce the tiny herniations of the intestinal wall that lead to diverticulitis, and their sheer size helps dissipate the abnormally high pressure that exists in some people — seemingly without cause — and which can lead to that disease. So, just as in cancer, the complex villains that cause diverticulosis may be foiled by a high-fiber diet.

The best news we found in this last regard is that the conservative (and widely accepted) medical textbook, *Current Surgical Diagnosis and Treatment* (Lange Medical Publications, 1977) in its most recent edition, agrees with us (it usually doesn't). It says there's controversy (it usually does). It says studies are not yet complete (it usually does). But it does recommend a bulky input to fight diverticulosis. And it agrees that fiber can help against colorectal cancer. We won't say we told you so.

Index

A

B

D

E

F

I

J

K

L

M

N

O

P

R

S

T

U

V